AN ABUNDANCE OF CAUTION

AN ABUNDANCE OF CAUTION

AMERICAN SCHOOLS, THE VIRUS, AND A STORY OF
BAD DECISIONS

DAVID ZWEIG

THE MIT PRESS   CAMBRIDGE, MASSACHUSETTS   LONDON, ENGLAND

The MIT Press
Massachusetts Institute of Technology
77 Massachusetts Avenue, Cambridge, MA 02139
mitpress.mit.edu

The MIT Press would like to thank the anonymous peer reviewers who provided comments on drafts of this book. The generous work of academic experts is essential for establishing the authority and quality of our publications. We acknowledge with gratitude the contributions of these otherwise uncredited readers.

This book was set in ITC Stone and Avenir by New Best-set Typesetters Ltd. Printed and bound in the United States of America.

Library of Congress Cataloging-in-Publication Data

Names: Zweig, David, 1974- author.
Title: An abundance of caution : American schools, the virus, and a story of bad decisions / David Zweig.
Description: Cambridge, Massachusetts : The MIT Press, 2025. | Includes bibliographical references and index.
Identifiers: LCCN 2024034442 (print) | LCCN 2024034443 (ebook) | ISBN 9780262549158 (hardcover) | ISBN 9780262380027 (pdf) | ISBN 9780262380034 (epub)
Subjects: LCSH: School management and organization—United States—Decision making. | Social distancing (Public health) and education—United States. | School closings—United States. | Schools—United States—Safety measures. | COVID-19 Pandemic, 2020—United States.
Classification: LCC LB2806 .Z94 2025 (print) | LCC LB2806 (ebook) | DDC 379.7309/052—dc23/eng/20241211
LC record available at https://lccn.loc.gov/2024034442
LC ebook record available at https://lccn.loc.gov/2024034443

10 9 8 7 6 5 4 3 2 1

EU product safety and compliance information contact is: mitp-eu-gpsr@mit.edu

To Eliana and Zev

Of all tyrannies, a tyranny sincerely exercised for the good of its victims may be the most oppressive. . . . Those who torment us for our own good will torment us without end for they do so with the approval of their own conscience.
—C. S. Lewis

CONTENTS

PREFACE

On March 18, 2020, a text exchange circulated among parents in my neighborhood. Someone shared the news that for the past few nights at 5:29 p.m., in a different part of town, there had been a communal "primal scream." The lockdowns had only recently begun, but everyone already had cabin fever and a general weariness and stress over it all. The text group unanimously decided to do it, too. And so each evening my family and many of my neighbors would gather on our porches and let loose. Rather than the famous nightly cheer of gratitude in the city for first responders that gained notice shortly afterward, this was purely the noise of suburban catharsis. Each night echoes of air horns and wooden spoons clanging on pots rang out from homes I couldn't see. Then, after a minute or so, with our voices hoarse and the last of the shrieks in the distance petering out, my family would go back inside, exhilaration dissolving, smiles fading, each of us retiring quietly back to our electronic devices.

After a week the novelty of the collective scream began to wear off and come 5:25 or so I'd often have to cajole my kids off their screens, to which they'd become hopelessly attached, to the back porch. We needed something else.

Near the end of March we started taking family walks after dinner to the riverfront, a fifteen-minute stroll down a steep road, past the shuttered library and the silent train station. This was the best part of my day, and something that we'd never routinely done before as a family. Throughout the mornings and afternoons we were all home but largely in our own worlds. But on these walks the four of us were together. There was an unspoken enchantment once we reached our destination, the sun softly setting somewhere beyond the Palisades, the Hudson River gently lapping on the shore. It was a rare offer of grace that the pandemic gifted to us. We were usually by ourselves, and when we did come across others everyone kept their distance.

One night in mid-April, though, we saw one of my son's good friends near the river with her mom and grandfather. We hadn't interacted closely with anyone outside the family for a month. My son and his friend immediately ran toward each other, charging across a field that rolled to the riverbank. Each parent called out for the kids to keep their distance from each other, but the command was halfhearted. Once united, they took off, chasing each other until they reached the rocky breakwater and danced along its craggy edge as silhouettes, dusk falling around us. Their far-off voices carried the distinct, high-pitched mirth of childhood.

A coil tightened inside me. The rocks, the river, nightfall speeding toward us. There was some unknown, remote, yet very real risk looming. But I had no intention of stopping them just yet. This was my little boy's life, a beautiful insouciance that had been crushed into nonexistence over the past month until this chance encounter with a friend.

Earlier that same week my daughter had a similar experience. I had texted the dad of one of her close friends: "E is getting pretty lonely and stir-crazy. Are you and Zoe free to go on a bike ride with E and me? I think it'd be good for her to see a friend, albeit at 6 feet."

We met on the dirt trail that runs atop the old aqueduct that snakes from the Bronx all the way to upper Westchester County, offering a slender rural escape through the many towns in between, ours among them. Within a few moments the girls were off ahead of us, riding side by side. I could hear them chatting animatedly the whole time, though I couldn't make out what they were saying. (Later, my daughter told me they had concocted an elaborate game. The details were confusing to me—it was one of the many worlds that kids disappear into but make little sense to adults. This type of thing, the spontaneous magic that only happens when a child is with a friend, didn't take place on Zoom.) My daughter beamed when we got home. And her spirits seemed to stay lifted, even for days afterward, like a neglected plant that had finally been given water.

For a month we had been existing within a miasma of fear. People were dying from a scary new disease, and my family and my neighbors were readily compliant with the governor's orders to stay home, and stay apart from each other until some unknown time when this thing was going to go away. And yet. This virus, which was a terror for the old, posed almost no threat to my kids or their friends.

Childhood is fleeting. My son had not been allowed to touch another child for a month—no arm around a friend, no roughhousing, no sitting next to each other on a sofa. This plan—keeping kids physically apart from each other for weeks, or months—did not seem sustainable or wise if they were in no great danger. I understood they could still get COVID and then pass it to my wife or me. But although our risk was higher, it was fairly clear, even then, that a healthy adult in middle age was also at very low risk. If parents had a medically frail child or lived with elderly or vulnerable people they could or even should keep their kids isolated with them. But what about everyone else?

The day after my daughter's bike ride, watching my kids in their rooms slowly wilting in the gray light of their school-issued Chromebooks, I thought about every other kid in my town and in the country, cut off from their peers because of mandated "remote learning," and I felt a visceral sense of injustice, which brought a growing sadness to me that gave way to gnawing frustration. How necessary was it to keep children away from each other for what was now more than a month? And how long was this supposed to go on? It's not normal or healthy to be confined to your bedroom day after day, week after week. And what about the families who didn't have comfortable homes or safe neighborhoods? Where were those kids—barred from school, and barred from being with each other— supposed to go all this time? It wasn't quite clear whether this injustice was just bad luck or the result of bad policy. I intended to find out.

Shortly after that night at the river I began to research everything I could find about the virus. I was in the middle of writing a book, but I put it aside. I could think of nothing else other than this bizarre new reality we found ourselves in.

For the better portion of a decade before becoming a journalist I worked for Condé Nast and other publishers as a magazine fact-checker, ultimately running the research department at an ill-fated glossy. In part from my training and experience in that role, and in part because of my disposition, I've long held most things I'm told to be suspect until proven otherwise. As a fact-checker I was taught that news articles, websites, conventional wisdom, even quotes from interviewees are often insufficient evidence behind a claim. You must always try to get to the primary source, digging further and further down. Time and again, something that seemed true turned out not to be so. This mindset has stayed with me as a journalist and in life generally. And it informed my motivation to get to the bottom of the pandemic policies regarding schools. In addition, from my previous work as a journalist and author, in which I had focused on the intersection of technology, culture, and psychology, I had years of experience reading academic papers and sorting through scientific findings. My greatest weakness as a writer is that I love research. I am obsessive about it, to the point that I never feel finished, even when I should be writing. There's always some new avenue to explore, some angle I may have missed. This makes me a very slow writer. But this voracious curiosity is an asset when I approach a new topic. I was well positioned to get started.

Because I'm not a scientist myself, siloed in a particular field and aware of the "right" and "wrong" questions, nor in competition with peers, I have no concern about appearing naive about a particular topic when I approach experts, which I do often. I've found most scholars and scientists are thrilled to talk about their work and answer questions, as long as they're respectful, interesting, and reasonably well informed.

In the early spring of 2020, I connected with the infectious diseases epidemiologist who authored a case study about a French student with COVID who attended three schools and didn't infect anyone else. I corresponded with specialists in Germany, Denmark, and Britain. There were very little data from the US. But that didn't stop me. I read reports from China, Iceland, the Netherlands. I reviewed data from Norway, Denmark, Sweden. Everything related to kids strongly pointed in one direction.

How was it possible that almost none of this was being covered in the US media or discussed by American politicians? I kept questioning if I was misunderstanding something, and I'd go back and reread my exchanges with the foreign experts. But then, toward the end of April news came out about European countries beginning to reopen their schools. I wasn't misunderstanding the data. The Europeans saw the same studies and evidence that I had seen, and they came to the same conclusion: Open the schools.

I initially had no intention of following this trail professionally. I simply was trying to make sense of what was happening in America. But it was clear that a very large story was not being told.

INTRODUCTION

In the span of one week in March 2020, the entire school system in America shut down. The academic year for more than 50 million students was over, blasting a hole in the calendar three months wide. 480,000 school buses, which until the week before had been carrying 23 million children each day, were parked neatly in rows on untold acres of asphalt lots. Cafeterias, which served 20 million free lunches to students each day, shuttered. Monkey bars and jungle gyms glinted silently under the spring sun, while beds of protective wood chips lay still beneath them in 100,000 abandoned school playgrounds. A master switch had been flipped by the governors of every state in the union in scattershot choreography, a vast, unrehearsed exercise of authority.

Just a beat later, an experiment called "distance learning" was implemented, albeit haltingly, on a continental scale, remote server farms streaming Google Classroom to children across the land. Isolated at home, with Chromebooks and iPads (for those fortunate enough to have them) propped on bedroom desks and kitchen tables, children spent hours alone every day, separated from their peers and teachers. "School" would now be attended through a screen. Parents of school-age children became their factotums, at once wardens of their confinement and their IT consultants, while moonlighting real jobs at home. Other parents were called to the front lines as essential workers, their children either foisted into ad hoc child care arrangements or, literally, left to their own devices.

Arts programs and athletics, the only safe outlets for millions of kids and teens, were also canceled. Children with special needs, including those with autism, Down syndrome, hearing and visual impairments, developmental disabilities, physical conditions such as muscular dys-trophy, behavioral and learning challenges such as ADHD and dyslexia, among many others, were unable to receive the in-person supports they required and to which they were entitled by law.

This did not last for a week or two. The school closures sustained through the end of the academic year, and in many parts of the country—almost exclusively progressive areas—schools, and the opportunities for kids to interact in person with their peers and teachers, remained either entirely out of reach or severely truncated and enfeebled for a full year or more.

It was a radical development, unimaginable in our lifetimes—until the moment it happened. And the harms and hardships felt by millions of kids and adolescents from extended closures were predictable, inequita-ble, and, for many, with lifelong consequences.

School closures, of course, don't only affect children. Many of the shared rhythms of our communities—whether in cities or rural villages, from Friday night lights to traffic patterns—pulse around schools, even for adults who are ostensibly disconnected from them. Their closure en masse was the rarest of public policies, one that knocked society off its axis, and the decisions that set it in motion were made incredibly quickly—and without a notion of their impact or when things would return to normal.

This book is an anatomy of that historic decision-making process and the many that would follow in its wake regarding schools during the coronavirus pandemic.

The characters who directed public discussion and the policy debate—from President Trump to Governor Cuomo, Anthony Fauci, and a sta-ble of public health experts-cum-pundits—functioned inside systems. Through a close look at their words and actions we see the machinery of decision-making and how policy was determined amidst ambiguity. We see how incentives that were misaligned with the interests of the public often drove decisions. We see how authority figures' influence was chan-neled through the media and, in turn, how the media influenced the authorities and regular citizens. We also see how the nature of news, and the muddling effect of the media's penchant for anecdotes and the spec-tacular, obscured mundane and nuanced reality. Lastly, we witness how ideological tribalism and groupthink overrode long-established values, specifically, how many progressives, professedly representing the party of science, completely disregarded overwhelming evidence about the safety of schools from around the world, in significant part, as a reaction to Trump and Trumpism.

Reassuringly, we also witness how through these failed systems and dynamics a few everyday heroes emerged.

This is a story of how we—as parents and communities—thought and behaved in an incredibly taxing and emotionally charged situation, one that regarded the well-being of what many would consider to be the ulti-mate concern for all people and cultures: their children. But if we take it as a given that societies, particularly those similar to our own, value chil-dren as we purport to, why was the response in American schools during the pandemic so different from that of so many nations in Europe?

Why were American schools, on average, closed or disrupted longer than those in Europe? Why were millions of children in California, Vir-ginia, Oregon, Washington, Maryland, and elsewhere in the US unable to set foot in a school building for more than a year, while many of their peers across the Atlantic resumed classes in the spring of 2020 and, with a few exceptions, continued attending school unabated on a normal sched-ule throughout the pandemic? Why did so many American schools, when they were open, impose far more restrictions—from excessive distancing to quarantines to, most controversially, masks on young children—and for longer durations than did their European counterparts? (If you think the answer is because all of the countries in Europe "controlled the virus," you are wrong. If you think it was because European schools were an oasis of HEPA-filtered air, you would also be incorrect.)

I have been fascinated, obsessed, enraged, and baffled by these ques-tions since the spring of 2020. And the evolving answers to these ques-tions are much of what animate this book.

The postmortem on school closures has largely divided into two camps: Many on the left argue that the prolonged school closures were a fog-of-war decision made on the best available information at the time. Many on the right argue that it was the malevolent influence of teachers unions, which operated out of self-interest and a lack of concern for the well-being of kids, that caused prolonged school closures.

But neither of these explanations is adequate.

The true story of what happened—why schools remained closed, despite a lack of evidence, and quite a bit to the contrary, that doing so would yield a net benefit for children, or society—is more complex and more important.

Through this story, school policies emerge as a window into the larger conversation around COVID-19 and, broader still, a prism through which to approach fundamental questions about why and how individuals, bureaucracies, governments, and societies act as they do in times of crisis. Ultimately, this is not a book about COVID. It's about a country ill-equipped to act sensibly under duress.

A mosaic of factors explains the gross and long-term imprudence in decision-making that resulted in catastrophic consequences for millions of children. But the foundation of it, and where we can look for wisdom and clarity during future crises, has to do with information—how it is presented to the public, and who is afforded a platform to present it. Trusted professionals in the health establishment failed to accurately interpret the evidence, and they neglected to convey the uncertainty and enormously consequential trade-offs around a range of actions and outcomes. For its part, the media shirked its core duty of investigating the facts and interrogating claims made by favored officials and anointed experts. As a result, much of the official guidance, and the policies that stemmed from it, was based on subjective *values* yet was presented to the public as objective science.

*   *   *

On July 29, 2020, Gallup released the results of a poll of more than 10,000 American adults. One of the questions asked was what people thought the distribution of COVID-19 deaths was among different age groups. The respondents overestimated the proportion of deaths for people age twenty-four and below by *40 times*. Not double. Not even ten times. But a 40-fold difference.

That age group composed just 0.2 percent of total COVID mortality, but respondents perceived it to be 8 percent. At the time, children under age fifteen accounted for an even more infinitesimal 0.04 percent of fatalities. For the duration of the pandemic, this basic age stratification of risk barely budged, despite schools finally opening full time, despite the Delta variant, despite the Omicron variant, despite summer camps and whatever else one wants to throw into the mix. More than a year after the survey, in the fall of 2021, people age twenty-four and below were 0.3 percent of total deaths. And all children through age seventeen accounted for 0.09 percent of COVID-19 mortality in the US. The number of pediatric deaths and hospitalizations from COVID were not just significantly but, in some cases, multiples lower than a wide range of other dangers to kids, from suicides to drownings to, by some accounting, in many seasons, the flu.

This distortion of risk assessment is not uncommon for humans in all sorts of facets of life. We ignominiously fear shark attacks, for example, which account for an average of one death a year in the US, yet blithely use our roadways even though more than 40,000 Americans die in vehicular accidents every year. But the gross misperception of risk to children during the coronavirus pandemic led to a consequence unprecedented in American history: barring healthy children from attending school.

There were additional reasons cited by authorities, the media, and others for school closures, notably a perceived risk to teachers and staff, and the potential for transmission to adults at home and in the community. But the alleged risk to children was always a key justification for closures and, when schools were open, for mitigation measures. Why were so many American parents so wildly off the mark in their assessment of the risks to children? And why, unique relative to its European peers, were school closures in America tolerated and even championed for so long?

Initially, and well into 2021, school closures, and masking and other mitigations imposed on kids for years, were vigorously defended by many officials and professionals as necessary. But as the pandemic wound down much of the media and left-wing establishment began to coalesce around a new narrative: that in hindsight those decisions were regrettable, yet they were understandable during a time of fear and uncertainty. I will show that that is a specious argument. Many other countries made far more sober decisions than the US did regarding children and schools. Those countries spanned a wide range of demographics, political leadership, and disease burden; there was no evidence that the US was epidemiologically different in any meaningful sense regarding schools. And US officials had access to the same information as everyone else at the same time.

To try to prevent disastrous decision-making during the next crisis, it is important that we not accept a narrative that is conveniently exculpatory, but false.

What led the US to be if not uniquely, then certainly exceptionally dysfunctional? I will reveal that American politicians, health officials, much of the broader medical establishment, and the media misled, lied to, and manipulated the public. Some of this was intentional, but much of it was due to political and social dynamics in the US that influenced what and how our leaders and much of elite society believed and behaved.

A NOTE ON LANGUAGE USAGE

Throughout the book, when I write that a school was "closed," I mean that students were not able to attend school in person, and "partially closed" signifies schools where students could only attend part time in person. I recognize that some people include remote learning under the umbrella of "school." But that form of learning—when a child is not in the physical presence of a teacher or peers—is not school in the traditional sense of how the term is typically understood or used, so I do not use it in that manner.

In the summer of 2022, Dr. Alasdair Munro, a pediatric infectious diseases specialist and member of the UK government's Transmission of COVID-19 in Schools working group, wrote in response to a claim that schools were not categorically "closed" just because they moved to remote instruction:

All available evidence suggests "remote schooling" failed even on the single function it is able to provide, which was education.

[Remote schooling] cannot even attempt to provide the vital health, social and safeguarding services that in-person school provides.

They were closed.

The World Health Organization put it succinctly in a report on schooling during the pandemic: "Schools deliver essential functions beyond education that cannot be delivered online."

Others, of course, are welcome to disagree with this usage. And it certainly is reasonable for remote learning to be considered a *form* of school in a general sense, just as "home schooling" is a form of school. But for clarity's sake, as a matter of semantics, let it be known that is how "closed" will be used in this book.

I

SEDUCTIVE MODELS
FEBRUARY AND MARCH 2020

1

REMOTE LEARNING WHILE
FLATTENING THE CURVE

By March 1, 2020, fears of the coronavirus in the US had begun to per-
colate into the public consciousness. Two Americans had died, and the
first case in New York City was confirmed. Still, it was early. The *New York
Times* ran a story headlined "Panic Shopping for Coronavirus Supplies,
but Brunch Is Packed," capturing the uncertain mood.

On Wednesday, March 4, the superintendent of my village's school
district, in New York's Hudson Valley, sent a mass email, oddly precise yet
opaque, informing the community that "a parent, whose children attend
school in our district, was physically present in a location that was closed
due to contact with a person who is under quarantine from the coronavirus." Out of "an abundance of caution," schools would be closed the
following two days for sanitization.

My kids were back in class the next week but, as cases and concerns
rose, by that Friday we were told schools would close again the following
Monday, March 16, through the end of the month. They did not fully
reopen until more than a year later.

In late March there was a flurry of emails and texts between parents
and school administrators about the failures of distance learning. Even
just a couple weeks into isolation, it seemed many children were list-
less and disengaged from the chaotic jumble of busywork and unhelp-
ful links to Wikipedia pages in Google Classroom that had become their
school. A Board of Education member told me privately that the teachers
union was refusing to amend its contract to mandate any recorded or live
stream instruction.

Another group of parents, however, was unperturbed. When concerns
were raised their general response was, "It's a pandemic! Don't complain
about remote learning. It'll sort itself out later."

My son, in third grade at the time, had always loved school and was a highly motivated student. That year he had been blessed with one of those special, veteran teachers who was a master of the craft. He was quirky, stern but fun, and regaled the kids with tales of his adventures around the world, while peppering his lessons with jokes delivered with a sophisticated, dry sense of humor. One wall of the classroom was covered by a world map pinned with tourist photos of the teacher in different locations where he'd been, which the students would often point to and discuss. During an event that parents attended I marveled at a three-foot-high stack of cases of Tab, the saccharin-laced soda I thought had been discontinued in the 1980s, piled in the corner of the room. It was a lively, weird, and memorable place. My son would come home from school each day reciting some new fact he had learned about hurricanes or Fabergé eggs.

Once schools closed, that all changed. While some teachers in the school were conducting a few live lessons online, even if just briefly each day, my son's teacher was not. Instead, sitting alone at a desk in his bedroom, my son was confronted each morning with a confusing list of assignments via Google Classroom, an online platform that presented him with reading materials or links to outside sites (often videos on YouTube) and instructions on how to access different software programs. English lessons were now conducted by Raz Kids. Math via IXL, and later through something called Zearn, a program my son found so tedious that it drove him to crying fits out of frustration.

A bright kid, he blazed through each day's work often in minutes and didn't know what to do with himself the rest of the day. My wife and I tried the best we could to keep him busy and engaged, but we both had professional obligations, so there was a limit to what we could do. I attempted to decipher poorly written guidelines for him on how to do one assignment or another, concocted projects like mini book reports, and bought him a math workbook, which he engaged with on his own for short stretches. Mostly, though, he became profoundly lonely, and poisonously bored. He desperately missed seeing his teacher and his friends.

My daughter's fifth grade teacher was impressively organized, creating color-coded daily checklists for the students, so they could stay on top of their copious assignments. The rest of "school" was an endless list of video lessons and software programs. Her teacher, who had three school-aged kids of her own, tried valiantly to keep the students on task, but, for my daughter at least, this model of instruction conferred too much autonomy and too much solitude to handle. Unfinished assignments piled up. Frustrations mounted. Eventually, later in April, the class had two to three live "meetings" each week, and, while an improvement, they weren't enough to resolve the issue: Sitting alone in a room for five-plus hours a day, staring at assignments on a screen, was not working. She watched YouTube for hours on end, which couldn't be blocked because so many of her lessons required viewing videos hosted on the site.

This, of course, was a picture of privileged suburbia. Many other kids, millions with special needs who required individual care from professionals, those in chaotic homes with abusive or neglectful parents, those with inadequate or no remote schooling on offer, or inadequate or absent electronic tools to access online schooling, and parents who had to work outside the home, were much worse off. But the government and public health officials told us this was an emergency situation, and there was no other appropriate course of action than to close the schools.

*　*　*

This all was a burden to be taken in stride. People were dying. Emergency rooms and ICUs just a short drive away were filled with patients suffering from a new and scary illness. We were told we needed to "shelter in place" for a limited duration to prevent the hospitals from being overwhelmed, and many of us complied eagerly.

I had friends who said things were going great. Parents were posting photos on my local Facebook group of the spectacular forts their kids had built and science experiments conducted and cookies baked. Moms (it usually was moms) posted tips for scheduling and education programs based on some pedagogical theory or other. This was a great time, they said, to take advantage of "project-based learning." A sense of guilt and inferiority hung over me. While my wife and I tried to get work done, my kids often devolved into whining and fights and, when my pleas for them to "go for a walk" or "read a book" were ignored, endless hours of screen time, an excess that prior to the stay-at-home order by Governor Cuomo would never have been allowed.

As March slouched in to April, most afternoons I'd go for a walk on the high school track with a friend and fellow parent (wearing masks and dutifully taking distanced lanes 1 and 4), and we'd speculate about when schools would reopen. Nearing May, I mused, Surely the kids would be back in class for the last two months of the school year. New cases in New York had been dropping dramatically, more than 50 percent since a peak on April 10. We had flattened the curve!

"Dave, they're not going back," he said, as we puffed through our masks rounding the end zone on that late April day. "The schools aren't reopening." I didn't quite believe him at the time, and I now realize it was with an optimist's denial that I kept thinking it would be just be another week or two.

Preventing hospitals from being overwhelmed was the initial justification for the general "stay-at-home" order in New York, which included closing schools. On a national level, the mission was made official on March 16, with the slogan "15 days to slow the spread." We were told if we all stayed home—with the exception, of course, of healthcare workers, delivery people, food service workers, police, and all others whose out-of-home work was deemed necessary to keep society functioning—that the threatening parabolic "curve" depicting the projected rise in cases would "flatten," and then, presumably, normalcy, at least to some extent, would resume. This meant, to my mind, sending kids back to school.

At the time, President Trump was fancifully downplaying the severity of the situation. Throughout February, March, and into April, he repeatedly announced, with a metaphorical wave of the hand, that the virus would just "go away." And he was seen by liberals and portrayed in much of the media as bungling the federal response. Among the fiascos early on there was a critical dearth of tests available, with reports from medical professionals around the country of people with symptoms unable to be tested. Moreover, kits from the CDC, which initially controlled nearly all testing, were flawed. And as hospitalizations began to spike in New York and other places, without the executive branch actively overseeing resource distributions, states found themselves in the absurdist situation of bidding against each other for medical equipment and supplies, such as ventilators.

Flattening the curve

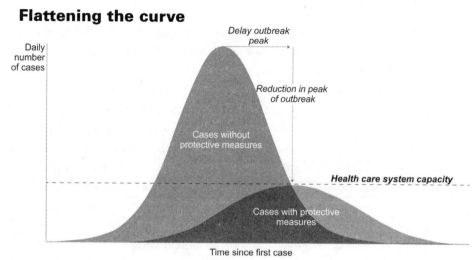

Source: CDC

One of many versions of the "flattening the curve" meme widely shared in social media posts, shown in television news segments, and embedded in news articles, ca. March 2020. Courtesy Christina Animashaun, *Vox* and Vox Media, LLC.

Trump grudgingly listened to and often contradicted public health professionals. Liberals, who had long been disgusted by the president, now found their disgust metastasized into fear- and indignation-driven rage. A new, contagious virus was circulating in the country and the guy in charge, a paragon of wishful thinking and unseriousness, was going to cause unnecessary mayhem and harm and deaths.

As in any classic story, an antipode to the villain was needed. A hero was called for. And New York's governor, Andrew Cuomo, emerged quickly in Act I to fill that role. Unlike the maleficent buffoon in the White House, Cuomo took the virus seriously.

At the end of March, in one of his no-nonsense speeches, which he and the media had regularly portrayed as overtly grounded in science and reason, Cuomo, projecting a paternalistic, calming authority, evoked a military metaphor, casting healthcare professionals as "soldiers fighting a battle for us." This was a war, he said, while warning: "This virus doesn't discriminate. It attacks everyone, and it attacks everywhere." The latter part of this statement was true insofar as anyone could become infected. But the former part, that the virus doesn't discriminate, was a demonstrably false statement, even early in the spring of 2020. Indeed, the coronavirus was fanatically prejudiced. It harmed the old and the vulnerable with a more than thousandfold higher incidence of severe disease and death compared to the young.

Yet raising the specter of danger to children, of course, was not exclusive to Cuomo. Two weeks before the governor's press conference, Michael Mulgrew, the head of the United Federation of Teachers, New York City's teachers union, posted a public letter to Mayor Bill DeBlasio excoriating him for "recklessly putting the health of students" in jeopardy by not closing the schools. Not only were school closures part of the overall shelter-in-place plan to reduce community transmission, they were also explicitly touted by politicians, and advocated for by many parents, teachers, and others as a prudent action to protect kids.

While Cuomo was sounding the alarm about the grave and immediate risk to everyone, including children, evidence from China, then Italy, and then throughout Europe, was remarkably consistent: children were largely unaffected by COVID-19. (The majority of COVID deaths in Italy, by early March, were in people over age eighty.) And, significantly, in regard to the risks they posed to teachers, children likely were less contagious than adults. This information was known even well before the March shutdowns.

On February 24, the *Journal of the American Medical Association* published a summary report by the Chinese Center for Disease Control and Prevention of 72,314 cases, which noted that just 1 percent of patients were under ten years old, and another 1 percent were aged ten to nineteen. Further, there were zero deaths in the youngest cohort. "Disease in children appears to be relatively rare and mild," a report published at the end of February from the World Health Organization stated. Children aged eighteen and under accounted for just 2.4 percent of reported cases, and of those cases 0.2 percent (or 0.0048 percent of the total) were categorized as "critical disease." Members of the investigative team "could not recall" instances of a child transmitting the virus to an adult.

Nevertheless, a rough consensus emerged among decision makers to shut down much of society, including every school in the country.

This was an extraordinary action. And a rich compendium of evidence casts doubt on any certainty that it was necessary or wise in all but a few locations. Still, the original school closures were largely harmless, and arguably reasonable (even if incorrect) under the circumstances. But they precipitated the grand folly that was to come: in dramatic contrast to their counterparts throughout Europe, American schools remained closed through the spring and for the majority of students—tens of millions of them—did not open fully for more than an entire year. And it's important to understand that the political, bureaucratic, philosophical, and social factors that led to closing schools initially both reinforced and reflected many of the dynamics that underpinned all future decisions on schools. The seeds were already planted.

2

GIGO

For two days in June 2006, a large gathering that included dozens of employees from the Centers for Disease Control and Prevention, executives from the National Institutes of Health and state and local health departments, representatives from multinational corporations like Delta Airlines and Exxon Mobile, and epidemiologists, infectious diseases experts and professionals from universities and institutions around the country convened at a four-star Atlanta hotel for a conference on mitigation strategies during an influenza pandemic. Jennifer Nuzzo, a young researcher at the Center for Biosecurity at Pittsburgh Medical Center, nervously prepared to deliver a presentation in the ballroom. A bright but junior epidemiologist (she was still eight years away from a PhD), Nuzzo was accompanied by D. A. Henderson, her mentor at Pitt and widely considered the most influential figure on disease outbreak policy in the country and possibly the globe. Henderson had a mile-long list of credentials and accomplishments, among them working as a bioterrorism adviser to multiple presidents. But, most famously and importantly, he had directed the World Health Organization's program that eradicated smallpox, a spectacular achievement that Henderson executed through a new tactical strategy known as "ring vaccination," inoculating strategic groups of people who were exposed to the virus. Its success required a keen understanding of how a virus spreads in real time and, critically, hands-on involvement of public health officials in the affected populations. Henderson was put in charge of the project as a young man, in 1966, in part because so many health officials had assumed the program was doomed to fail and no one more prominent wanted to take on the task.

"So there I am," Nuzzo said, recounting the event to me, "arriving at the conference with this legend. And all these people are approaching us. Julie Gerberding, the director of the CDC, made a beeline to him, and then turned and introduced herself to me."

With the War on Terror in full force and overall biosecurity a preoccupation of then-president George W. Bush, a call had been put out for a formal preparatory plan for pandemics. The authors of the plan, a small team comprising administrators from various executive branch departments, such as Homeland Security and Agriculture, included Dr. Carter Mecher, a physician and medical officer at the Veterans Administration, who presented an early version at the Atlanta conference and at a smaller National Academies meeting. The presentations were essentially a road show, in which the authors tried to sell their plan to the audience of experts. Much of their presentation would ultimately turn into the US government's official pandemic playbook from the CDC, released the following year, with the ungainly title "Interim Pre-pandemic Planning Guidance: Community Strategy for Pandemic Influenza Mitigation in the United States—Early, Targeted, Layered Use of Nonpharmaceutical Interventions." An updated version, released in 2017, retained and built on much of the contents of the original, including guidance on school closures.

As Mecher and his colleagues presented to the room, Nuzzo had an uneasy feeling. Everything in their plans was based on models: projections on how influenza might spread, projections on how many people might get sick or die, and projections on how certain nonpharmaceutical interventions (NPIs)—such as social distancing, personal protective equipment, and school closures—would mitigate that spread. If certain measures were implemented early enough, the model showed specific reduced trajectories of transmission.

Models are a useful and necessary part of epidemiology; they're one tool scientists use to try to predict what will happen. But the Achilles' heel of models is that they are always based on sets of statistical assumptions, which are then plugged into mathematical formulas that spit out results or ranges of results. The formula itself might be valid, but if you insert the wrong numbers then you get the wrong result. Researchers tartly call this problem "garbage in, garbage out." (The problem is so pervasive and foundational to computing that the phrase, often referred to by its acronym GIGO, dates back to military computer programmers in 1957.)

Let's take a detour for a moment to look at an example of this problem. A modeling paper called "To Mask or Not to Mask" by researchers at Arizona State University, published in April 2020, made a variety of claims, including that an 80 percent adoption of even weakly effective masks in a low-transmission area could reduce COVID mortality by 24 percent to 65 percent. The authors arrived at this conclusion by assuming masks had, at worst, a 20 percent effectiveness. Where did they get 20 percent from? They cite another modeling paper, "Mathematical Modeling of the Effectiveness of Facemasks in Reducing the Spread of Novel Influenza A." This paper, however, cites a study that found surgical masks can have a performance as poor as just 15.5 percent effectiveness at blocking virions. The study also found that, depending on particle size, nine out of ten N95 masks, which are supposed to block 95 percent of particles, failed to meet that benchmark. Some of the tests in the study also used aerosolized salt, which has different characteristics from viruses. And, importantly, the study was conducted in a laboratory on manikins, with the masks "sealed to the manikin's face." The authors noted the obvious: "in real life leaks may lead to considerably increased penetration." Considering most of the public during the pandemic did not wear N95s, but wore surgical or cloth masks, and considering that penetration of an infectious dose of a virus through a mask is not synonymous with penetration of salt particles, and that a manikin in a lab is not the same as a person wearing a mask in a grocery store or on a train, the assumption of baseline effectiveness that lay at the foundation of the ASU model's conclusion was completely untethered from reality. Moreover, the authors didn't define what 80 percent adoption meant. Did that mean wearing masks just in the community or also inside one's home? Did it assume that 80 percent of grade school kids would have perfect compliance for seven hours a day in school? The authors didn't say. Nevertheless, the ASU modeling paper was cited in hundreds of subsequent academic papers and multiple governmental reports; it was shared on social media by immunologists, primary care physicians, and academics, one of whom said this was "proof" about the effectiveness of masks; and it was featured in the news with headlines like "ASU Study Predicts Widespread Mask Use Could Save

Thousands of Lives." (Making matters worse, a model is a simulation. It is not a "study." Yet news articles often refer to models as studies, leading the public to perceive an inflated degree of certainty from their findings.)

The ASU masking model was based on a relatively simple set of inputs. Models of the effect of school closures, however, are wildly fraught. They rely on a near-infinite number of uncontrolled variables, from assumptions about how much or whether kids interact with each other outside of school to the rate of transmission in homes—perhaps the two most important unaccounted for variables that undermine the assumed benefit of school closures throughout the pandemic.

Models can tell a compelling story, except you don't know if it's fiction.

"They weren't explaining how they put together the models," Nuzzo said. While the presenters were casually saying, "If you implement X, Y, or Z" you will get a certain result, some of the audience members were looking at each other with raised eyebrows, as if to say, *"But where are you getting X, Y, and Z?!"* An infectious diseases specialist turned to Nuzzo and quietly said, "Models bury assumptions."

One of the presenters said that their models assumed the NPIs would be implemented before something like 1 percent or 0.5 percent of the population would be infected by the virus. From the presenter's view this appeared to be a minor point. But if the effectiveness of the NPIs depicted in the model was reliant upon their implementation before a specified percentage of people were exposed to the virus, getting that specified percent correct mattered *a lot*. Nuzzo knew it was unlikely that authorities would be able to track how many people were infected early on in an epidemic (which, due to inadequate testing capabilities, is exactly what happened in the US at the beginning of COVID), so there would be no way to know what percentage of the population had been exposed before implementing the NPIs. Moreover, the models themselves, even beyond questions about their inputs, were run on computers ahead of the presentation, and no one knew how exactly the formulas were designed. The whole thing was a black box.

In other words: The presenters were suggesting that American cities and states that implemented NPIs, including closing schools, would achieve certain results based on projections from models that didn't account for information and behaviors in the real world. It was like a football coach showing his team a complex offensive play and insisting it would result in a touchdown, without acknowledging that each of the opposing team's defensive players might not do what he expected them to do. Even the most elegantly designed plays by the best coaches often turn out ugly on the field. Like their human counterparts, the scientific models were a beautiful ideal.

Nuzzo said that at the meeting no audience members publicly criticized the models. Without pushback the models looked great. The decision makers were persuaded, and the White House went ahead with authorizing publication of the playbook.

Unlike the modelers, Nuzzo and Henderson came from an opposite tradition of gathering and analyzing empirical data. In the early 2000s, before her appointment at the Pittsburgh Medical Center, Nuzzo worked for the City of New York, monitoring its tap water. In exchange for its exemption from requiring filtration plants, New York City has surveillance programs that include epidemiologists who monitor things like the sale of diarrhea medications or the rate of GI-related emergency room visits. A spike in one or more of these factors could signal that something might be wrong with the water. After 9/11, Nuzzo's duties reclassified toward tracking bioterrorism threats. "I kept wondering, 'Is today the day NYC gets poisoned?'" she said. Nuzzo didn't deal in assumptions. She aimed to keep people safe by tracking data on the ground (or in the water, as it were).

Similarly, a key reason for Henderson's success was that he understood the value of being personally engaged with people, knowing how individuals and groups behave and interact, rather than relying on abstractions and giving orders from a distant office. To vaccinate people you need to reach them physically, you need to persuade them this medical product is safe and necessary, and you need to be strategic about who gets vaccinated when. During his time at the WHO, he repeatedly traveled, sometimes at personal risk in war zones, to countries afflicted with smallpox to oversee the vaccination efforts. Later in his career, as dean of the school of public health at Johns Hopkins, he altered the curriculum to send more students following his footsteps into the field. "D.A. was an operational guy," Nuzzo said. Understanding the dynamics of disease spread requires understanding people socially and psychologically as much as, if not more than, biologically.

In the 2007 official pandemic preparedness report, which launched from the presentations made at the Atlanta meeting, school closures are not the only tool in the box, but their prominence is unmistakable, their expressed necessity immutable. They are mentioned in the summary. They are mentioned in the introduction. They are mentioned in the conclusion. They are mentioned in the majority of pages of the document. They are the hammer. Why?

The NPIs, and specifically the focus on school closures, in our nation's pandemic planning guides originated in no small part from the work of Robert Glass, a complex systems modeler, who brought his work to Carter Mecher while he and partners were developing the playbook. Mecher, known for his creative thinking and innovations at the VA, was thrilled by Glass's elegant, neoteric models and incorporated them into the guide. Glass got the idea and the first inputs for his models from Laura, his fourteen-year-old daughter. She, with the elder Glass's help, had made computer simulations of how to slow the spread of a pandemic for a school science project. Laura and then her father worked from the premise that kids and teens socialize and interact more than anyone else, so if schools are closed and kids stay home, the virus won't be able to spread. Children and teens, they wrote, "form the backbone" of viral spread in an epidemic. In a paper detailing his involvement in the 2007 report's development, Glass remarkably asserted that if the pediatric stay-at-home compliance were 100 percent "adults could continue to go to work with business as usual to keep the economy rolling." By simulating the closure of schools, he and his daughter had conjured a "simple straightforward solution" to halting the spread of a virus, he wrote.

The Glass models that so captured Mecher and helped form the foundation of our government's official pandemic response guide feature a series of complex color-coded diagrams, charts, graphs, and tables depicting in various ways how a virus spreads among people, and how implementing NPIs, most important of which being school closures, arrests the transmission. But these seductive models are based on a long series of assumptions, the most important of which is that schools are a prime source of transmission and that closing them, in particular over long periods, would thwart transmission. (Among the scenarios modeled is one in which children and teenagers remain home "for the duration of the pandemic.")

Remember "garbage in, garbage out"—it's critical that the numerical assumptions in Glass's models were accurate; the effectiveness of the NPIs that our government was supposed to implement in the real world on real people was dependent on it. So where are the figures in the Glass models from? In many instances in Glass's paper the references for his assumptions linked not to empirical data but to *more models*. For example, one of Glass's references is a modeling paper called "Strategies for Mitigating an Influenza Pandemic." This paper, by the highly influential modeler Neil Ferguson—a name that will resurface in our story later—is also directly referenced by the 2007 government report. Ferguson's model assumed that 37 percent of transmission occurs in schools and workplaces, with schools having twice the transmission rate as workplaces. These figures are very important—they are the basis of the model, and the foundation of its projections about the effect of school closures. So, where did Ferguson get these figures? The answer is not in the main paper. To find the source of the figure one has to spelunk deep into the paper's supplement, where you would discover the following text:

"It is necessary to make assumptions about the proportion of transmission which occurs in schools and workplaces, as data do not exist. . . . Our assumption is that 37% of transmission occurs in these contexts, with the within-school transmission coefficient being twice that of the within-workplace coefficient. However, *this choice is arbitrary*" (italics added).

If you need to take a moment to let the previous sentences sink in, I understand. When I first found this passage I felt like a cartoon character rubbing his eyes at seeing a mirage. I had to read it three times before I believed it was real.

So: The expected effect of school closures listed in the playbook was based on Glass's model, which was based, in part, on Ferguson's model, which was based on *a made-up figure*.

Glass's models also are based on the assumption that children and teenagers are more infectious than adults. Glass and his co-authors wrote that children and teens have closer contact with others, and are less likely to wash their hands or control coughs. The citation given for the latter claim was a paper called "A Bayesian MCMC Approach to Study Transmission of Influenza." Yet this paper contained no information about pediatric coughs or hand washing. Instead it was populated with, yes, *more models.* To give you a sense of the complexity of the models, below is one of the many gnarly formulas in the paper:

$$P(v, \Psi \mid \Theta) = \prod_{i \in I} d_{\mu_i, \sigma_i}(\Psi_i - v_i) \prod_{i \in I - \{1\}} \lambda_i(v_i) e^{-\int_{v1}^{vi} \lambda i(t)dt} \prod_{s \in S} e^{-\int_{v1}^{15} \lambda_s(t)dt}$$

(It may be true that kids are less likely to wash their hands or stifle coughs. Or it might not. And if it is true about kids, to what extent is it true? Are they 10 percent less likely to wash their hands and cover their coughs? 20 percent? 50 percent? And how much of that lower percentage translates to what percentage increase in disease transmission?)

Although the Bayesian paper didn't contain information about the relative rate of controlling coughs, it did model children's role in infectious disease transmission. So, where did the assumptions for the models in this paper come from? It's impossible to know because there were no citations given next to the assumptions in the models. However, among the references listed there are, you guessed it, *yet more models.* To wade into this material is to experience the unreality of a never-ending matryoshka doll, forever revealing yet another doll inside of a doll.

These details might seem picayune. But they're not. The public was told that closing schools was one of the most, if not *the* most effective means of controlling the spread of the coronavirus. If that claim were based on models that were based on incorrect numbers—which, given that some of them are made up, is quite assured—that's a big problem. Remember the ASU mask paper. The model made a baseline assumption of 20 percent effectiveness of masks, which was based on another model, which was based on a lab study on manikins in which the authors stated that masks in the real world would likely perform worse than masks did in their lab, and didn't even address cloth mask effectiveness. Since Ferguson's input of 37 percent and that schools had twice the transmission rate of workplaces was just a guess, it's possible that the real number for schools is 50 percent or maybe just 5 percent. If the transmission rate in schools is far lower than what the models assume, that's an error of great consequence, as it obviously changes the calculus about whether closing schools, particularly over the long term, actually achieves the benefit that the modelers and policy makers and public health pundits continued to claim, and that much of the public was led to believe.

To be clear on one thing: None of this means that school closures do nothing to slow the spread of a virus. There is of course an intuitive logic behind the idea that if you close schools, along with many other aspects of society, virus transmission will be slowed. And the evidence is good that, if done early enough in conjunction with other extremely intensive interventions, school closures may be effective for a limited time. However, there was no factual basis behind the assumption that closing schools should have been the cornerstone of viral mitigation policy. There was no quality evidence to support the idea that closing schools or severely truncating attendance for months, let alone for a year or more, while other aspects of society were open, would have any meaningful benefit. And, indeed, no uniform evidence ever emerged that areas with prolonged school closures or hybrid schedules were correlated with a reduction in transmission or deaths.

Closing schools or limiting capacity might superficially seem like a logical way to reduce transmission. But from a review of the scientific literature—even just dipping a toe beneath the surface of assumptions—it is clear that other than for a very brief time period, while in conjunction with other severe NPIs, this logic is flawed. As I have and will continue to point out throughout this book, our intuitions are often wrong, and medicine and public health are not immune from this poor record of prognostications and understandings of the world.

There are many reasons why assuming that closing schools would be an effective mitigation strategy was unfounded. It is one of our greatest public health failures that officials made this assumption, and as a result children were kept out of school for as long as they were. Transmission among children outside of school was warned about as early as summer of 2020 by experts at Harvard's T. H. Chan School of Public Health, Johns Hopkins University, and elsewhere, but largely to no avail.

In brief—and this point will be referenced repeatedly throughout the book—children, and their caregivers, do not stay home all the time. And the longer the closures lasted the less that people isolated. During a pandemic some children will go to daycare, others will meet up with friends, others will be cared for by relatives. Many parents will work outside the home and will bring a virus back to the family, and so on. The possibilities for transmission outside of a closed school are numerous. While some portion of families had the desire and ability to keep every household member in extreme isolation for close to a year—until vaccines were available for adults—that was not the norm. And families in which at least one parent had to leave the home for jobs were certainly not able to isolate. As early as the end of April 2020, one-third of US adults said they were deemed essential workers and were already working outside the home. (Seventy percent of those essential workers leaving home did not have a college degree. So, on average, those who were less educated—and likely less financially well off—had the greatest proportion of compelled exposure.)

There is also a very provocative biological consideration specific to a novel coronavirus that Mecher and the others did not take into account. It is true that children have higher rates of endemic respiratory viruses. But, as Dr. Shira Doron, an infectious diseases specialist at Tufts University, wrote in a 2023 paper on how to handle the next pandemic: "What if the paradigm—that children interacting in schools universally drive respiratory pandemics—is based on incorrect assumptions about the relative importance of in-school contact patterns for driving population spread, particularly in the longer term?" Instead, Doron and her coauthors wrote, an alternate explanation for these well-recognized transmission patterns for endemic respiratory viruses is that children are always a more immune-susceptible population relative to adults. In other words, the authors explained, it's possible that the reason endemic respiratory virus transmission appears to be driven by children is *not* because of their in-school contacts or behavior, but rather because children, as a whole, "have not had time to acquire immunity to these endemic viruses to the extent adults have." Children's elevated rates of transmission with flu and other viruses might be primarily due to biology, not social conditions such as schools. Even during novel influenza pandemics, the authors wrote, evidence suggests that adult immunity from prior exposure to related flu strains provides protection.

It may very well be that there is nothing inherently more virulent about COVID-19 than influenza, RSV, or any number of other respiratory viruses. The only reason more adults got very sick or died from COVID, relative to other viruses, it's theorized, is not because SARS-CoV-2 itself is intrinsically more dangerous, but rather because, unlike other viruses, adults had never been exposed to it in their youth. Unlike many past epidemics, which disadvantaged children, this time everyone was in the same boat—adults were equally as immune naive as children, yet children were, with rare exception, fine, because their bodies, once they pass infancy, appear to often handle initial exposure to pathogens safely in a way adults' bodies often do not. (There are innumerable of examples of this, from chickenpox to tuberculosis. It's been termed the "honeymoon period" by researchers.) As the pandemic wore on and people were repeatedly exposed to SARS-CoV-2—either through vaccines, the actual virus, or both—the risk of severe disease and death declined with each exposure because the body was no longer facing a novel threat. While there are exceptions, this process is a basic truth of immunology. And it helps explain why children, relative to adults, early on were less likely to get infected or be symptomatic, and less likely to transmit the virus.

This biological reality suggests that focusing on contact patterns among children—as Mecher, Anthony Fauci, and other public health officials had done—versus those among adults, was unlikely to yield the predicted reduction in COVID transmission.

*   *   *

But it gets worse. Setting aside that the models were based on a downward spiral of dubious assumptions—an aside that, granted, is like a forensic report of a building collapse setting aside that the structure's foundation was laid in loose sand—no one followed the government's plans anyway.

The 2007 report suggested that in the most severe pandemic categories, in which deaths are projected to be in excess of 900,000 or in excess of 1.8 million in an unmitigated environment, schools should close for up to twelve weeks.

The 2017 playbook premised school closures on three objectives:

(1) in the very early stages of a pandemic, for *up to two weeks*, school closures would buy time for authorities to assess the transmissibility and severity of the virus;

(2) in areas with outbreaks school closures, for *up to six weeks*, would slow the spread so healthcare facilities could prepare additional resources for the expected increase in demand; and

(3) closures, for *up to six months*, would allow time for a vaccine to be
     produced.

During March of 2020 the entire US school system blew past number
1. Following those two weeks areas with early outbreaks, notably the New
York metro area, saw case and hospital rates decline dramatically within
six weeks of onset—the criteria for objective 2—yet schools continued to
remain closed. And as far as objective number 3 goes, that option was premised on the notion that creating flu vaccines for new strains typically
takes up to six months. *Yet there was no such expectation* for the development and availability of a vaccine for this "novel" virus. At the fastest, it
was thought it might take around a year, and even that speculative timeline was dismissed as too optimistic by experts such as Anthony Fauci,
perhaps the most influential health official in the country.

It was impossible for the authorities to credibly claim they were following the playbook for any of its school closure objectives.

It is important to recognize that COVID, of course, is different from
influenza, so the government should not have been expected to precisely follow influenza playbooks when they were dealing with a different pathogen. Indeed, at two separate press conferences in February CDC
officials said they would adapt recommendations from the playbook to
current circumstances. Yet they said they intended to be "very aggressive" with NPIs, and cited school closures. The adaptation went in the
wrong direction. Relative to many flu epidemics, COVID's lower risk of
sickness for children, and children's initially lower likelihood of getting
infected and transmitting the virus, if anything made school closures
less appropriate than the playbook suggested.

Let me elaborate:

Health professionals and policy makers frequently cited the 1918 influenza pandemic as a template for NPIs for the COVID pandemic. Yet while
1918 could offer some lessons for 2020, that pandemic's virus behaved
differently from COVID in some instrumental ways, which made 1918 a
very poor example to follow. Incredibly, a nearly completely overlooked
fact is that, according to a study cited by the CDC, 95 percent of deaths
from the 1918 pandemic occurred in people under age 65. Yes, you read
that correctly. This age stratification of risk is effectively the *opposite* from
what it was for COVID. Yet a key justification for extended school closures

during the COVID pandemic (in addition to attempting to reduce overall transmission) was for the safety of students.

This isn't to say COVID posed zero risk to children, but rather that its risk—which was known since the spring of 2020—was on par with myriad other potential dangers to kids. After all, in the past schools were never preemptively closed for weeks or months because of circulating influenza viruses, even though in many seasons the flu posed a greater risk to children than COVID. Saying that closing schools was, at least in part, needed for the protection of children was disingenuous.

Knowing who is most—and least—at risk should, of course, influence policy and the burdens placed on various populations. Sure enough, that is what the CDC 2017 report recommended—it called for identifying strategies for particular groups who are at high risk. In a March 2020 *New York Times* piece, Jennifer Nuzzo highlighted this exact point—unlike influenza, she wrote, COVID did not generally appear to cause severe illness in children, nor did kids appear to drive the spread of COVID. As such, it was "likely that school closings will have little effect on its spread."

All this is to say: If officials were going to veer from the playbooks, it should have been in a direction of *less* aggression toward schools and children. Yet they did the opposite.

That the early—and continued—response to COVID in the form of NPIs, specifically school closures, was untethered from the government's official pandemic plans matters greatly. In the obvious and superficial sense this is because it showcases a failure of panicked officials to follow blueprints that had been laid by the health establishment. But, more importantly, as we will see, that failure dovetailed with an ignorance and dismissal of a rich literature on both the inescapable harms that would result from the closures and on the evidence of their lack of benefit over the long term.

3

RED DAWN

As the coronavirus was just beginning to take off in the US, an email chain, nicknamed Red Dawn (a cheeky reference to a 1980s movie in which a group of Americans resisted Soviet invaders), featured a lengthy dialogue between Carter Mecher, then at the Department of Veterans Affairs, and ultimately dozens of other officials at the Department of Homeland Security, the CDC, Health and Human Services, the Department of Defense, the State Department, and former government officials and outside experts at universities and other institutions, in which the spirit of the playbook he had authored was debated and largely championed. The email chain is a fascinating window into what these people in positions of power were thinking, and how they intended to influence policy.

Throughout the chain, which continued in various permutations from January 2020 through March 2020, closing schools was repeatedly mentioned as a critical tactic to control the spread of the virus. This act would be part of "targeted layered containment," or TLC, which Mecher, and Tom Bosset, a former Homeland Security adviser, explained meant implementing multiple interventions at once. "The biggest misunderstanding about coronavirus interventions is they are an à la carte menu of options to be selectively implemented. This is dead wrong. They ALL must be implemented. For instance, close schools AND cancel events," Bossert wrote (the all caps are Bossert's). School closures in Japan, Hong Kong, Singapore, and China were mentioned over and over by multiple people throughout the chain.

In a March 10 email, Mecher ran through a list of arguments against closing schools: kids potentially are not prime vectors for transmission, and their illness is mild; closing schools is too disruptive to parents, who will be forced to stay home; a large number of children depend on schools for meals; and if they're not in school, kids will have more time to mix with family members and other kids at "the mall." The last point, that even with schools closed children would still interact with each other (and adults)—whether at the mall, daycare, or in any number of other contexts—would prove to be a very important point later in the pandemic, because it negates the assumed benefit of transmission reduction of both full school closures and partial closures in so-called hybrid schedules.

Mecher then dismissed each of the concerns he raised, writing, "We close schools for 1 week for spring break and the world does not fall apart. The nutrition of children does not suffer. Why not close for two weeks and then reassess." He ended his email: "Many of you have kids, do any of them hang out at malls? In my neighborhood I don't even see kids outside—they are all inside texting, on Instagram, playing games with their friends online or whatever they do these days." The only place kids all go to together, he noted, was school.

The nation was facing what appeared to be a looming catastrophe, and the White House was widely perceived to be in denial. The general tenor of the emails is one of increasing urgency. Mecher warns of impending "chaos and panic." To a large measure, it was up to the elite participants in this exclusive dialogue to protect the country. The feeling among them is that it's better to act, to do more than is necessary. Eva Lee, a renowned modeler at Georgia Tech, and an active writer in the chain, concludes that if the NPIs are successful that they will be underappreciated because people wouldn't know the horror that was averted. Interventions must be done before it's too late, she says, otherwise the results could be "catastrophic." By design, she says, "successful mitigation is often undervalued." Lee said the NPIs of school closures and telework from home could perform "beautifully and effectively," and included line graphs of models she made of ninety-day projections showing a near vertical rise in infections if no interventions were taken, contrasted with several gently ascending lines representing dramatically reduced rates of infection if schools, or schools and businesses, closed early enough. The differential between the representation of unmitigated versus mitigated spread looked like a sketch of ski trails: a triple black diamond versus a bunch of bunny slopes. What would happen after ninety days was not addressed.

By mid-March, articles from news outlets around the world were telling of a nightmare scenario playing out in northern Italy, where doctors in overwhelmed hospitals were being forced to ration care and deprioritize elderly patients. Mecher, along with many others in the chain, had grown impatient with and angry at the authorities' inaction. "I don't pretend to have perfect knowledge of the extent of disease in the U.S. There is a lot of uncertainty," he wrote. "But given this uncertainty, isn't the safest approach to close the schools until we know more? We can always reopen the schools. If we delay our response and the outbreak takes off like Italy we will have made a terrible gamble with the lives of Americans, over what, an extended spring break?" In a shift from his comments from just a few days earlier, he no longer suggested the closures would be for just a week or two. "I don't think the intent is to close schools for only 2 weeks," he wrote. "Longer term school closure will be necessary." Yet recall the objectives of school closures listed in the playbook: close schools for up to two weeks to provide authorities time to assess the situation. For schools to close in an area for longer than two weeks, as Mecher was now suggesting, the playbook indicated there would need to be outbreaks in that area. Yet on March 13, outside of pockets in New York, Washington State, and a few other places, much of the country was not in the midst of outbreaks. Even the author of the original playbook, himself, was going off script.

On Thursday, March 12, Governor Mike DeWine of Ohio announced that all schools in his state would close the following Monday and stay closed until at least April 3. (Notably, DeWine waited until three days later to announce closures of bars and restaurants, a portent of the attitude toward placing schools first for disruption and last for normalcy that many governors around the country would follow for the next two years.) By the next day, sixteen states announced school closures, with many governors stating they'd last two to three weeks. Governor Andrew Cuomo of New York announced on March 16 that schools throughout his state would shut down two days later until at least April 1. Part of Cuomo's closure included exempting schools from the state's requirement of 180 days of instruction each academic year. This exemption would prove to be critical. With no legal obligation to open their doors, schools could remain closed or in hybrid schedules for as long as any district administrators desired or unions demanded, long after the rest of society had returned to relatively normal.

Surprisingly, despite not being among the first governors to make this decision, Cuomo still had to be pushed into announcing his state's closures. According to a source with intimate knowledge of the highest level of the Cuomo administration, who spoke on the condition of anonymity due to concerns over professional consequences of speaking publicly, Cuomo may have started his state's closures even later if it weren't for Bill DeBlasio, New York City's mayor. "DeBlasio told Cuomo he intended to close the city's schools. Being scooped by the mayor was intolerable to Cuomo, so he jumped in front to announce school closures at the state level first," said the source during several conversations with me in early 2022. "I don't remember any coordination from the federal government or CDC for closing schools. There were many inquiries coming in from local officials to Cuomo asking if he would close. It became a drumbeat." The broader closures in New York, of nonessential businesses, the canceling of all nonessential gatherings of any size for any reason, and so on, didn't begin until the evening of March 22.

DeWine, Cuomo, and numerous other governors ordering school closings *before* shutting down many other major aspects of society was, in many ways, the original sin. It wrongly implied that schools, and children in particular, were the primary source of transmission, and, despite whatever verbal assurances given to the contrary, implied that children were at great risk. The *action* of closing schools, and especially that they were first, spoke louder than words. For reasons that will be discussed later, this initial impression would prove to be intractable for many people.

4

MORE ASSUMPTIONS

While the authority to close schools resides with governors, the CDC's comments preparing the public for the likelihood of societal shutdowns gave whatever political cover was necessary for the closures to happen. Millions of people had also begun altering their behavior voluntarily. Many thousands of flights were canceled, conferences terminated, the NBA season was suspended, and by mid-March restaurants in Boston, New York, and Seattle saw their patronage drop by more than 60 percent compared to the previous year. So there was, at least in parts of the country, a sense among politicians that there likely was a public desire for more formal restrictions. And given the Red Dawn chain's highly placed insiders, including staff at HHS, CDC, and DOD, the plans advocated in the emails were circulating among the halls of power in DC and beyond. Moreover, the models, including the flatten the curve meme and, specifically, those from a highly influential team at Imperial College London—referenced by Eva Lee in the Red Dawn chain, and referred to by coronavirus task force officials—which gave frightening predictions communicated in visually arresting, simplistic graphs were, naturally, seized upon by the major news outlets and circulated on social media. The models were in the ether; their predictions were now part of the narrative.

There are a few facts to highlight about the Imperial College pandemic models, the most influential of which, released on March 16, were part of a paper called Report 9:

First, the models were cataclysmic, predicting more than two million deaths in the US by the end of August of that year if their recommended mitigations, including school closures, were not implemented. Second, they were cited by Dr. Deborah Birx, the head of the White House coronavirus task force, as informing her policy recommendations. Third, the media, from the *New York Times* and the *Washington Post* on down, widely reported on the models. On March 16, the *Times* ran an entire feature about the ICL models, including one of ICL's line graphs depicting millions of deaths in the US over the next few months in the absence of "drastic action" to slow the spread. The article noted the ICL paper concluded that, despite enormous costs to society, this was "the only viable strategy."

Lastly, the models were created by Neil Ferguson, the renowned modeler who, you may remember, based earlier projections on arbitrary figures for school transmission, and whose work Robert Glass relied upon for his models, and who was cited directly in the CDC's pandemic playbook.

Given the authorities' explicit reliance on the models, the *Times* piece contained one of the most revealing statements, made by Ferguson, of the entire pandemic: "*We don't have a clear exit strategy. We're going to have to suppress this virus—frankly, indefinitely—until we have a vaccine.*"

The ICL report makes a distinction between suppression and mitigation. The latter is defined as measures taken that are intended to slow transmission, but not halt it completely, to reduce peak healthcare demands and protect those most at risk of severe disease. Suppression, by comparison, requires implementing NPIs on a societal scale of sufficient breadth and intensity so as to lower the reproduction number (known as the R0) below 1, meaning each existing infection causing fewer than one new infection, leading to a decline in case numbers, theoretically down to zero.

Neither the *Times* nor *Washington Post* pieces investigated or questioned any of the assumptions underlying Report 9's predictions or its methodology, nor was the feasibility or cost-benefit of the overall strategy detailed.

It's hard to overstate how important the "15 days" press conference on March 16, along with Report 9, and the uncritical reaction to it, was. An immense metal baton was jammed into the spinning gears of society. And the justification given by Deborah Birx, the leader of the pandemic response in the US, along with the support of the president, was a model that terrified much of the country into submission. One would think there would have been teams of scientists and other experts scrutinizing every detail of the model, loudly and publicly debating its every fine point, with an army of reporters at our top news organizations joining the interrogation. But that's not what happened.

Yet it's critical to understand Report 9, and how Ferguson and his team modeled the effect of school closures, particularly over the long term, since this model was a foundational justification for that policy.

The report states: "Per-capita contacts within schools were assumed to be double those elsewhere in order to reproduce the attack rates in children observed in past influenza pandemics." Without a careful eye, one could read past that sentence without pause. Yet it should have caused health officials, such as Birx, and policy makers, to hit the brakes. After all, much of Imperial College's modeled predictions about the effect of school closures hinged on this assumption. What was it based on? No details were given in the report. However, a 2005 modeling paper, "Strategies for Containing an Emerging Influenza Pandemic in Southeast Asia," published in the journal *Nature*, coauthored by Ferguson, was cited as the source of this claim.

Yet when I read that paper there was nothing in it related to per-capita contacts within schools being double those elsewhere. I decided to reach out to Ferguson.

He told me, "Our assumption of contact rates between children in schools being twice that of adults in workplaces reflected preliminary results from contact rate surveys underway at the time," which ultimately were published nearly three years later in a *different* journal, *PLOS Medicine*. Yet the *PLOS Medicine* paper, the actual source for Report 9's claim about pediatric contact rates, raised a series of concerns. To name one, it "deliberately oversampled" children. I left our exchange without a clear sense of the validity of this critical assumption in Report 9.

This is complex, esoteric stuff, so I had a substantial degree of humility about my confusion. I wanted to speak with someone specifically from the epidemiological modeling field to make sure I was not mistaking my lack of satisfaction in getting a clear answer for there not being a clear answer.

An epidemiological modeler named Alexander Washburne agreed to talk with me. Washburne has a PhD in computational biology from Princeton, and among his past work are models on the epidemiology of pathogen spread and analyses of zoonotic spillover of bat viruses to humans. Washburne intimately understands this material. He also produced models at the start of the pandemic on disease spread of COVID and was involved in numerous large private email threads among epidemiological modelers, including those considered the most prestigious in the field, from Cornell, Harvard, Princeton, Oxford, and elsewhere.

Washburne's main concerns are that ICL, in its *Nature* papers, and in Report 9, applied statistics from different countries to each other, such as those from the UK onto Southeast Asia, which introduces all sorts of potential distortions. The *PLOS* paper, he said, showed that kids have approximately 30 percent more contacts than adults. However, when you drill into the data, you see that Italians had more than double the numbers of contacts as people in Denmark, and more than 60 percent more than the contact rates of Britons. "This massive heterogeneity in contact rates likely impacts the relative importance of schools as sites of transmission across countries," Washburne said.

Another striking pattern, Washburne said, was how Report 9's conclusions were determined by hidden but critical assumptions, and these assumptions were often arrived at in a circular manner. For instance, in one of Report 9's citations—a 2008 paper coauthored by Ferguson, which estimated the effect of school closures—the authors translated contact rates to transmission rates, which required assumptions about immunity. But children have a different immunological history with flu than adults. If, for example, there's twice the incidence of flu in kids versus adults, it's not clear if kids have twice the contact rates of adults, or if they have the same contact rates as adults but adults are twice as immune (half as likely to get sick upon contact). "To model the impact of school closures, they needed both the contact rates and immunity of kids, but these were both estimated endogenously from their model," Washburne explained. His concern dovetails with the theory Shira Doron and her coauthors proposed about COVID transmission among children being lower than it was among adults because the entire population lacked immunity, which is not the case with strains of influenza in which children appear to have higher transmission.

If you have a mild headache right now or your eyes have glazed over, in a way that's the point about why the models can be so dubious. They are fantastically complex, built upon assumptions, which makes them extremely sensitive to any even minor hidden assumptions, all of which affect the model's predictions. "What your questions to Ferguson reveal, with models built upon models," and myriad assumptions, Washburne said, is "a house of modeling cards." He summed it up by saying, "I don't think they had a firm, empirical understanding of transmission within US schools."

At the end of my exchange with Ferguson, he said something surprising, and humble: "The biological susceptibility of children to infection with COVID and their likelihood to transmit was more complicated than we assumed in Report 9. Young children (under 12) were substantially less susceptible to infection (even measured via serological surveys) than older children and adults in the first wave." In other words, *according to its senior author*, the initial model—which informed Deborah Birx's policy recommendations that ground much of America, including, crucially, its more than 50 million children, to a halt—was based on an incorrect assumption about the transmissibility of the virus among kids. School closures, therefore, would not have the effect on transmission reduction that was predicted.

*   *   *

On February 25, 2020, Nancy Messonnier, the director of the CDC's National Center for Immunization and Respiratory Diseases, led a press conference to address the developing coronavirus crisis. Messonnier warned the public that without vaccines NPIs would be the most important tools in the country's response. "What is appropriate for one community seeing local transmission won't necessarily be appropriate for a community where no local transmission has occurred," she said. The school closures that would be implemented the following month, and that endured through the end of the school year in nearly every one of the roughly 13,800 school districts in the US, many of which had wildly different infection levels, showed this directive was not followed.

At the time of the initial closures, in mid-March, vast areas in the US were absent any known cases. Still, to the extent that a planned response to influenza was an appropriate universal pandemic guide, this action was aligned with Objective 1 in the CDC playbook—a two week closure of schools for authorities to gain time to assess the severity of the pandemic. Given the news being reported of care rationing in northern Italian hospitals (a claim, it should be noted, that was disputed by Italian authorities), following Objective 1 to avoid that horror was not unreasonable.

Jennifer Nuzzo told me, "Italy spooked us. We did not want to be Italy. The governors all saw China and Italy lock down and decided to follow their example." My source with intimate knowledge of the highest level of the Cuomo administration similarly said that the news from Italy, as well as the example from Wuhan, made shutting down society—a previously unthinkable action—possible in the political and public imagination.

Though the news from Italy had a definitive impact, it was China's draconian lockdown that both inspired and permitted public health leaders through much of the world to follow (to varying degrees) its lead. In June 2020, Dr. Stefan Baral, a physician and epidemiologist at Johns Hopkins University, with an expertise in global control of infectious diseases, wrote a commentary for the journal *Annals of Epidemiology* in which he and coauthors referenced the World Health Organization's heralding of China's remarkably aggressive response, and how the media and public health authorities around the globe then quickly fell in line, lauding this approach. When I spoke with Baral he made his position clear: "I have no doubt that there was an effect of what happened in China on the response in other settings," he said. By following China, Baral told me, the WHO, the US, and other countries followed a model where the more intense the reaction, the "stronger" the leadership was perceived to be. This shifted the dynamic from a public health response to a political one. These political pressures "affected public health leadership in new ways that forced their hand to be more aggressive than I think many would have otherwise chosen, given the data in front of them." Dr. Monica Gandhi, an infectious diseases specialist at the University of California, San Francisco, who has extensive contacts throughout the CDC and other governmental health agencies, told me that US officials sought to emulate the strict lockdowns they witnessed in China. The Chinese model directly influenced federal decision makers.

As late as January 24, 2020, when news of the Chinese lockdowns shocked the world, Fauci said, "I can't imagine shutting down New York or Los Angeles." He added, alluding to the long-held epidemiological evidence, "Historically, when you shut things down it doesn't have a major effect." Yet, just a month later, in February 2020, Anthony Fauci dispatched Clifford Lane, a top deputy at NIAID, on a WHO mission to China. According to remarks Fauci made in a court deposition, Lane was "very impressed" with China's response, including its use of "extreme social distancing." The infection can be controlled, Lane had reported back, though he acknowledged that to do so would come at a great cost. To bring our outbreak under control, Lane said, the US may have to act as extreme as China. Fauci said he had every reason to believe Lane's assessment was correct.

It will forever remain an unresolved counterfactual, but it is an open speculation among many epidemiologists and others that had China not locked down the rest of the world might not have done so either. China, governed by an authoritarian regime that rules the country with tremendous top-down power, does not share the same attitude toward personal liberties as do Western democracies. And neither the 2007 nor 2017 playbooks, nor the pre-2020 consensus within the public health field favored a lockdown of society of the breadth that we would experience. On a countrywide scale, from both an epidemiological perspective and a human rights perspective, closing all nonessential business, closing all schools, prohibiting social interactions and nonessential travel, and so on, was not considered feasible or wise. "Prior to COVID-19 there was a strong global health discourse that argued against lockdowns and similar mass quarantines," said Nicholas Thomas, an associate professor in health security at the City University of Hong Kong, in a *Bloomberg* interview in January 2021. "The containment of a city hasn't been done in the history of international public health policy," said Shigeru Omi, who headed the World Health Organization's Western Pacific Region during the SARS outbreak in the early 2000s, in a January 2020 interview, also in *Bloomberg*.

We should plant a permanent signpost here that it's possible the entire pandemic response pushed by Birx, Fauci, and public health leaders within the US and around much of the world—with a few notable exceptions— never would have happened were it not for China's initial example. After all, the arrival of a new infectious virus was not unprecedented—but the response to it was.

Since we lacked the ability to test, Nuzzo said, shutting schools, along with other facets of society, initially made sense. The problem, in Nuzzo's mind, was not closing down in March; it was that there was no plan. By "no plan," Nuzzo was referring to two interrelated problems: (1) all the potential harms of closures, and (2) the challenge of unwinding interventions once they were implemented.

Authorities acknowledged yet dismissed the first problem. In Messonnier's press conference, she mentioned the CDC's 2017 pandemic report directly, said that school closures were part of the plan, and recognized that they were likely to be associated with unwanted consequences such as missed work and loss of income. "I understand this whole situation may seem overwhelming and that disruption to everyday life may be severe. But you should think about what you would do for childcare if schools or daycares close," she advised. There was no mention of how the government might aid families during school closures, or, for example, about what a single parent with a job as a cashier in a grocery store and a four-year-old at home was supposed to do. Rather, in just one line amid a lengthy speech, people were told to simply "think about" it. To government officials and many others at the time this was a regrettable but entirely reasonable approach—a presumed temporary loss of wages and childcare issues were lower-order concerns compared to the coming onslaught of a pandemic.

Yet what was positioned as a secondary issue—a mere abstraction, warranting just a brief mention—led to catastrophic consequences for millions of children, and their families. By a year later, my kids, along with tens of millions of other children, were still trudging through remote learning, either as their exclusive form of schooling or through so-called hybrid schedules during which they could only attend classes part time. Teachers in much of the country had been prioritized for vaccines—making them eligible for protection before some other, more vulnerable populations—yet schools in half the country still weren't open full time, and in many places weren't open at all. Randi Weingarten, the high-profile head of the American Federation of Teachers, the second largest teachers union in the country, said in a February 8, 2021, *New York Times* interview that she hoped things would be "as normal as possible" *by the following fall.* Class action lawsuits in multiple states had been filed on behalf of children with special needs on the claim that the conditions of IDEA, a federal law that requires certain services (such as physical and occupational therapy, supplemental aids and equipment, etc.) for children with disabilities, were not being met in a remote learning model. Opinion pieces with titles like "Remote School Is a Nightmare, Few in Power Care," had been appearing in major news outlets since the previous summer. Working parents, especially mothers, were dropping out of the workforce in staggering numbers due to childcare obligations caused by school closures. An analysis by the US Chamber of Commerce found that nearly 60 percent of parents who left the workforce did so for this reason. The psychic toll on parents and children was never and can never be calculated. It won't show up in statistics, but it was real for millions of families. A sentiment expressed by Kaitlyn Fontano, a mother quoted in a *Wall Street Journal* piece, was typical. With her kids in virtual school from March to November, and her husband back in the office, she was left alone to manage and endure "stress and craziness on a day-to-day basis." Fontano said this made her "not be the person and mother that I wanted to show up for my family." When asked about the impact of school closures on her, Kathleen Brown, a nurse and mom of a nine- and ten-year-old, said the unpredictability of remote learning, with its technical problems and wonky schedule, was like "trying to make a routine out of a blender." In her home heads banged on the dining table in distress. Millions of children, especially those without resources for tutors or parents to oversee them during the day, were losing ground with their academics and, worse, suffering from isolation and frustration, and, for an increasing number of them, depression from spending their days alone in front of an electronic screen. News pieces circulated about children without a home internet connection sitting on a concrete curb outside of a Taco Bell, and others in the parking lot of a McDonald's, using the dashboard of their parents' car as a desk, to access the fast food chains' WiFi for remote learning. Untold numbers of other children became "lost," having dropped out of school entirely. Putting aside whether school closures had arrested or even stalled the spread of the virus, these consequences, still pervasive a full year into the pandemic, were not adequately anticipated or prepared for by those in power who advocated for school closures.

But they should have been.

Even a rudimentary understanding of chaos theory—most famously illustrated by the so-called butterfly effect, in which the flutter of the creature's wings could ultimately lead to a storm across the globe—which dictates that even small actions can lead to enormous unforeseen consequences, would have given pause to health officials before they hit the giant red button on schools.

Worse still, damaging effects of school interruptions were not unforeseen. They were explicitly warned about in the academic literature. Exhibit A is a 2006 paper called "Disease Mitigation Measures in the Control of Pandemic Influenza," in the journal *Biosecurity and Bioterrorism*, written by Jennifer Nuzzo, D. A. Henderson, and two other coauthors. "There is simply too little experience to predict how a 21st century population would respond, for example, to the closure of all schools for periods of many weeks to months," the authors wrote. "Disease mitigation measures, however well intentioned, have potential social, economic, and political consequences that need to be fully considered by political leaders as well as health officials. Closing schools is an example." The authors went on to warn that closures would force some parents to stay home from work, and they worried about certain segments of society being forced to bear an unfair share of the burden from transmission control policies. They wrote:

No model, no matter how accurate its epidemiologic assumptions, can illuminate or predict the secondary and tertiary effects of particular disease mitigation measures. . . . If particular measures are applied for many weeks or months, the long-term or cumulative second- and third-order effects could be devastating.

Nearly a decade and a half before the pandemic—in a stark rebuke to Mecher's approach, which was championed by the CDC, Birx, and other powers that be—D. A. Henderson, possibly the most celebrated expert in the history of managing the spread of infectious diseases, had called out with unambiguous clarity the major harms that would come to afflict many families in our country as a result of school closures. Yet, from the spring of 2020, health officials who directed our pandemic response ignored, did not prepare for in any effective manner, and did not sufficiently inform the public of any of the consequences. Desperate and afraid, the officials had opened a bottle of medicine while disregarding the skull and crossbones on the warning label.

And the portents were not just in Henderson's and Nuzzo's paper. A 2011 paper by researchers from Georgetown assessed the decision-making behind and consequences from several hundred brief school closures enacted during the 2009 H1N1 pandemic. The authors noted that the childcare costs to families were substantial, and that hardships from closures were inequitable. "Officials considering closure must weigh not only the total amount of disruption but also the extent to which social costs will be disproportionately borne by certain segments of society," the authors wrote. Even the CDC playbooks themselves warn of some of these issues. Both the 2007 original and the updated 2017 reports cautioned that school closures could lead to the secondary consequence of missed work and loss of income for parents who need to stay home to take care of their school-aged children. This effect, the latter report noted, would be most harmful for lower-income families. With prescience, and comic understatement, the authors noted that school closures would be among the "most controversial" elements of the plan.

While many of the disastrous harms of school closures were warned about by Henderson, the most august epidemiologist of the last fifty years, the second of Nuzzo's points—that unwinding interventions is often incredibly difficult and there must be a plan on how to do so—was also a well-established reality.

Just as public health experts are biased toward intervention, they, along with the public, are also biased toward keeping interventions in place. This is a known phenomenon within the literature of implementation science, a field of study focused on methods to promote the adoption of evidence-based practices in medicine and public health. Westyn Branch-Elliman, an infectious diseases physician with an expertise in implementation science, at Harvard Medical School, told me that de-implementation is generally much harder than implementation. "People tend to err on the side of intervening, and there is often considerable anxiety in removing something you believe has provided safety," she said. There also is a sense of inertia and leaving well enough alone. It's not unlike legislation—oftentimes repealing a law, even an unpopular one, poses bigger challenges than whatever barriers existed to getting it passed. While the initial school closures may have been justifiable (even if off-script in many locations), there was no plan on when and how to reopen them. And not having predefined and largely agreed-upon goals for reopening meant there would be limited recourse against a public who had been led to believe this intervention was a net benefit, even long after evidence showed otherwise. The lack of an exit plan—or "off-ramp" as many health professionals would later term it—would prove disastrous for tens of millions of children in locations where social and political pressures prevented a reversal of the closures.

Without sufficient acknowledgment of the harms of school closures, or adequate planning for unwinding this intervention, officials showed that their decisions to close were simply reactive, rather than carefully considered. The decision makers set a radical project in motion with no plan on how to stop it. In effect, officials steered a car off the road, threw a cinder block on the accelerator, then jumped out of the vehicle with passengers still in the back. No one was in the front or even knew how to unstick the pedal.

As a defense, politicians and public health professionals repeatedly invoked the phrase "we're building the plane as we fly it." This metaphor was useful for them because it conjured a sense of permanent chaos, freeing policy makers and their advisers from being held responsible for not setting goals or timelines on ending school closures. But the metaphor was false. People like D. A. Henderson and others had already built the planes. And researchers and clinicians like Branch-Elliman knew the data from inside the "black boxes" from planes that had remained fixed on ill-fated courses in the past. A small number of experts had warned of these harmful inevitabilities, in both academic literature but also in public forums—such as Nuzzo's March 2020 *New York Times* piece—but their voices were drowned out, dismissed, or ignored.

5

(WRONG) LESSONS FROM THE PAST

There is one other critical example early on beyond that of Italy that spooked politicians, public health officials, and regular citizens alike. However, this cautionary tale, which was one of the most widely cited lessons on the effectiveness of NPIs, came not from other countries shutting things down during the COVID-19 pandemic but from the past. And it exemplifies why we need a full reckoning of the initial school closures, however reasonable they may have been, to understand why the subsequent extended closures were not reasonable.

"I know people talked about this before, but I just looked at a chart. You look at the pandemic of 1918, you compare the two cities of St. Louis and Philadelphia," said Ohio governor Mike DeWine in a March 15 TV interview to justify his closure of his state's schools. "The national experts say, 'Every day counts so much. You cannot wait. You've got to move very, very quickly,'" he said. Philadelphia waited too long to act and suffered greatly for it. That same day, during a press conference on his state's closures, DeWine showed a graph depicting Philadelphia's folly versus St. Louis's wisdom. The image, which would come to be shared in countless social media posts, depicted death rates over time for the two cities. Philadelphia's was a sharp spike like a witch's hat; St Louis's was soft, rolling hills. The message of the visualization was clear: close early and prevent a deadly peak. "We all want to be St. Louis," DeWine said.

NPR, the *Washington Post*, CNN, and the *New York Times* were among the long list of news outlets that covered the Philadelphia versus St. Louis story. It's such an influential comparison that Mecher referred to it in the Red Dawn chain on three separate occasions. With NPIs timing matters, he wrote. There's a narrow window and "Italy missed it."

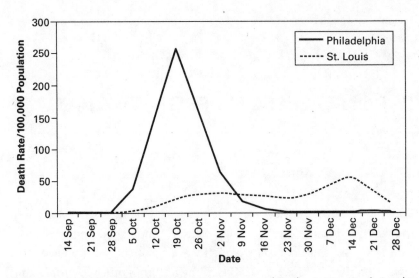

Philly vs. St. Louis. From "Public Health Interventions and Epidemic Intensity during the 1918 Influenza Pandemic." © 2007 National Academy of Sciences, USA.

If a strict society-wide stay-at-home order is put into effect early enough, it can blunt an immediate rise in cases and help prevent hospitals from being overwhelmed. This action, no doubt, can weaken a surge. But the problem with the St. Louis versus Philadelphia paradigm is that policy makers, public health authorities, and the media excluded a crucial detail. What was seldom mentioned by officials or in news accounts is that lockdowns, along with many other NPIs, are what Branch-Elliman, the implementation scientist, calls temporizing measures. For a highly contagious respiratory virus they merely *delay*, but do not stop, the inevitable. This is an established phenomenon within implementation science, part of what is referred to as voltage drop—interventions are *expected* to yield lower benefits as they move from efficacy (the ideal) to implementation (the real world). This is especially seen as a factor of time, as fidelity to interventions wanes. Many children can stay isolated for a week or two, but by six weeks, let alone six months, all but the most hermetically cloistered will interact with others. Without an effective vaccine, you're going to end up in the same place, Branch-Elliman said.

In April 2020, Robert Barro, an economist at Harvard University, published a report with the National Bureau of Economic Research, a nonpartisan, influential think tank that counts nearly three dozen Nobel laureates as past and present members. In his paper Barro categorized NPIs as school closings, prohibitions on public gatherings, and quarantine/isolation. His analysis of the 1918 pandemic found that when implemented early NPIs indeed "flattened the curve." But his analysis also found something else: the effect of NPIs on overall deaths over time was so small it was statistically insignificant.

Looking through the table of forty-five large US cities included in Barro's paper one is confronted with some striking comparisons between other cities that cast the Philly–St. Louis example in a different light in regard to the value of school closures in a pandemic over the long term. Chicago didn't close schools *at all*, yet its overall excess death rate was nearly the same as that of St. Louis, which had one of the longest durations of school closures. Milwaukee's schools were closed for half as long as those in St. Louis, yet it had a *lower* excess death rate. Kansas City and Denver had around the same school closure durations as that of St. Louis yet had roughly 70 percent higher excess death rates. It's easy to see, even with just a cursory view of the data, the evidence behind the conclusion of Barro's analysis: school closures in 1918, over the long term, did not reduce excess mortality.

Barro's findings from 1918 echo those from a long list of other studies, reviews, and meta-analyses on school closures enacted in subsequent pandemics. A 2009 World Health Organization report noted that if schools are closed during a pandemic, staff and students must stay home, a demand that of course is only feasible on a short-term basis. The report noted: "If students congregate in a setting other than a school, they can spread the virus and negate the intended effect of school closures." A 2011 National Institutes of Health review concluded that in a pandemic lasting months or years the proportion of cases averted by school closures "remains uncertain." A large-scale review, published in 2014 by the Canadian National Collaborating Center for Infectious Diseases, concluded that early school closures may blunt the short-term impact of an outbreak but that the total number of people infected "may not be appreciably affected" by the closures.

The Philadelphia versus St. Louis narrative, with its arresting visualization of different death rates, along with the "flatten the curve" meme also circulating at the time, that so captured politicians, the media, and the public, left out the ending of the story. Just as the models (based upon models based upon assumptions) that undergirded the close-the-schools approach in the pandemic playbook didn't adequately account for interactions outside of school or the second order effects of school closures, the Philly–St. Louis example, too, gave a superficially persuasive yet ultimately specious justification for school closures, which ended up lasting far longer than whatever short-term benefit they may have conferred.

It's important to emphasize that Barro's paper came out in April 2020. National and intergovernmental agencies' reports that also cast serious doubt on the effect of long-term school closures had been published long ago and were accessible to anyone who cared to look. Yet this evidence was absent from the narrative.

* * *

There is one other potential key issue related to 1918. The Spanish flu pandemic, despite being referenced repeatedly throughout the COVID-19 crisis, may be the wrong pandemic to use as an instructive antecedent for NPI policy. The title of the 2007 government report, which contains the text "Community Strategy for Pandemic Influenza Mitigation," gives a hint why. So does the title of the 2017 report: "Community Mitigation Guidelines to Prevent Pandemic Influenza." One word unites both reports and the 1918 pandemic: influenza. Yet the COVID-19 pandemic, of course, was based on a coronavirus. This matters in several potentially significant ways, yet, oddly, no one, from governors to journalists to public health officials, seemed to notice.

A doctor doesn't use a rheumatoid arthritis treatment protocol for a patient with type 1 diabetes, even though they are both autoimmune diseases. While influenza and the novel coronavirus are both respiratory viruses, they interact differently with the population and in particular with children. Yet policy makers and the experts who influenced them referred to models and historical examples based on influenza, as if it were the same as the coronavirus.

Intriguingly, there may be an analogue for the COVID-19 pandemic, but it's not 1918. It's 1889. Often referred to as "the Russian flu" or, at the time, "la grippe" (the French name for influenza), there is compelling evidence that the pandemic of 1889–1891 may have, in fact, been caused by a coronavirus.

"As in Covid-19 and unlike in influenza, mortality was seen in elderly subjects while children were only weakly affected," wrote the authors of a paper comparing the two pandemics, which was published in the journal *Microbial Biotechnology*. The similarities between the 2020–2021 and 1889–1891 pandemics are remarkable: Evidence from the 1889–1891 pandemic suggests there was multi-system disease, which included loss of taste and smell; presymptomatic transmission; occasional symptomatic reinfection; men fared worse than women; obese people and those with comorbidities didn't fare as well; and, most saliently, children did not have it "so severely as adults," suffering less and recovering faster. "The physicians observed a 'peculiar immunity of young children' untypical for influenza" and "peak mortality in the Russian flu pandemic was with the elderly, substantial mortality was also seen in adults but children suffered only mild symptoms." For good measure, a technique called a "molecular clock analysis" of two modern coronaviruses suggests that a coronavirus jumped from an animal to humans in the 1890s.

Moving forward toward the modern era, it has been well established that coronaviruses in general share these characteristics regarding children. Nearly all children get infected with seasonal, endemic "common cold" coronaviruses, which are almost never severe for them. Yet there is much evidence of those same coronaviruses resulting in significant morbidity and mortality in long-term care facility patients.

Numerous papers on the coronavirus-based SARS epidemic from 2003 feature similar evidence regarding the pediatric population as the accounts from 1889, such as fewer than 5 percent of cases were found in those under age 18, and that there was less transmission among children. Descriptions from papers published in the journals *Emerging Infectious Diseases*, the *Journal of Medical Virology*, the *Pediatric Infectious Disease Journal*, and *BMJ* attest to this: "The disease seems to be substantially less severe in children than in adults," "Young children appeared to have milder disease with a shorter time to resolution," "Transmission of SARS from pediatric patients appears to be uncommon but is possible," and "There is only one published report of transmission of SARS virus from a pediatric patient." Even the CDC noted that regarding SARS "the role of children in transmission is likely much less significant than the role of adults." There are similar findings for MERS, another coronavirus epidemic, which arrived in 2012. Like SARS, MERS infected very few children, around 2 percent of reported cases. In a review published by the Italian Society of Medicine and Natural Sciences, the authors wrote: "Although children are well known to be a source of viral respiratory infections, they did not seem to play the role of 'reservoir' in the diffusion of MERS-CoV." Further, they wrote that MERS was milder in children than in the adult population, and most cases were asymptomatic.

Phrases like "but we don't know for sure" about the effect of COVID on children were frequently invoked as a reason to keep schools closed. (This phrase was recited so often by parents and others that I thought about using it as the title of this book.) As time went on the logic behind this phrase wore increasingly thin. But even at the onset of the pandemic the coronavirus was far less exotic than media reports and public health officials made it seem.

Euzebiusz Jamrozik is a physician and bioethicist at the Monash Bioethics Center in Australia, and at Oxford University. Jamrozik's research focuses on philosophical and policy issues related to infectious diseases, and he has been a member of the World Health Organization Ethics Working Groups on infectious diseases. When I spoke with Jamrozik during the pandemic one of the first things he said was, "Please avoid using the word 'unprecedented' when talking about the coronavirus." It feeds into the narrative of framing this virus as alien and mysterious, he said, which leads to a justification for more extreme mitigation measures imposed on children. Most people before the pandemic had never heard of coronaviruses, he said, even though they've been with us, circulating in society, for eons. The acronym COVID (COronaVIrus Disease), which is the name for the illness caused by the virus SARS-CoV-2, was also new and strange sounding, versus the familiarity of "the flu." Even use of the word "novel," which was frequently inserted as a prefix before "coronavirus," while technically correct, built in a layer of fear. "My view is that once we knew we were dealing with a coronavirus," Jamrozik told me, "our assumption should have been that, like seasonal COVIDs, SARS, and MERS, this virus would be mild in children but severe in older adults. And that is exactly what the early Chinese data showed."

To be clear, the epidemiology of SARS and MERS were very different from that of COVID-19, and the SARS and MERS data on children were limited because the number infected was so small. Moreover, the evidence that 1889 was a coronavirus, though compelling, is not proven. Nevertheless, taken together this evidence strongly buttressed the data the World Health Organization and China published in February 2020 regarding children and COVID. The coronavirus in 2019 was novel, but it was still a coronavirus and all of the evidence—from the distant past, recent history, and the immediate data from China—gave no reason to doubt, and every reason to believe, that it was following the same pattern as all other coronaviruses in regard to having a benign course for nearly all children.

The old medical adage for diagnosing and treating patients, "When you hear hooves think of a horse, not a zebra"—meaning the wisest course of action, least likely to cause unnecessary harm, is to assume that a patient's symptoms conform to the most obvious diagnosis unless proven otherwise—should have guided our policy. Instead, politicians and the media kept referring to the zebra. As a result, schools were initially closed and remained closed, in part, based on the notion, against all evidence and clinal logic—and greatly perpetuated by the media and politicians—that children were facing a unique degree of danger.

* * *

As much as the gross imprudence of insisting on a zebra was part of the justification for school closures, it is more so the models—which showed a catastrophic rise in cases if severe interventions, including, especially, closing schools, were not implemented—that were the main driver of our restrictive policies related to schools.

And if you haven't been sufficiently persuaded about the dubiousness of models guiding so much of our pandemic response there is one more devastating note. While health officials and the media often cited individual research teams, such as the one out of Imperial College, along with a highly regarded program called the Institute for Health Metrics and Evaluation (known as IHME) from the University of Washington School of Medicine, they were only the most famous players in the forecasting space. Many other entities—including groups at Ivy League universities, government agencies, and industry teams—were also modeling cases, hospitalizations, and deaths. An ensemble of forecasts from all of these groups, called the COVID-19 Forecast Hub, was extremely influential. So much so that it was not only referenced by the CDC but its forecasts were actually published by the CDC each week.

I first learned of the ensemble from Steve McConnell, who runs a company that does software forecasting. (He helps companies predict how long it will take to create a software product, how many people will be needed on the project, and other details.) The fascinating and surprisingly meritocratic thing about the ensemble is that any person or entity could have their forecasts included as long as the forecasts met certain eligibility criteria. McConnell, who lives in Washington State and was well familiar with IHME, saw early on how wildly off the mark the predictions were from that team and many others. Although his background was in software, McConnell reckoned the techniques he used in that work should be applicable to pandemic forecasting. He figured why not give it a try himself, and threw his hat into the ring.

An analysis of the performance of more than two-dozen modelers from April 2020 through October 2021 was ultimately published in the journal *Proceedings of the National Academy of Sciences*. The results are astonishing—and unmooring. Three of the top four most accurate modelers were from outside the public health field. Among the three was McConnell. The other outsiders at the top were a team from a management consulting firm called Oliver Wyman and a Canadian physicist named Dean Karlen.

It is important to slow down here and let the facts deeply sink in: A team from a management consulting firm, along with—to be frank, two random guys—McConnell and Karlen, outperformed teams with researchers from Johns Hopkins, MIT, Duke, Columbia, the University of Michigan, the famed IHME, and the US Department of Energy's elite Los Alamos National Laboratory, among others. It is hard to imagine a more damning indictment of public health "experts" than this outcome. In particular, the fact that a team of people at IHME—who have spent entire careers working in public health—were bested by a physicist and by a man who runs a software development consulting business, is hard to wrap one's head around. It's as though an auto mechanic and a scrimshaw artist started performing open heart surgeries, and achieved better outcomes than a dozen of the top cardiothoracic surgery teams in the nation.

As of 2017, IHME had received more than 400 million dollars from the Bill and Melinda Gates Foundation. IHME has hundreds of employees, and it produces some of the world's most influential forecasts and analytics related to all matters of global health, from AIDS to health policy and planning. This isn't to suggest, necessarily, that IHME doesn't do excellent work in any number of areas. But its predictive models for COVID—the single most important public health disaster in generations—were less accurate than those from McConnell, Karlen, Wyman, and several other groups. Deborah Birx mentioned IHME's models repeatedly in the spring of 2020, warning of escalating deaths if the citizenry didn't do as it was told. News outlets from CNN to *Politico* to PBS to the *Times*, all referenced IHME. Birx talked confidently and reassuringly about how her own team's models matched IHME's projections.

All the while, few journalists challenged the models, inquiring how they were made. They simply *reported* them.

While the predictions made by inept professional modelers held great emotional power over much of the public and policy makers, there was, perhaps, some limit to the sway of the models on their own. It was China's actions that showed Americans, and the world, that the NPIs prescribed in the models as necessary to prevent calamity could actually be implemented on a vast and brutal scale. It was through the surreal example of Wuhan, a city of 11 million people, being locked down by an authoritarian regime, and the terrifying news stories coming out of Italy, that the until-that-moment fantastical notion of ordering millions of citizens to shelter in place across the US transmogrified, like the script of a dystopian thriller coming to life, from the unthinkable to an alarming reality.

Considering that this turn of events—no matter how heretofore outlandish—also reflected the playbook's early objectives, not to mention much public sentiment, some degree of social distancing was arguably a reasonable temporary response. And in a few locations this action may have helped avert a crisis in hospitals.

The problem, however, was that fundamentally flawed models guiding policy, in addition to politicians and media misrepresenting both the risks to children and what school closures would actually achieve, ensured that school closures would not be temporary.

THE ILLUSION OF THE PRECAUTIONARY PRINCIPLE

APRIL THROUGH JUNE 2020

6

EUROPE

On March 31, Deborah Birx gave a joint press conference with President Trump, Anthony Fauci, and Vice President Mike Pence. Birx, calm and stern, appearing at the lectern wearing an elegant silk scarf, an accessory that would go on to become her trademark for seemingly every public appearance, delighting reporters from the *Washington Post* to *Vogue*, and even earning a dedicated Instagram fan account, projected sophistication and confidence. A former HIV/AIDS director at the CDC and later a global AIDS ambassador, Birx, a cosmopolitan scientist and diplomat who had worked under administrations of both parties, was seen as neither a Trump lackey nor a shopworn DC creature like Fauci—her presence, at least early in the pandemic, lent an air of presumed reasonableness and objectivity.

She opened by saying that the American people were going to have to do "things for the next 30 days to make a difference," and then thanked the modelers from Harvard, Columbia, Northeastern, and Imperial, and later presented a model from IHME. "It was their models that created the ability to see what these mitigations could do." She said the models showed that 1.5 to 2.2 million people in the US would die from the virus, but if people would social distance and stay home, and if schools were closed, this fate could be avoided. Pence, Trump, and Fauci all repeatedly mentioned that another thirty days of mitigations would be critical. Fauci said doing this was inconvenient but that it would "be the answer to our problems." Birx and Fauci mentioned the words "model," "modelers," and "modeled" nearly thirty times.

The "15 days to slow the spread" campaign, which began fifteen days earlier, had morphed into forty-five days. In New York, despite the shelter-in-place order, cases rose vertiginously anyway before peaking in mid-April and then followed a steady decline—a trajectory later memorialized as a bizarre piece of folk art ordered by Governor Cuomo in the form of a giant foam sculpture dubbed "the mountain." Nearly every other state had far more modest bumps and molehills. California has double the population of New York State yet saw around just one-tenth the number of daily cases during the same time frame.

This shift from fifteen days to forty-five days was a fairly extraordinary development. After all, objective 1 from the government's playbook—close schools for two weeks to assess the situation—had already been met. And most of the country outside the New York metro area was nowhere near meeting objective 2, allowing schools to close for up to six weeks if there were active outbreaks. Yet this 200-percent extension of "lockdown" measures, an untethering from the government's formal playbook, went largely unchallenged by the media.

On school closures, we were now officially off-script, never to return. The plans that Bush had commissioned some fifteen years earlier, and that Carter Mecher and many others had crafted in various iterations, were scrapped. Policy for American schools during the rest of the pandemic would be one incredibly long improvisation. For all the talk of the pandemic being "unprecedented," the virus's spread and virulence, as opposed to our response to it, fit well within parameters that had been planned for. During this type of crisis the government was supposed to operate akin to a classical orchestra—have a conductor, follow the written music. Instead, we got a jam band with a two-year-long ad-libbed guitar solo.

As flawed as they were, the pandemic plans were made in a sober, nonemergency context, were detailed and methodical, and did at least make passing mentions of the risks of school closures. Crisis planning—be it in medicine, business, defense, law, engineering, you name it—is considered critical to minimizing errors and harms and maximizing a chance at a more favorable outcome when in the midst of a crisis. There is a reason why airplane pilots are drilled in their training to memorize certain protocols to follow during various emergencies. During an emergency people panic. And during an emergency, if we can help it, we don't want to wing it. Instead, we rely on plans. This is a core feature of humans: We make plans for the future, and we make histories of the past to help inform us about what to do in the present. With that said, deviating from a play-book is not wrong in and of itself. But if the public health authorities and policy makers were going to call an audible they needed to provide a persuasive reason why they were doing so. This was not done.

Remember, at the press conference Birx and the others gave no explanation for veering off the plan (which had been invoked weeks earlier), and in particular for keeping schools closed, other than, as Fauci said, that the models showed continued mitigations "would be the answer to our problems." But there was nothing epidemiologically unique about the COVID pandemic relative to the planning scenarios that suggested it required a different, more aggressive policy in regard to school closures. As I noted earlier, if anything, relative to influenza, the more benign course of COVID in children, and the stunted transmission among them that was initially observed, suggests that if there were to be any deviation it should have been in *the opposite direction*, toward fewer mitigation measures imposed on children. Indeed, this was the conclusion most of Europe came to.

By early May schools in the Netherlands, Norway, Finland, France, Switzerland, Germany, Spain, and more than a dozen other nations had opened. A number of countries only opened lower schools. Others, such as Germany, saw certain areas open secondary schools for older grades. Whatever the specifics, it was seen as imperative for at least some of the schools to open. "This decision was made in line with health authorities of the Royal Netherlands Institute of Public Health and the Environment (RIVM), who consider the opening of schools to be sufficiently safe," an article in the *Brussels Times* on April 23, reported, "as children play a relatively small role in the spread of the virus." While Americans were being begged and cajoled into social distancing, encouraged to treat each other as radioactive, at the end of April Switzerland's head of infectious diseases said that kids were permitted to hug their grandparents. Denmark announced the same policy a few days later. Most of the US, by contrast, was still locked down, including the closure of the entire school system for some fifty million children, which—with the exception of a few districts in Montana and Wyoming—would remain so through the rest of the academic year.

Many of these European countries had not "controlled the virus," as some closure advocates often mentioned as a reason why schools could open there but not in the US. By mid-April the seven-day averages of cases per capita in France, Denmark, and Spain were, respectively, above, below, and the same as that in the US. Moreover, crucially, the elevated US numbers were heavily skewed by high rates in certain regions. Most of the country was far below the average.

In addition to the early data from China, more evidence began to roll in from around the world reinforcing the conclusion that COVID was not a great or even modest risk to children. In early May, in Italy, where more than 200,000 people had been infected, about 2 percent of cases involved children or teenagers. Two out of the country's roughly 30,000 recorded deaths from the disease involved people under the age of nineteen.

Data from New York City at the same time showed seven deaths for those under eighteen years of age, out of more than 14,000 in total. Six of the seven children had underlying conditions, and the health status of the remaining case was unknown. The death of a child with underlying medical conditions is no less tragic than that of a healthy child, but this was extremely relevant information for parents to understand the risks to their children. Nevertheless, when discussing COVID policies for children, American public health authorities and the media would almost entirely ignore this point for the duration of the pandemic.

While the data from New York City were relevant and useful, if one wanted more information about what was happening stateside the CDC published a much larger American data set on April 8. It is a remarkable document, and its evidence regarding children was ignored.

The paper, published in *MMWR*, the CDC's house journal, analyzed the records of 1,482 Americans hospitalized with COVID from March 1 to March 28 in fourteen states, including major population centers such as California and the early hot spot, New York. It found that 0- to 4-year-olds, and 5- to 17-year-olds each accounted for 0.4 percent of the total hospitalizations. These data echo what was seen earlier in China, and should have been reassuring to those who felt statistics from outside the country were not as reliable or applicable. But here's the most important part: considering there generally was around a week or so lag from infection to hospitalization, this dataset reflects COVID transmissions that occurred from roughly the last week or so of February through the third week of March—a time span while schools were still predominantly open. Not only that, but during this time the schools had *zero* mitigation measures—no masks, no distancing, no barriers, or anything else. The American public health authorities knew, from April 8 on, that school-aged kids and adolescents accounted for 0.4 percent of COVID hospitalizations *while schools were open.*

There's something else extraordinary and telling about this report. It was covered by a long list of media outlets, from NPR to the *Atlantic* to NBC. In all of the news articles that covered the study that I reviewed the framing was about COVID's disproportionate risk to men, Black people, and people with obesity and other underlying conditions. Not one of the news items mentioned the dramatic and reassuring statistics regarding kids and adolescents. Considering at the time of the study's publication the entire American school system was shut down, in part because of a purported risk to children, this was an extremely pertinent fact to report. But it was ignored.

These facts—that not only was COVID graciously sparing most children, but of the few who were seriously affected nearly all had significant medical vulnerabilities—were known from the beginning.

Studies and reports out of Iceland, France, the Netherlands, and Canada all brought similarly encouraging news regarding COVID and children. A report from Australia's National Center for Immunization Research and Surveillance found that among eighteen confirmed cases in fifteen schools, just two children became infected. And of great relevance regarding the safety of schools, the report found that "no teacher or staff member contracted COVID-19 from any of the initial school cases."

A joint press release in late April from three associations of French pediatricians stated that the "risk of infection for adults is mainly due to contact between adults themselves (teachers, staff, and parents grouped out of school)." It encouraged the return to school even for children with chronic diseases, as "delaying this return appears to be of no benefit for the management of their illness."

And, of greatest importance, by late May and early June there was more than a month of empirical evidence directly related to schools. Two weeks after Danish schools opened on April 15, Christian Wejse, a scientist in the Department of Infectious Diseases at Aarhus University, Denmark, said, "There are no signs whatsoever that the partial reopening has caused a bigger spread of infection." An official from Denmark's disease control agency also said there was no impact from schools opening.

Most dramatically, on May 17, education ministers from the European Union gathered on a conference call to discuss the reopening of schools. Children, in different grades depending on the location, had been back in class for three to four weeks in twenty-two European countries, and it was announced that there was *no evidence of a significant increase in COVID infections or a negative impact from reopening schools.* Pause and reread the previous sentence. This is the moment, to my mind, that has to be reckoned with.

In March and April, even if from a transmission standpoint and per the playbook guidelines schools in nearly all of the US *should* have remained open, or, at most, not have been closed for longer than a couple weeks, from a practical standpoint leaving them open was likely not feasible. There was great fear and uncertainty among much of the American public at the time, and it is likely many teachers simply would not have shown up, and many parents would not have sent their children. (I knew multiple families that pulled their kids out of school even before the schools closed in March.)

The first question to reckon with is not necessarily why schools closed initially, as problematic as that decision may have been. The question is why schools opened in Europe when they did, but did not do so in the US. Further, the second, far more damning question is why American schools remained closed even after this May 17th EU meeting. Regarding American school policy during the pandemic, this may have been the most portentous moment of the entire pandemic.

In much of the US, where the academic calendar typically runs toward the end of June, there was still at least a month left for kids to return to school following this news. But the momentous announcement at the EU meeting was not on the front pages of our nation's papers, nor did it blare across cable news screens. It was not the subject of popular discussion. And it was not referenced by our politicians or public health officials. At the time, any acknowledgment of this momentous determination—which was made not in an obscure journal, or a blog post, but in an *official meeting of the European Union*—was, as far as I can tell, completely absent from the entirety of the American media and public health apparatus. It was as if we had taken a time machine to the eighteenth century and word from the continent, reliant upon a ship at sea to be relayed, hadn't yet reached us. Not only did we not open schools when they did, but even a month *after* the Europeans opened their schools, when our inadvertent guinea pigs then gave the "all OK" signal, we still didn't open.

But we didn't even need an official word from the education ministers' meeting. The data were obvious and available to every public health official in the US. Here is a graph showing what happened to cases in Europe after schools reopened there in the spring of 2020.

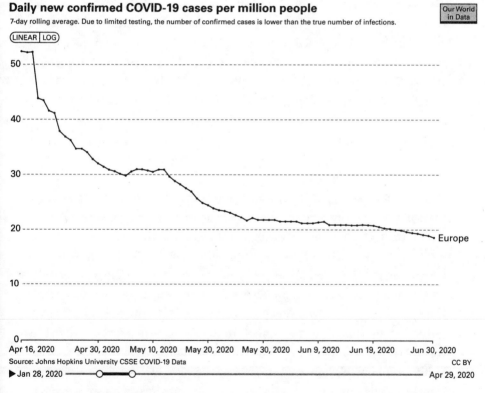

Daily new confirmed COVID-19 cases per million people

7-day rolling average. Due to limited testing, the number of confirmed cases is lower than the true number of infections.

Our World in Data

LINEAR | LOG

Source: Johns Hopkins University CSSE COVID-19 Data

CC BY

Apr 16, 2020   Apr 30, 2020   May 10, 2020   May 20, 2020   May 30, 2020   Jun 9, 2020   Jun 19, 2020   Jun 30, 2020

▶ Jan 28, 2020 ——————⊙━━⊙———————————————————————————— Apr 29, 2020

Seven-day-rolling average of new confirmed COVID-19 cases per million people, Europe, April 16, 2020–June 30, 2020. Courtesy Johns Hopkins University CSSE COVID-19 Data, processed by Our World in Data.

It is impossible to look at the data, showing the long downward slope of cases *after* schools had opened, and draw any conclusion other than what the EU ministers had drawn: opening schools there had no observable negative impact.

One European country of note did not reopen its schools in the spring. That's because they never closed. I am of course talking about Sweden, the famous (or, as much of the American media framed it, infamous) outlier among Western nations for applying only the lightest of grips on its citizens as a reaction to COVID. As they did in the spring of 2020, Swedish lower schools would remain open during the entirety of the pandemic.

The Swedish children were not masked, and there was no specific distancing requirement. There was no systematic test and trace program in place, and schools did not all install sophisticated HVAC systems with HEPA filters. Rather, the schools generally had no air filtration systems at all. Some classes opened windows, though this was not required. The main interventions were an emphasis on practicing good hand hygiene and for kids who were ill to stay home.

Yet there was no evidence of a rash of school-related outbreaks. And cases in the country remained relatively stable until a brief bump in June. There was no mass testing throughout Sweden at the time, so it is likely that cases were undercounted, though that was the circumstance in America as well.

While Sweden certainly has different cultural and social dynamics from many areas in America, the Swedish cases per capita were on par with rates in the majority of regions in the US. And the average class size in Swedish lower schools was nearly identical to that in the US (twenty versus twenty-one). Remarkably, by the end of May there was a report of just one "outbreak" at a Swedish school, in which eighteen teachers tested positive. (There was no evidence that the infections occurred as a result of transmission in the school, though it is certainly possible that was the case.) Still, out of 105,000 teachers employed by lower schools, and 1.2 million children aged six through fifteen, there would have been numerous obvious outbreaks if children were maximally infectious and schools were a high-transmission environment, as was feared.

This was not a small sample of three schools in the mountains of Tibet. This was more than one million children and tens of thousands of teachers, a significant portion of whom were in greater Stockholm, a densely populated city. Yet the evidence was ignored or waved away.

In the summer of 2022 I interviewed Anna Ekström, Sweden's minister of education during the pandemic. She told me that, for a considerable time, she spoke with her European colleagues several times a week, and early on spoke every day with her counterpart in Iceland, a country that also never closed its primary schools. What were the challenges? The successes? What things worked? What didn't work? Ekström, as the leader of Sweden's schools, had a font of information to share about what was happening in her country. No officials from the US ever contacted her.

Not only was the evidence about schools in Sweden in particular, but also those in Europe, readily available but ignored by American decision makers, an active effort was made to avoid it.

Did the results from Sweden and, later, almost two dozen European countries mean that schools yielded zero contribution to the spread of the virus? Of course not. Is every European country epidemiologically matched to the US or specific cities or regions of the US? Of course not. But it was clear, as early as May 2020—from the observable data itself for anyone who cared to look, and from the official statement acknowledging as much in the EU meeting—that schools, even with minimal mitigation measures, were not meaningfully contributing to transmission, let alone triggering an explosion in cases.

This evidence damningly, dishearteningly, only continued to mount through the summer and the fall via the tens of millions of kids in school in Europe and, later, in large portions of the US, while thousands of American schools, nevertheless, remained closed.

How was it possible that this real-world evidence was ignored?

DEEP DIVE: PEANUTS, LEMONS, AND EVIDENCE-BASED MEDICINE

This wasn't the first time the American medical establishment, and the public guided by it, remained fixated on expert consensus while blind to empirical evidence, causing great harm as a result. Twenty years earlier, the American Academy of Pediatrics published what would prove to be disastrous recommendations for children, which only recently were fully recanted.

In the late 1990s, reports of child anaphylaxis—a potentially life-threatening condition, when the body goes into shock—related to peanut allergies began to surface in the pediatric allergy community. "It's not clear that there actually was a change in anaphylaxis rates," Dr. Ronald Sunog, a pediatrician in Massachusetts, and the author of a book about pediatric allergies, told me, "but the news began to make caregivers nervous." Medical authorities in the field assumed that to play it safe infants should avoid the food. Starting in 2000, as a precautionary measure, official guidance from the American Academy of Pediatrics and the NIH began to recommend against early exposure to peanuts, telling parents to delay introduction until age three.

Despite the peanut lockdown, the rate of peanut-related anaphylaxis rocketed during the following dozen-plus years; some children even died. As a result, schools, camps, child birthdays, playdates, and even airplanes became high-tension peanut-free zones in the process.

Yet, at the same time, something strange was happening outside the US. During this entire era, and the preceding three decades, a small, industrialized country was experiencing a very different peanut phenomenon. Since the late 1960s, Israeli infants had been gobbling a snack called Bamba, essentially peanut-flavored Cheetos, by the fistful. And the incidence of peanut allergy in Israel was near zero. The children in Israel, for the most part, had the same genetic makeup as many children in the US. And there were no obvious clinically relevant external contrasts between the countries. The only difference in the nature-nurture spectrum was that Israeli babies, near universally, were fed a peanut-derived snack very early, during infancy, while American children were not.

The benefits of early exposure to various microbes and environmental substances had already been a widely researched and discussed theory by then. And multiple studies showed that, for example, consumption of fish during infancy was associated with a reduced allergic response in subsequent years. Yet the American pediatric medical establishment kept recommending that young children *avoid* peanuts to reduce the likelihood of peanut allergy, when real world evidence that doing the opposite—that early exposure to peanuts was not only not harmful but was protective—was occurring the whole time out in the open.

Israel was a modern, industrialized nation, with an advanced medical system and physicians active in the global research community. The situation in Israel was known. But it was dismissed.

It took *seventeen years* before the US, after waiting for the results from a multiyear controlled study inspired by the Israeli evidence, reversed its recommendations. To this day, more than twenty years after the dubious AAP recommendations came out, there are still doctors and parents who erroneously—and dangerously—believe that avoiding peanuts in early childhood is the appropriate course of action to prevent peanut allergy.

The American guidance was not only wrong, but diametrically so. By avoiding exposure at a key moment in immunologic development, American children were *more* likely to develop the peanut allergy. The recommendations actively harmed untold numbers of children and conceivably led to some of the peanut allergy-related deaths.

"The post-mortem of the food allergy guidelines," Dr. Mark Gorelik, a pediatric allergist and immunologist at Columbia University, told me, "suggests that the lesson here is that without robust evidence, even the most reasonable of assumptions, prescribed for the most cautious of reasons, can result in large-scale unanticipated adverse effects."

The medical community's penchant for expert opinion over empirical evidence has a long history. British sailors suffered from scurvy, the disease resulting from a lack of vitamin C, for years because of this phenomenon. While at sea in 1747, a Scottish physician in the Royal Navy named James Lind led what is considered by some to be the first randomized trial. He took twelve sailors with scurvy, "as similar as I could have them," split them into six groups, and for two weeks gave each of the pairs of men one of six daily treatments: a half-pint of seawater, a garlic and herb paste, vinegar, cider, diluted sulfuric acid (the navy's official treatment at the time), and two oranges and a lemon. The two men given the fruit recovered; the others didn't.

A few years later Lind published his study results as part of a massive treatise and reiterated them in subsequent books. In addition to Lind's findings, for hundreds of years there had been reports by sailors of the medicinal effects of oranges and lemons against scurvy. Even the famed explorer Vasco da Gama wrote of this in 1498. Yet the Royal Navy refused to accept what Lind saw, and what so many sailors knew, and instead continued to prescribe sulfuric acid. Some senior officers and naval physicians, knowing from firsthand experience, sided with Lind. But it took more than forty years, only after lemon juice had been demanded for a long voyage and none of the sailors got sick, for the navy to finally accept citrus as a remedy for scurvy.

Lind's results and how he reported them were not as precise as a modern trial or prescription, and in addition to his correct findings with citrus his treatise also included some faulty inferences. But although his conclusions and methods were imperfect, there's a salient point about his scientific approach. He wrote: "It is indeed not probable that a remedy for the scurvy will ever be discovered from a preconceived hypothesis; or by speculative men in the closet who never saw the disease."

Like Nuzzo and Henderson, Lind drew a distinction between the assumptions of experts and the value of seeing how things operate in the real world. Lind noted that his work was to be founded "upon attested facts and observations, without suffering the illusions of theory to influence and pervert the judgement." This approach is the foundation of empiricist epistemology—in other words, experience (primarily through our senses) as a basis of knowledge.

This isn't to say observational evidence alone should guide all decisions. Effects that seem obvious when looking back may have been harder to spot or to conclude at the time, which is why experiments are often necessary. Still, as Dr. Sunog told me, "I don't need a randomized controlled trial to know that the sun will rise in the sky tomorrow morning."

Sunog's comment may appear flippant but it gets at an issue of profound importance: How do we evaluate evidence? Or, more philosophically, how do we know what is true? Scientific findings are validated with what's known as a hierarchy of evidence, meaning different types of evidence—randomized trials, case studies, laboratory data, and so on—are valued at different levels. Not surprisingly, there is some disagreement in the scientific community about how exactly the hierarchy should be structured. But the one commonality is that expert opinion typically is near or at the very bottom.

Jeremy Howick is a clinical epidemiologist and philosopher of evidence-based medicine at Oxford University, and an adviser to the National Institute for Health and Care Excellence (the British version of the FDA). He studies how and why different forms of evidence are used to approve various interventions and treatments. I asked Howick to explain why he thought officials in the US discounted or ignored the evidence from schools in Sweden and more broadly many countries in Europe. He began with an example:

Dr. Benjamin Spock was a pediatrician and wildly successful author of the book *Baby and Child Care*, first published in the 1940s, which has sold more than fifty million copies. To reduce infant mortality, Spock advised parents to have their babies sleep on their stomachs, based on his reasoning that if babies are on their backs and they vomit they could choke. Plainly, Spock's influence was vast, and for decades untold numbers of parents followed his advice. Yet Spock's guidance for sleeping in a prone position was based on his expert opinion, which was based on an assumption (however intuitive it may have seemed). It did not account for the real-world evidence that in countries where babies traditionally sleep on their backs the rate of SIDS (sudden infant death syndrome) had historically been low. In the 1980s, a series of comparative studies, echoing what had already been seen empirically, found that, indeed, contrary to Spock's advice, back sleeping resulted in a lower incidence of SIDS. ("Healthy babies, unlike drunk or drugged adults, are quite skilled at swallowing and spitting," Howick wrote in his book on evidence-based medicine.)

The examples of the medical and public health communities siding with expert opinion while discounting actual evidence are near limitless. Research papers and books on evidence-based medicine often use a pyramid to depict the hierarchy of evidence. Meta-analyses and systematic reviews—the most trusted, most reliable forms of evidence, which analyze results from many randomized trials or other studies—are often at the top. Then come individual randomized trials, then cohort studies, in which different groups are compared to each other. Then there are layers of other types of studies. Then, all the way at the bottom—the lowest, least-reliable form of evidence—is expert opinion. An opinion, even if there is a purported consensus, is still just an opinion. It's not science, and it doesn't supersede evidence to the contrary. Yet we seem to keep falling into this trap.

In Howick's view, in the beginning of the pandemic it was reasonable to close schools because evidence was still limited. But once there was evidence that schools could be open without additional harms—as was seen in Europe by late spring—it no longer was reasonable to keep them closed. Moreover, American authorities didn't just ignore but willfully refused to look at the other side, Howick said. It was an extraordinary leap. "Sure, isolating someone might prevent them from getting the virus, but they didn't look at the harms of being out of school." He continued, "It was like looking at the supposed benefits of a drug without looking at its safety profile."

Numerous physicians, bioethicists, and other scholars I interviewed—some of whom will make appearances later in the book— echoed Howick's views. Dr. Tracy Beth Høeg, a physician and epidemiologist who authored a number of studies related to children and COVID during the pandemic, including one on school transmission that was published by the CDC, is worth quoting at moderate length here because her statement to me encapsulates their views:

School closures, sports closures, masking, asymptomatic testing, vaccine requirements—the burden of proof should have always been on showing that the benefits of these interventions outweighed the harms. None of the above passed any sort of rigorous or thoughtful risk benefit analysis in the US or elsewhere. Children, almost inexplicably, faced the harshest restrictions totally out of proportion to their disease risk.

Howick has written about how financial conflicts of interest are often powerful enough to upstage evidence when it comes to deciding whether interventions are safe and effective. What we see with financial bias is that attempts to counteract it with purely evidence-based tools are destined to be ineffective. But this dynamic is not exclusive to finance, Howick said; rather it is about power. Whatever interests have the power, be they financial or otherwise, greatly affect how evidence is perceived. Indeed, there is a whole field of scholarship called the sociology of scientific knowledge that studies how sociological forces influence the scientific process, including what ends up being considered as evidence.

Howick's paper on the topic points to the work of Bent Flyvbjerg, a widely cited emeritus professor at Oxford University's business school, who has written extensively about power and rationality in decision making. Most of us like to think of ourselves as rational actors, public health authorities especially so. And yet Flyvbjerg's work details how "power defines reality."

We are all familiar with Francis Bacon's adage "Knowledge is power." But the inverse, "Power is knowledge," is perhaps more important, as Flyvbjerg explained. Using a single, long case study of an urban planning project, Flyvbjerg vividly showed how, in a democracy, powerful interests get to determine the framework for what is considered rational, and thereby what counts as reality. American politicians, public health authorities, and other vested interests (which we will get to later) defined preventing children from attending school—in many places on a part-time basis or entirely for more than a year—as rational, even though, as Howick notes, this went against the evidence. A significant portion of the citizenry went along with this, many liberals vehemently so, because the public health and medical community set the parameters of what was rational—they defined reality. The mistake in the US was the presumption that various authorities are objective interpreters of evidence, or determiners of what even gets to be considered as evidence, free from their own biases.

In 1689, John Locke warned about this in his magnum opus on empiricism, *An Essay Concerning Human Understanding*. Locke referred to the concept of "borrowed principles," by which he meant regular people believing whatever the experts have to say, "never venturing to examine" the principles on their own, and winding up believing things that are absurd merely because they are fashionable among the elite.

When schools were open in Europe and, later, in many states, it was obvious this did not lead to any overt elevation of COVID rates either in the schoolchildren or their communities. Many American school administrators, teachers unions, journalists, and regular citizens nevertheless listened credulously to the policy makers, their advisers, and the public health pundits who either ignored this reality or dismissed it for some theoretical reason or another. This deference to the experts, even when it was clear their positions conflicted with what was plain to see, was the error that John Locke had warned about 330 years earlier.

While there have long been scientists like James Lind, the norm of validated evidence throughout history has tended toward anecdote and expert opinion. Amazingly, it wasn't until the 1990s, with the arrival of evidence-based medicine (EBM), that a formalized process for assessing medical evidence came about. In the immediate decades prior to that time the norm was what were known as "consensus statements," where groups of experts in a specialty got together and put out statements about various medical interventions. EBM challenged this idea by saying rather than having guidance based on so-called consensus opinions, guidance should be based on hierarchies of evidence alone.

"While mechanistic evidence is useful," Howick said, "when push comes to shove, observational evidence is superior." This type of systematic approach is foundational to EBM, and, indeed, the scientific method.

The idea that schools were going to be the locus of infections, and that closing them was a crucial and beneficial action, was based on models, which were based on often dubious assumptions. The idea that HEPA filters and masks were essential interventions for making schools "safe" was based on mechanical studies or lab results that didn't account for real world environments and human behavior. The idea that six feet of distance (a contrived metric) between students was critical—which compelled schools to operate on hybrid schedules to comply with the spacing requirement, resulting in students attending classes, at most, half the time—did not account for how an infectious dose of the virus actually spread in a room, or account for all the interactions and potential transmissions outside of school.

On one side of the ledger were all of these expert assumptions; on the other side we had actual evidence to the contrary. The schools in Europe were open, and they were not the source of explosions in cases. The schools in Europe did not, as a general rule, have HEPA filters or other sophisticated HVAC systems. Many of the children were not wearing masks, especially those in primary grades. And the prescribed distance between students was often, at most, one meter (roughly three feet).

In essence, during the pandemic, the purported benefit of school-related NPIs endorsed by the American public health and medical establishment represented a regression back to "listening to the experts" over looking at evidence in a structured, hierarchical way. By late May of 2020, and even more so by that fall, they continued to value lab studies and simulations over what was seen in real schools, with real children—an epistemology that favored theory over empiricism.

Alas, this approach to public health was in line with a long historical precedent, from lemons to peanuts. But the scale of implementation and impact, on full public display, was never before seen. For a society-altering campaign of this magnitude the public health and medical authorities did not engender it on their own.

7

THE MEDIA, PART I

New York is a large state, covering some fifty-four thousand square miles, with more than four million children. On May 1, New York governor Andrew Cuomo announced that in order to keep "children and students and educators safe," schools across his state would stay closed for the remainder of the academic year. "We must protect our children," he said.

NPR, CNN, ABC, NBC, and the *New York Times*, along with every other major media outlet, covered Cuomo's announcement. Not one of their articles mentioned that schools throughout Europe, including those in areas with similar case rates to much of New York, were opening. Not one of the articles mentioned that the governor provided no metrics as a specific justification for the closures. Conversely, each article included Cuomo's warnings about the risks to children and educators and did so without providing sufficient context on the evidence about what the absolute risks were.

Unlike its traditionally interrogative role, much of the news media instead unquestioningly supported and amplified the narrative defined by the public health experts (and by the politicians who ostensibly were guided by them). Abstractions such as "safety" and "protecting children" went unchallenged as to their specific meaning.

But functioning as a megaphone, rather than a filter, was only part of the media's complicity in creating the juggernaut of misinformation. Much of the prestige media, including, most damagingly, the *New York Times*, deliberately and repeatedly emphasized supposed dangers to children and, specifically, the role schools would play in potential harm to students and the community.

When discussing American media, I'm focusing on the *New York Times* because the *Times* is arguably the most influential media outlet in the country among the cultural elite, in particular journalists and decision makers at other media outlets. Therefore, the *Times* also serves as a good proxy for the prestige media in general, since coverage of major news stories in the *Times* often sets the tone and direction for other mainstream outlets (and when the *Times* is not leading, it tends to echo the rest of the legacy media).

The *Times* had an almost relentless obsession with framing its articles on the topic of COVID and children around the potential dangers to children, children's potential to cause vast death by transmitting the virus to others, and how schools specifically would serve as the launching pad for the calamity.

A week before Cuomo's announcement about the need to close New York's schools to "keep students and educators safe," the *Times* published a brief write-up of a call Trump had with governors in which he suggested some schools should reopen. The only comment in the article on Trump's suggestion was that it was unbidden and ran "counter to the advice of medical experts." Yet, like the coverage of Cuomo's announcement, there was no mention that schools were reopening throughout Europe. Nor was it discussed why European medical experts had reached the same conclusion as Trump (even if they arrived there through a different process) and the opposite conclusion of the unnamed American experts the *Times* was referring to.

The following day, on April 28, the *Times* ran a story titled "Despite Trump's Nudging, Schools Are Likely to Stay Shut for Months." Passing mention was made of Denmark and Germany opening schools, but this action was dismissed by the claim that those countries had made "faster strides in testing and contact tracing." No explanation was given about what "faster strides" meant exactly.

That Swedish schools had been open, and without a mass testing program, was not mentioned. The article also represented one of the early forays into not just whether schools should open but *how* they should open. It cited Chinese students wearing masks and using glass desk dividers, and the disinfecting of basketballs. Like the reports centered on opening in general, the coverage of mitigation measures provided no evidence of their effectiveness.

On May 5, Apoorva Mandavilli, the main COVID beat reporter for the *Times*, authored an article with the ominous subtitle "Cases Could Soar in Many U.S. Communities If Schools Reopen Soon."

This article, tweeted approvingly by journalists at NBC News, the *Wall Street Journal*, and other outlets, as well as public health pundits like the physician and bestselling author Eric Topol, former New York City council members, and school superintendents, led a narrative shift. The low risk to children was acknowledged; the new driving concern, as the article noted, was whether they pass the virus on to adults.

Given the article's headline, "New Studies Add to Evidence that Children May Transmit the Coronavirus," it opened with a leading question: "What role do children play in keeping the pandemic going?" Before the text began, there was an arresting photograph of workers in protective gowns, booties, hoods, and full-face respirators with protruding breathing cartridges on each side, spraying down the hallways of a French school with "disinfectant." There was no mistaking the tone, even without reading all of its 1,700 words.

The first "study" the article referred to was not a study, but a model that simulated the benefits of school closures. The second study was not published or peer reviewed; rather, a German researcher posted it on his website. The study, as Mandavilli relayed it, purported to show that children had viral loads as high as or higher than adults, suggesting they were as infectious as adults. Yet the study was met with great criticism by some scholars, including Dr. Alasdair Munro, a widely cited pediatric infectious diseases specialist in the UK, who contended that when the data were analyzed properly they actually showed children had lower viral loads. Published papers are often met with collegial criticism, but at least they have the imprimatur of a journal, indicating they underwent an editorial review process. This paper wasn't even published, so the bar should have been set extremely high for it to be the linchpin of Mandavilli's thesis. To validate such a work in a mainstream publication would entail including a rigorous unofficial peer review, with a variety of experts sharing reactions to it in the article, with the majority concurring with the results, which Mandavilli did not do. Absent such a process there is a great risk of reporting invalid results.

It took more than a year for the German researcher's paper to be published officially, after revisions. The peer-reviewed version concluded that the researcher's data showed children had *lower* viral loads than adults.

In Munro's Twitter thread where he critiqued the original paper, he noted that children indeed can get COVID. Munro added that "of course" outbreaks will happen. But, he said, children were barely affected by infection and that schools were likely lower risk than adult work environments.

More than that, numerous studies showed children at that time were far less likely to be infected. A large study in Iceland, published on April 14, found in randomized population screening, "no child under 10 years of age had a positive result." In targeted testing, children under ten had roughly half the positive rate of the rest of the population (6.7 percent versus 13.7 percent). The European Academy of Paediatrics reviewed the Icelandic data and concluded that none of the cases were infected by a child younger than ten, "whereas infections from adults to children were quite common." Similar conclusions were drawn from a study of families in the Netherlands. An Australian study, published on April 26, found that in fifteen schools, of 128 staff members deemed close contacts of eighteen confirmed cases, composed of nine students and nine staff, zero contracted COVID. A French study published on April 11, which included a positive child who attended three different schools and did not transmit to anyone despite close interactions within schools, "suggests potential different transmission dynamics in children," wrote the authors.

None of these studies offered definitive proof that children were less likely to be infected or contagious. But the data, especially from Iceland, which were based on 46,000 tests, were strongly suggestive and called into question the claims in Mandavilli's article on the unpublished German paper. These studies, and others with similar conclusions, were all accessible before the *Times* article was published. Yet none of them were included.

There was one small mention, via a quote from Jennifer Nuzzo, who was the lone voice in the article to caution about school closures, of a Dutch study that said, "patients under 20 years play a much smaller role in the spread than adults and the elderly." But this statement was discounted in the next sentence because the study only looked at household transmission, potentially biasing the results. More broadly, Nuzzo's few comments, in which she advocated for taking a holistic view of the impact of school closures, and wrote that decisions to reopen should not be based solely on attempts to prevent transmission, were entirely overwhelmed by the lengthy focus on the modeled simulation, the faulty unpublished German paper, and by quotes from various experts expressing dire warnings. Marco Ajelli, the author of the simulation, estimated that without closing schools the number of infections tied to a case (known as the R0) could rise and the effect would be "devastating." Bill Hanage, an epidemiologist at Harvard, said if the assumptions about children's transmission were wrong the consequences would be "disastrous."

The *New York Times* had planted a flag. The meme of children as potential silent superspreaders had officially begun.

The contrast of the coverage of children by European media also was underway. For example, the week after Mandavilli's article, the *Irish Times*, one of Ireland's top news sources, published a piece that began, "Children are not substantially contributing to the spread of COVID-19 in their households or in schools," citing an analysis from Ireland's health information agency. Munro also coauthored a paper with Dr. Saul Faust, a pediatric immunologist and infectious diseases specialist in England, in the prominent British medical journal known by its acronym *BMJ*. It was published the same day as Mandavilli's article and titled "Children Are Not COVID-19 Super Spreaders: Time to Go Back to School." Munro's paper noted that school closures were implemented around the world based on the presumption that since children were drivers of influenza transmission, they were potential silent spreaders of SARS-CoV-2 as well. Yet, the paper noted, there was no evidence behind that presumption. "Governments worldwide should allow all children back to school," Munro and Faust wrote. It's hard to envision a more radical divergence in how children and schools were covered than between these pieces in the *New York Times* and *BMJ* on May 5, 2020.

The *Times–BMJ* split on May 5, 2020 is a microcosm of the larger phenomenon of American media coverage of the pandemic versus that of media coverage outside the US. A fascinating study of this exact comparison was published as a working paper by the National Bureau of Economic Research in late 2020. Researchers at Dartmouth College and Brown University conducted an analysis of 20,000 news articles and transcripts of TV news segments on the pandemic from both American media and foreign English-language media, spanning seven months of 2020. Using a computational technique called sentiment analysis, which categorized pre-coded language for positive or negative tone, they found that pandemic coverage overall in US major media outlets was far more negative in tone than coverage in non-US major sources. They also found that the negativity was "unresponsive to changing trends in new COVID-19 cases." Among topics analyzed, the researchers looked at schools coverage specifically. They found that *90 percent* of school reopening articles in American mainstream media were negative, compared to only 56 percent for English-language major media in other countries.

On May 10, the week after Mandavilli's "cases could soar if schools open" article, the *Times* ran a 1,700-word feature on Europe reopening its schools. The article exemplified the type of resource-intensive piece that only a richly funded and deeply staffed organization like the *Times* could publish. The reporting was conducted on location by the *Times*'s Berlin bureau chief. The article included interviews with some half-dozen people and featured multiple commissioned photographs, including those of masked German teens sitting in class, unmasked Danish children in primary school, and a German girl giving herself a COVID test. Its subtitle: "Restarting classes is central to reviving economies. But one question haunts the efforts: Just how contagious are children, and could they be the next super spreaders?" The article touted the unpublished German paper with its false conclusion "by the country's best-known virologist and coronavirus expert," once again, as Mandavilli's article did, erroneously referring to it as a published study. The article did not include one reference to or mention of why American schools were not opening. It was as if opening schools in the US were impossible, a foregone conclusion not even worth discussing in the context of the more than ten countries cited in the article.

The following day the *Times* published an article about schools reopening in the UK. The framing was not subtle. "Many parents are too concerned about the spread of the coronavirus to let their children attend," the subtitle fretted. The final line of the article quoted a parent: "He wants to be there all the time, but what can I do? If he became sick, if anything happened to him, I would just die."

This appeal to emotion and anecdote continued with the arrival of a COVID-associated inflammatory syndrome in children, called MIS-C. On May 17, the *New York Times* ran a 2,000-word profile of a previously healthy fourteen-year-old boy, relaying the terrifying saga of his battle with the syndrome, detailing his heart failure and pain that was like "straight-up fire" injected into his veins. The text was burnished with photos of him unconscious and pale in a hospital bed, requisite wires from various monitors dangling down to his body like a macabre mario-nette. On May 21, the *Times* ran an opinion piece titled "My Son Survived Terrifying COVID-19 Complications. If Schools Reopen, How Many Kids Won't?" The account had a happy ending, with the son leaving the hos-pital after four days with his "immune system functioning beautifully," but the writer still warned, "Our children are in far more danger than we realized." Elaborating on the title's rhetorical threat about schools reopening, the piece included the line, "It is already well recognized that if schools reopen, they could become vectors of disease."

The following day the *Times* ran yet another news piece about MIS-C, delivering harrowing details of "tubes fed down" a child's throat and an interview with a teenage patient who said he was incredibly frightened about potential injury to his heart. Even though Cuomo had already closed schools for the academic year, the lead-in to this disturbing con-tent was the suggestion that the syndrome could impact the reopening of schools, presumably to plant seeds of concern for the fall.

That same week the Royal College of Pediatrics and Child Health (the UK's version of the American Academy of Pediatrics) released a message from its president, Dr. Russell Viner. In the post he wrote, "One issue I don't believe is relevant to the discussion around schools is that of the newly-described inflammatory syndrome." In an interview with the BBC Viner said the syndrome was "exceptionally rare," and that it shouldn't stop parents from letting children exit lockdown. "The majority of chil-dren who have had the condition have responded to treatment and are getting better and starting to go home," he said. The BBC article featured interviews with multiple experts and referenced cases in several coun-tries. There were no sensational specifics about the patients, and school was never mentioned in the piece.

The difference between the MIS-C pieces in the *Times* and the BBC's coverage called to mind a big budget American disaster film, mayhem at every turn, and an understated British drama.

A week before Viner's post, I had corresponded with Dr. Charles Schleien, the chair of pediatrics at Northwell Health, the largest hospital and healthcare system in New York. Since New York was then the nexus of MIS-C cases, and because of Northwell's size, Schleien was well positioned to speak about the syndrome. At the time it was estimated roughly 15 percent of New Yorkers had already been infected. Though the cases of MIS-C were scary, I knew from discussions with a pediatric specialist at a major university hospital in New York City, who had personally cared for patients with the syndrome and who was in contact with colleagues around the country who had also done so, that almost all were entirely treatable, and the syndrome represented something on the order of 0.017 percent of pediatric cases of COVID. According to the pediatric specialist, Northwell and the university hospital likely saw more MIS-C cases than any other institutions in the country, or the world. In a conversation with Schleien, I said it seemed parents and pediatricians should be aware of the syndrome so children with symptoms could be brought for treatment as soon as possible to achieve a good outcome. But I asked whether, as a public health hazard for children, relative to all the other illnesses they can contract, it warranted the alarming coverage on TV, in the *Times*, and elsewhere. "I've actually been making the same point to individuals and media outlets, trying to calm down the hysteria around this new childhood illness," Schleien said. "When you look at the simple arithmetic, many serious childhood diseases are worse, both in possible outcomes and prevalence." Since children with the syndrome are not contagious, and it is unusual to contract, Schleien agreed with Viner that it was not relevant to any discussions about schools.

On May 21, Governor Cuomo gave a press conference in which he said he was still mulling over whether he would allow children to attend camp in New York that summer. Cuomo said he was waiting on more information about MIS-C to decide. The next day the *Times* ran a piece with the headline "Parents Need a Break. But Is Summer Camp Too Risky?"

Firsthand accounts from expert clinicians seeing patients, and the data on prevalence, indicated an entirely different reality from what American media was reporting and politicians were saying. To review: the chair of pediatrics at the largest hospital system in the state said the coverage and fear around MIS-C was overblown. These thoughts were echoed by a pediatric specialist at a top New York City children's hospital. For good measure the head of Britain's leading pediatric society also downplayed the incidence and concern around the syndrome. And if MIS-C weren't relevant for schools, as each of these experts suggested, how could it possibly be relevant for camp, where kids spent most of their time outdoors? Moreover, children were in school in much of Europe and there was no indication MIS-C was more prevalent there than in the US, where schools were closed.

Millions of children in New York had been cooped up in their homes for months. In normal years camp was a cherished reprieve for many of them, including thousands of disadvantaged city kids who relied on philanthropic programs like the Fresh Air Fund to take them away from concrete and into the country. This summer they needed it more than ever. Of course no one would want children to be put in harm's way, but by all accounts MIS-C did not present a unique risk relative to all the other risks children face every day. Cuomo's public health officials certainly had access to Schleien, other top doctors, and data from the state's major hospitals and reports from experts abroad like Viner. Yet it seemed the governor of New York's only sources of information were the *Times* and related media.

With just a modicum of research, and by speaking with the most informed experts on the issue, I was hearing a completely different story from what much of the American press and politicians were telling us about MIS-C, and, for that matter, a different story about kids and COVID overall.

Cuomo ultimately barred all overnight camps from operating in New York State that summer. Survey results from the American Camp Association found that only 486 out of 1,489 overnight and day camps participating in the survey (out of an estimated 15,000 camps in the US) opened in the summer of 2020. If the survey was roughly representative of camps overall, two-thirds of camps in America shuttered during the summer of 2020. Dovetailing with the three months of school closures that preceded the summer, this represents five months of organized in-person interaction and activity being canceled for millions of children.

The same day as the *Times*'s news piece on MIS-C, the paper ran a feature titled "Coronavirus Cases Fall in Europe's Capitals, but Fears Over Reopening Linger." Its subtitle reinforced the frame: "Although declines in the numbers of new infections and deaths have brought relief in Europe's major cities, there is uncertainty about how much people can now relax." The message from the past couple months had been if cases were rising that, obviously, was cause for great concern. And now the message was when cases fell, that too was cause for concern. Hollywood, again, is instructive. You grip your seat when the monster chases the hero and, if the production is done well, you grip your seat during the lulls too, anticipating the next emergency. The media, perhaps most masterfully the *Times*, showed there was no news or information on COVID that couldn't be molded into a narrative of danger, keeping the audience in a perpetual state of fear.

All the while, it's important to note that by the middle of May the theoretical harms of opening schools could then be contrasted with the actual and manifest harms of their closures. Most of the discussion about the harms of school closures focuses on the "lost year" of the 2020-2021 school year. Yet it's important to be aware that great harm was incurred in the spring of 2020 alone. In some ways it's the forgotten spring. Experts were already cataloging evidence of increased child abuse, many lower-income children were no longer getting a subsidized or free lunch at school, and millions of parents observed their kids slowly withering from months of isolation. Learning loss from the three months of closures, which should have been expected from years of evidence of the so-called "summer slide," was obvious to many parents and educators, and a report from the US Government Accountability Office later confirmed the loss. While plenty of kids were doing fine—more often in stable homes with plenty of resources and space—millions of their peers were suffering physically, academically, psychologically. And a distressing number were disappearing from the system entirely. An April survey of teachers found that one in five students never logged in or were sufficiently disconnected that they were deemed to essentially be truants. The rate was one in three for kids from low-income families.

* * *

Within the first few weeks of the pandemic I began reading studies in journals and some governmental reports about COVID. I had no professional interest in the topic, and I was more than a year into writing a book, for which I was under contract. I was not dismissive of the virus—in the opening weeks, I admit, we wiped our groceries down. But from my training as a fact-checker, and my skeptical disposition, I couldn't stop myself from digging a little. The tenor of the news reports I was seeing didn't match with the scientific data. In particular, the framing around kids and schools seemed strangely disconnected from the evidence. Soon I was unable to concentrate on my book, and spent all of my time reading scientific papers and conversing with infectious diseases doctors, epidemiologists, and other experts abroad. The picture that began to develop was very different from what news outlets, by and large, were portraying. But I was in the media, too! And so, as I saw it, there was only one option.

On May 1, I pitched a piece to a science editor at the *Times*. I had published several articles with the *Times* before, including the number one most read piece in the paper (about newlyweds stranded at a five-star resort in the Maldives when global lockdowns began) less than a month earlier. Although I was bringing something to light that pushed against the mainstream view in the US, I had a track record with the paper and had plenty of evidence. I noted that the initial spike in hospitalizations had passed, and that states were beginning various processes to reopen. Yet none of them included plans to reopen schools. Why? Moreover, a growing number of countries, particularly in Europe, were opening their schools. Supporting these decisions abroad, I explained, were research and papers from at least seven countries, published in respected journals, including the *Lancet* and the *New England Journal of Medicine*, and by national governmental institutions. I included a bulleted compendium of evidence I hadn't seen compiled anywhere else, with linked studies and reports from Iceland, Holland, Italy, Canada, China, France, Australia, and Switzerland that showed children were at extremely low risk, and were less likely to transmit the virus as well.

The editor replied that they were already covering this story, so they were going to pass. I got rejections from a list of other outlets, many of which I had written for in the past. Succeeding as an independent journalist is not easy. I never assume anything I pitch will be accepted. But this was disheartening, and at least a little surprising. It's rare to find an unoccupied lane on any topic, let alone a major news story. And this was a heavily sourced feature on one of the most important topics of the day, covering information that had not been widely reported. Yet I was met with a near total blackout. Finally, amid my pitches, I found a sympathetic editor at *Wired*, a magazine known, of course, for its tech coverage, but which also published general science-based journalism. The piece, titled "The Case for Reopening Schools," ran on May 11.

The week leading up to publication, while I did additional research and went through rounds of rewrites with my editor, I was in a mild state of panic. Since the *Times* editor said they were covering the story I knew I had to move fast. The evidence existed, it was glaring, and, with some rare exceptions, notably a piece in the *Wall Street Journal* by a London-based reporter that referenced some of the studies I had also compiled, no one seemed to be covering it. While I did interview several experts, none of the information I had was secret. I wasn't using any embargoed studies (a common practice by journals, when they send not-yet-published studies to media but disallow coverage until a specified date). I didn't have an inside track with public health officials. Basically, for any journalist willing to put forth the effort the information was readily accessible. Yet it was absent from the public conversation. Obviously either the *Times* or someone else was going to publish a similar roundup of all of these studies that I had compiled and point out the wild dichotomy between schools opening in Europe and not in the US. Every day, several times a day I nervously checked the *Times*, the *Washington Post*, and a handful of other sites, waiting to see myself get scooped by a massive article listing much of the evidence I had put together.

Yet something strange happened. No one wrote that article.

Instead, as noted earlier, that month the *Times* ran the piece based on the unreviewed (and later discredited) conclusions of the German paper warning of dire pediatric infectiousness, and the subsequent lurid articles on MIS-C.

Something else surprising happened. When the *Wired* article came out, a bunch of major figures on the Right—Rand Paul, Brit Hume, Ann Coulter, and others—tweeted it, which I somewhat expected, considering it matched their political viewpoint. But, interestingly, a smattering of doctors, academics, and people with PhDs in public health, economics, and so on, who were not associated with the Right, also tweeted it. But virtually no one in the middle seemed to notice it. The people I usually aligned with, mainstream journalists and your basic professional-class Democrats, were nowhere to be seen.

As far as I could see, no one took issue with any of the sources cited in the piece. The only criticisms I saw online were mainly replies like "F U, Rand Paul!" or "We screwed up our pandemic response, that's why schools can't open!" These reactions provided no evidence about what screwing up the response actually meant or how that rebutted the source material cited in the article. Seeing how the media coverage had been playing out thus far during the pandemic I, of course, was not so naive that I thought there would be a groundswell of support for the piece and that it would single-handedly shift the public debate. Yet I felt a deep disappointment. Reasonable people could disagree about whether the schools in the US should open or not at that time, but there was close to zero dissent among politicians or in the framing by legacy media outlets on the topic. The narrative was set.

8

IT'S GOOD TO FEEL LIKE YOU'RE DOING SOMETHING

By June, with schools already opened for millions of children around Europe for more than a month, I began to focus not just on the obstinance of American school closures, but on the mitigation measures that were, and were not, in place in those European schools that had opened. Toward the end of June I wrote a second piece for *Wired*, warning against extreme measures—which had no evidence of effectiveness—that were going to be imposed on children when school was set to reopen (at least in some parts of the country) that fall.

In the piece, I wrote that on May 16, the Centers for Disease Control and Prevention released guidance that

conjures up a grim tableau of safety measures: children wearing masks throughout the day; students kept apart in class, their desks surrounded by 6-foot moats of empty space; shuttered cafeterias and decommissioned jungle gyms; canceled field trips; and attendance scattered into every other day or every other week. Reports suggest that certain US schools may even tag their kids with homing beacons, to help keep track of anyone who breaks the rules and gets too close to someone else.

The CDC's preliminary guidelines form an extraordinary document, calling for measures heretofore never employed in American schools. While compulsory masking of children as young as age two for an entire school (or childcare) day became normalized in the US, it's worth pausing for a moment to appreciate how radical a departure this policy was from any NPIs, especially mandated ones, we'd seen in schools in the past. The previous guidance could be summarized as "wash your hands, cough into your elbow, and if you're sick stay home." Of course public health authorities and politicians argued that COVID presented a unique and especially dangerous threat, warranting more extreme measures, including masking children all day every day. But, as it was with the closures themselves, there was no solid evidence base behind any of these interventions. By the authorities' own admission, they didn't know which of these interventions worked or to what degree. It was sold as the Swiss cheese model: try everything and hope that the holes of each slice don't line up. As a result of this approach, children were forced to endure the varied harms from each of these interventions even though it wasn't known which intervention, if any, yielded any benefit. It was also apparent early on, from the data from China and a long list of other countries, that it simply was not the case that children were at great or even modest risk, certainly not beyond the risk for influenza, a virus for which none of these interventions were imposed.

This doesn't mean COVID presented zero threat to children. Nearly all of them ultimately got infected, most of whom had little to no symptoms at all or, at most, the equivalent of a bad cold. An extremely small portion of children, mostly those with underlying conditions, got seriously sick, and a smaller number even died. But during the decade before the pandemic alone, more children died of the flu in several individual seasons than died of COVID over each of its first two years. And these types of measures were never imposed on children for the flu.

If it was accepted that children were at extremely low risk from serious disease, then the case for masking them rested on the notion that masks would help prevent, to a significant degree, children from transmitting the virus to adults. Yet there were two problems with this supposition. First, the early data, as noted, suggested that children were far less likely to transmit the virus than adults. Second, there was zero evidence that community mask mandates, and specifically mask mandates in schools, were effective.

I'm not going to catalog here all of the literature on community and school mask mandates that arose during the course of the pandemic (which is in aggregate, even with a generous interpretation, conflicting, low quality, and weak). What I'm interested in exploring is the decision-making process that happened in real time, with the information available at that time.

Public health authorities, including the surgeon general, the head of the CDC, and, most influentially, Anthony Fauci, initially told the public to not bother wearing masks. Fauci wrote in an email (which was made public through a Freedom of Information Act request) dated February 5, 2020: "Masks are really for infected people to prevent them from spreading infection to people who are not infected, rather than protecting uninfected people from acquiring infection. The typical mask you buy in the drug store is not really effective in keeping out virus, which is small enough to pass through the material." On February 29 the surgeon general, Dr. Jerome Adams, tweeted: "Seriously people—STOP BUYING MASKS! They are NOT effective in preventing general public from catching #Coronavirus." During an interview on the TV news program "60 Minutes" on March 8, 2020, Fauci said, "People should not be walking around with masks. When you're in the middle of an outbreak, wearing a mask might make people 'feel' better"—he used air quotes on "feel"—"and it might even block a droplet, but it's not providing the perfect protection people think it is." He added that there are unintended consequences of wearing a mask, such as fiddling with it and continually touching your face. Less than a month later, on April 3, the CDC revised its guidance, and Fauci and other officials immediately went along with it, urging face masks—including those made from old t-shirts or bandanas—to be worn in public settings. As late as April 1, the CDC guidance was, "If you are not sick: You do not need to wear a facemask unless you are caring for someone who is sick (and they are not able to wear a facemask)."

Articles by the *Associated Press*, the *Washington Post*, and a website called factcheck.org, defended Fauci and the CDC's change in guidance by saying that "new information" had emerged on how the virus spreads, specifically that it does so among asymptomatic people. Of the change, Fauci said, "we fully realized that there were a lot of people who were asymptomatic who were spreading infection. So it became clear that we absolutely should be wearing masks consistently." What new information came to light during the three-and-a-half weeks between the "60 Minutes" interview and the guidance change is not clear since Fauci did not cite any studies or sources behind this claim. Yet there were numerous sources of evidence before the "60 Minutes" interview of asymptomatic transmission of SARS-CoV-2. Among them was a research letter published in February in the *Journal of the American Medical Association* that suggested its likelihood. A study published in February in the *Journal of Infectious Diseases* reported the likelihood of asymptomatic transmission citing a patient "with limited mobility who was exposed only to asymptomatic family members." A letter in the *New England Journal of Medicine* on January 30 suggested that asymptomatic persons are potential sources of infection. A US government official was quoted in a February 3 article in *Science*: "This evening I telephoned one of my colleagues in China who is a highly respected infectious diseases scientist and health official. He said that he is convinced that there is asymptomatic infection and that some asymptomatic people are transmitting infection." That US government official was Anthony Fauci.

There is also a wealth of scientific literature on the potential of asymptomatic spread of other respiratory viruses, specifically influenza, so it was not as if asymptomatic spread was an unusual or unexpected phenomenon that would have taken health officials by surprise. Anthony Fauci himself even coauthored a paper in the *Journal of Infectious Diseases* where he wrote that "for many common respiratory viruses such as influenza" and RSV, a barrier to herd immunity is asymptomatic transmission.

It is unequivocal and undeniable that when they gave their initial guidance to not to wear masks Fauci and officials at the CDC knew asymptomatic transmission was not only possible but likely. It was conceivable, as Fauci suggested, that *more* information about asymptomatic transmission came about during the few weeks between the *60 Minutes* interview and the change in guidance a few weeks later. But, again, no evidence was cited.

For such an important policy, with a wide-ranging impact on public life in America—not the least of which on schoolchildren—that was a 180-degree shift from the previous recommendation, one would expect the authorities to have referenced a wealth of high quality evidence showing a high rate of asymptomatic transmission that would have emerged during that short interim. The reason none was cited was because it didn't exist.

In June 2020, Dr. Maria Van Kerkhove, head of the World Health Organization's emerging diseases and zoonosis unit, said that transmission from asymptomatic people was "very rare." This conclusion was based on a number of countries doing very detailed contact tracing, she said. (The next day, after criticism from some health professionals, WHO officials walked back her statement, and Van Kerkhove said it was a "complex question.") Even as late as January 2021, according to a much-cited paper in *JAMA Network Open*, the best "evidence" of high rates of asymptomatic transmission was mere conjecture based on models based on low quality observational studies. (Much of the later statistics on asymptomatic index cases were from household transmission, an environment of course in which people sleep in the same beds, eat meals, sit on sofas, and so on with each other for long stretches—far different from typical interactions outside the home.) And the authors of that paper had the benefit of a retrospective look at all of the accrued data, which was not available to Fauci and the others at the time of their claim. Conversely, a sophisticated test developed at Stanford University that spring, called minus strand PCR, that—unlike observational studies and models—definitively could determine whether a positive asymptomatic person was infectious, found as early as July 2020 that 96 percent of people who tested positive without symptoms did not even have the biological capability of transmission to others. And as one of the authors of that study explained to me, simply having the technical capability of transmission does not mean it was likely. Meaning, the actual rate of transmission from infected people without symptoms was lower than 4 percent.

But the real issue is that the prevalence of asymptomatic transmission was beside the point. Whether a large percentage of people was transmitting asymptomatically or not, what actually mattered was whether, or to what extent, community mask mandates worked. What was the evidence on the effectiveness of community mask mandates? Before the pandemic systematic reviews (formal interpretations of many studies on a particular topic) published by Cochrane, the prestigious British review organization, concluded that wearing a mask outside of a healthcare environment "probably makes little or no difference to the outcome of laboratory-confirmed influenza compared to not wearing a mask," and that the use of an N95 or respirator "probably makes little or no difference" compared to a surgical mask. Even an analysis by the CDC itself of community masking evidence before the pandemic, in which the authors identified ten randomized trials of community mask use, found "no significant reduction in influenza transmission with the use of face masks." (Just to make sure there is no ambiguity about the state of evidence, please read the previous two sentences again.)

To make matters worse, Fauci and other officials encouraged cloth masks, which could be purchased on websites like Amazon or Etsy, or even made from T-shirts at home. Consequently, cloth masks, which offered *less* protection than surgical masks, and which had no formal standards or approvals by accredited governmental organizations, were the dominant form of mask worn in the community and in schools for at least the first year of the pandemic. The evidence of benefit of cloth masks was so poor that the only randomized trial on cloth masks before the pandemic, performed on healthcare workers, found that people wearing them had significantly *higher* rates of influenza-like illness than participants in the control group. Penetration of cloth masks by particles was almost 97 percent.

In short, there was no new randomized trial, typically the "gold standard" of evidence-based medicine, on masking published in the three weeks between the change in guidance. And Fauci, the CDC, and the surgeon general did not cite any other, lesser quality new evidence published during that time frame that would have overturned the conclusions from all of the existing literature on community masking.

In a later interview, in July, with the *Washington Post*, explaining the initial guidance to not wear a mask, Fauci said, "Back then the critical issue was to save the masks for the people who really needed them because it was felt that there was a shortage of masks." Once the shortage was resolved, and authorities decided you could use plain cloth as a mask, Fauci said, then he felt comfortable recommending widespread mask usage. Preserving masks for healthcare workers was a noble aim. But the supply issue was unrelated to the claim about gaining new information on asymptomatic transmission, and the degree of asymptomatic transmission didn't change the existing evidence relating to community masking.

Science changes, and public health guidance should change along with it. The problem wasn't that the guidance on community masking changed. It's that the authorities presented no quality evidence to justify the change. This was an extremely odd and arguably catastrophic communications strategy behind telling more than three hundred million people to do something that was the opposite of what you had told them just a month before. While a sizable portion of the population was eager to go along with the new guidance, it should be no wonder that a different and also sizable portion of the population was not. The discord among the citizenry wasn't helped when Trump, while announcing the new CDC guidance, said that wearing a mask was voluntary and "I don't think I'm going to be doing it."

Fauci, CDC officials, and other health authorities were aware, or should have been aware, of the prepandemic scientific literature that showed a lack of evidence of benefit of community masking. For them to recommend a change in guidance and say, with certainty, that this was an effective intervention was essentially fraud.

It's hard to overstate the damage from this episode. Had Fauci and the CDC said "There is no evidence this will help but we ask everyone to give it a try," that would have been one thing. But that's not how it was presented. On the contrary, not only was this presented as true, that community masking would lower transmission, but it was moralized. *Your mask protects me, my mask protects you*, the public was told. No evidence existed to support that claim on a population level, and in fact there was much evidence to the contrary. But after Fauci's and the CDC's about-face the rest of the American public health establishment fell in line, and then, in turn, so did much of the public. An anomaly on the world stage, and at odds with recommendations from the World Health Organization and the European Centre for Disease Prevention and Control, the US even forced two-year-olds to wear masks for six or more hours a day, for years, and among much of the prestige media and the public this policy—which would have been considered extraordinary, absurdist, and cruel under any other circumstance—went entirely unchallenged. There also was, and still is, as I write this more than three years after the beginning of the pandemic, no evidence that masking toddlers made any difference in the outcomes of the pandemic. More than ten million children under age six (the WHO age cutoff) in Europe were not required to mask, as they were in the US, and there is no evidence that this led to worse outcomes in Europe.

In April 2023, after years of adamantly promoting the importance of community masking and school mask mandates, Fauci said during an interview with the *New York Times* that at the population level masks only "work at the margins."

I've focused on the details behind the change in mask guidance because this episode is emblematic of two very important dynamics that directed American school closure policies and school mitigation policies that would follow in its wake for the next two years. The first is that humans in general, and particularly people in positions of authority, have an instinct to act when confronted with a potential harm. Broadly, this falls under an "action bias"—within medicine this phenomenon is referred to as intervention bias. The second is that the instinct to act is so strong that as long as some intervention is implemented, empirical evidence of its benefit is seen as not necessary and evidence showing a lack of benefit or even harm may be ignored.

There is a rich literature from philosophy to psychology that explains that people, understandably, want to feel they have some control over their environment and their destiny. Indeed, scientists, such as Kevin Ochsner, the chair of the department of psychology at Columbia University, have argued that there is "a biological basis for the need for control." Because of the inherent responsibility of their role, this instinct is amplified for those who oversee others' well-being, whether it's a physician caring for an individual patient, or a public health official making guidance for millions. The person with authority wants to feel that they can influence outcomes, that they are "doing" something. And intervention—prescribing action—even without evidence of its benefit, satisfies that desire.

Despite the rise of EBM, there is a virtually endless list of medical practices, including the prescribing of certain drugs, administration of tests, and implantation of medical devices, that began without evidence of benefit, or continued after evidence showed a lack of benefit or even after evidence showed a net harm. There is a well-documented problem of physicians ordering tests, prescribing medicine, and performing procedures without evidence of benefit. The motivations for this can be financial, a "CYA" protective action in a litigious society, or because misinformed patients demand them. But this also happens because physicians, like all of us, want to feel helpful. It's estimated that more than 30 percent of antibiotic prescriptions are unnecessary, despite the fact that, among direct harms to patients, this fuels an increase in antibiotic-resistant bacteria.

For years, thousands of harmful metal-on-metal hip replacements were implanted in patients because the FDA allows use of devices that have no clinical trials as long as manufacturers showed they were similar to other devices that were approved, even if the approved devices were recalled for being faulty. If you're an orthopedist and you have a patient with a busted hip, financial incentive aside, you likely don't want to say, "Sorry, there's nothing I can do." You want to try *something*.

When I talked with Branch-Elliman, the Harvard infectious diseases physician and implementation scientist, trying to understand where her critical view on the effect of pandemic interventions came from, she recounted for me a study of nearly 80,000 patients she conducted on prophylactic antibiotic use for surgeries. "It was my most famous paper before the pandemic, the third most cited article in *JAMA Surgery* that year," she said. "I'm interested in norms that are based on assumptions. I always want to know if the assumptions are true." Branch-Elliman and her coauthors found not only that longer duration of antibiotic use did not reduce surgical site infections, but that it was associated with an increase in kidney injuries and C. diff infections. Nevertheless, this practice continues.

"When you're looking at only one outcome you become hyper focused on improving that outcome, but that doesn't mean you're improving everything," she said. "With the antibiotics study, doctors weren't looking at the overall patient outcome, they were looking at the infection rate, but patients were having other negative outcomes."

This phenomenon is arguably far worse with public health interventions, since they generally don't have to pass the (albeit, as detailed above, often inadequate) regulatory hurdles that drugs and devices have to pass. "Public health authorities make recommendations for policy action, yet these are not based on high quality evidence," wrote a group of epidemiologists and public health scholars at the University of California, San Francisco, in a 2018 paper titled "The Discordance between Evidence and Health Policy in the United States." A 2015 study, published in the *American Journal of Preventive Medicine*, of nearly one thousand public health practitioners found that a quarter of them reported programs continuing after they should have ended. A 2012 analysis found more than 150 healthcare practices in use that were potentially ineffective or even unsafe. A 2019 study of misimplementation of public health measures concluded that decisions about continuing or ending a program "were often seen as a function of program popularity and funding availability as opposed to effectiveness."

Americans of a certain age will all remember D.A.R.E. (Drug Abuse Resistance Education), the campaign intended to teach young people to say "no" to drugs. The program began in the 1980s, and by 1994 was the most widely used school-based drug prevention program in the country, with the government spending three-quarters of a billion dollars on it that year. Numerous studies at the time, including meta-analyses, found the program to be ineffective, yet it continued anyway. Worse, its likelihood of success seemed dubious from the start. D.A.R.E sprang from two programs of experimental curricula that were "neither fully developed nor equally successful," the authors of one analysis wrote. The program grew into a $750 million per year colossus, even though its benefit was suspect from its original implementation.

We'd like to believe that public health officials are making cold, objective decisions about our care, and if a major initiative is enacted with significant downsides that there is definitive evidence behind its effectiveness. Yet a wealth of research has shown that time and again programs are initiated or continue simply because they're popular, because there is ample funding for them, or because practitioners need to feel like they are "doing something," none of which necessarily have any relation to evidence of their effectiveness.

The need for authorities (and likewise many regular people) to feel like something is being done is most relevant, perhaps singularly so, to explain implementation of many of the NPIs during the pandemic, including the early reversal on community masking guidance.

A study published in the journal *Implementation Science Communications* on public health agencies' "inappropriate continuation of programs that are not evidence based" found that one of the reasons state health employees continue ineffective programs is because of a desire to act. The authors believed this factor to be so critical that they titled the paper "It's Good to Feel Like You're Doing Something." The authors wrote: "Practitioners discussed the idea that it feels good to know that at least something is being done to address a public health concern, *even if the program is not effective"* (italics added). Seen through this lens it's easy to understand why Fauci and others felt the need to implement measures—in this instance community masking—even without sufficient evidence behind them. As public health officials in charge of the pandemic response, they had to feel like they were doing something, even if there was a lack of evidence or, worse, evidence to the contrary that it would be beneficial. But we don't need a study to tell us this. Many of us would rather drive an hour out of our way to avoid forty minutes of sitting in traffic. We need to feel like we are moving forward, even if we know "forward" is an illusion. This tendency is so strong that emergency medicine physicians have to refer to an axiom to help them fight against it: "Don't just do something, stand there."

It would also be preposterous to not acknowledge that those in power, from public health officials to politicians, know that they benefit from the mere *appearance* of helping. If the authorities can appear proactive, and give regular people a tool to make them feel that they have some semblance of control, even if it may be illusory, over a dangerous infectious virus then it's a doubly effective policy. It's a fairly obvious observation, but worth noting that psychological studies going back decades have shown that the mere perception of control, when desired, affords positive effects on mood.

Despite a dearth of evidence to suggest that community masking was going to make an appreciable dent in transmission rates, health officials' and many citizens' desire for a semblance of control over a situation that appeared to be getting out of hand led to the masking guidance that ultimately became one of the most divisive policies in the country for years.

Like most of the school-based interventions, including, most importantly, closures and hybrid schedules, masking requirements for American children—at great odds with the recommendations from the WHO, the ECDC, and policies in many countries throughout Europe—were based, in part, simply on the impulse to do something. This was not an anomaly within the history and present of medicine and public health practice, but, alas, an expected outcome of human nature.

9

OUT OF AN ABUNDANCE OF CAUTION

In its communications regarding nearly every single intervention in my kids' school district—from school closures to plastic desk barriers to masks to distancing to deep cleanings—the administration repeatedly invoked the justification that it was being done "out of an abundance of caution." In lengthy emails, in board of education meetings, and in slide presentations the phrase was often employed as a preamble, a closing statement, or somewhere in the middle of a block of text. It didn't matter where, as long as the phrase was included. The terminology, and the notion that an action was being done "to be safe," all but shut down any allowance for debate, discussion, or dissent. When it came to children, who wouldn't want to be cautious! We were confronted with a deadly virus and even if we weren't sure a measure was going to help, it was worth trying, and continuing. Even if evidence showed no benefit, even if evidence showed harm, it was *still* worth it.

Many people felt this was the precautionary principle in action, what the average person might define as something like "better safe than sorry." Close the schools, and keep them closed until we know it's "safe." And for schools to open a list of measures must be employed to keep them "safe." But the precautionary principle in general is a fundamentally misunderstood precept, and its supposed application toward school policy, specifically, was not what people think it was.

First, the "abundance of caution" that justified so many actions merely appeared as a precautionary measure, but in actuality was based on a poorly grounded cost-benefit analysis that goes back to the models. As we know, the models purported to show a specific, quantified benefit of reducing cases and deaths by employing a variety of measures, most consequentially school closures. This framing served as the scaffold for much of the pandemic policies that would follow. "Models create false cost-benefits," Branch-Elliman, said. Models give precise statistical outputs, yet, ironically, they are based on assumptions. And during the pandemic, the more time that passed, the more harm that was incurred by following guidance based on assumptions of benefits of an intervention that were overstated.

I had several lengthy discussions about the precautionary principle, models, and ethics, with Eric Winsberg, a philosopher of science at the University of South Florida and University of Cambridge, who has written extensively about the policy and ethical implications of models. "If I'm missing scientific facts then I don't have a way of calculating how many lives will be saved by closing schools, or how much learning loss will happen," Winsberg told me. "It's basically immoral to put out a model that purports to show something that it's not showing," he said.

In a cost-benefit analysis, the relevant question is not simply whether school will cause any infections at all; it is whether open schools will cause *more* infections than students would otherwise get in the community and at home, and, if so, how many more, and for how long, Winsberg explained. And once the answer to that has been ascertained, then, if there is a known benefit of closures, the question is whether it outweighs the harms, bearing in mind that the harms differ among different people. Branch-Elliman noted that it's possible the initial closures did reduce transmission by some unknown amount, but that benefit likely vaporized quite rapidly. And what she and Winsberg, and some other prominent voices (who we'll get to later), argued is that people who are not in the laptop class—many of whom are from less privileged circumstances—were disproportionately vulnerable to transmission during school closures and general societal shutdowns because work for many of them was outside the home.

In an interview with the *Washington Post*, in a unicorn of an article in March 2020 that questioned the epidemiological benefit of school closures, Jennifer Nuzzo shared similar comments. She said there were not great data to support school closures as an effective tool to stop viral spread. "Any benefits school closures may have will not be achieved if kids recongregate or if kids are left with elderly grandparents, or if

closures make it hard for health-care workers and other essential person-
nel to show up and meet society's basic needs," she said.

Beyond the particulars of whether the closures conferred the benefits
they were purported to confer, is the reality that the cost-benefit analysis masquerading as a precautionary act that resulted in school closures
showed a moral confusion and a logical inconsistency with past decisions around schools. Let's say there was a reasonably good way of calculating how many lives would be saved versus how much learning loss,
weight gain, depression, and so forth would occur if schools were closed
for certain durations of time. And then we got people together to represent the public interest to decide: How much of these harms is worth one
death? Neither "science"—nor precaution—provides an answer to this.
But we know the answer is not zero, because a certain number of kids
die every year from school violence; some likely die traveling to or from
school; some even kill themselves as a result of bullying that takes place
at school; and so on. We accept that some unknown number of kids will
die in normal years every year from going to school, yet schools remain
open nonetheless and parents send their kids in. So then the question
is: what number above zero is a tolerable risk in order for kids to be
in school?

Most importantly, a cost-benefit analysis must answer moral questions about different outcomes, yet those types of questions are rarely
answered by quantifiable causal claims.

Indeed, the Imperial College model at the start of the pandemic, known
as Report 9, which directly informed Deborah Birx's policy recommendations, explicitly notes this limitation. Recall that the Report 9 model dif-
ferentiates between suppression and mitigation—essentially, an attempt
at stopping spread versus slowing spread—with the former requiring far
more intensive NPIs. The report held that mitigation might reduce peak
healthcare demand by two-thirds and deaths by half, still resulting in
hundreds of thousands of deaths. Therefore, for the countries that were
able to achieve it, "this leaves suppression as the preferred policy option,"
the report stated. Except, the report noted, the social and economic costs
of such a strategy would be "enormous," and might "themselves have
significant impact on health and well being." Despite the report's recommendation for suppression, which would require "social distancing of the

entire population," and its citing of school closures as the most effective
of other options, it contains the following statement: "*We do not consider
the ethical or economic implications of either strategy.*" (If a documentary
is ever made of this book, now would be a prime moment for a record
scratch on the audio track.)

The public health authorities, along with regular people, believed
they were operating according to the precautionary principle by closing
schools "out of an abundance of caution," yet there was no evidence to
quantify how much, if any, benefit there was of keeping schools closed,
or, when taking into account the harms of continued time outside of
school, even if there were a reduction in cases from a school closure,
whether that yielded a net benefit relative to the harms that would result
from the closure. Is it worth keeping an entire city of children out of
school for a month if that yields one fewer transmission? What about ten
transmissions? Or a hundred? Is it worth closing an entire city's school
system for two months if that means one child won't go to the hospital? And how, exactly, could it be assumed that the child wouldn't get
infected outside of school? None of this was accounted for. For two weeks
it may have been reasonable to suggest that even if there wasn't a known
benefit of a closure, the consequences to most kids of being out of school
for that duration are so benign that, at the worst, it would be a wash.
But as time slipped to three, then four weeks, and then the remainder
of the academic year (let alone the following school year for millions of
American children), it was fallacious to continue to say that closures were
persisting "out of an abundance of caution." There was a pretense about
known benefits of closures, yet no such knowledge existed. Jean-Jacques
Rousseau, the Enlightenment thinker (whose writings, incidentally, were
influenced by John Locke) warned about the harm of assuming you know
more than you know:

*Remember without fail that ignorance never caused any harm, that error alone is fatal,
and that we do not go astray by what we do not know, but by what we believe we know.*

"It's worse to use models that falsely appear to give a cost-benefit,"
than to be honest about what you do and don't know, Winsberg told me.
"If the authorities had said, 'We don't actually have any evidence about
whether or to what extent school closures will benefit the kids or adults,

or what harms they will cause, but we think it's worth trying,'" Winsberg said, "then it's far easier to reopen them than if you used a model showing a ton of people dying." Echoing Rousseau, Winsberg's point is that false information, and projecting an air of certainty when there isn't actual certainty, is more harmful than no information.

The problem wasn't just that the models got things wrong. The problem was relying on models to begin with.

Had we not relied on the models, American officials still may have arrived at the conclusion to close schools, and even to keep them closed after they were open elsewhere. But doing so would have compelled the authorities to produce an argument for this action. Admitting uncertainty also would have encouraged more of a public conversation about values, and an acknowledgment of the empirical evidence—that schools were not driving transmission (and that many kids were suffering harms from being out of school)—that began to accrue. Instead, schools remained closed based on feelings and assumptions, and in a belief that modeled outcomes were more credible than actual outcomes being witnessed in real time—the exact opposite of science.

In the 1930s, the philosopher Alfred Korzybski famously warned in his book *Science and Sanity* that "a map is not the territory." By this he meant that we should not conflate the representation of something with the thing itself. This seems like eye-rollingly obvious advice, and yet Korzybski understood that over and over humans have shown a tendency to do exactly that. The modelers, and the rest of the public health establishment, believed their forecasts (the maps) more than the evidence that was occurring in the real world (the territory).

Remember, Branch-Elliman talked about how de-implementation is very hard. Once an intervention or practice is in place, it is very difficult to remove it, even after evidence arises that shows it's not helpful, and even that it may be harmful. Her comments are borne out by the studies of the public health professionals who said programs were kept in place even after it was clear that they weren't beneficial. Perhaps it's part of the desire to "do something." Perhaps it's inertia. Perhaps it's financial or other bad incentives. Whatever the cause or combination of causes, once an intervention is set in motion, it does not come to rest easily. After an intervention is implemented, the psychological burden then shifts to needing to see proof that the risk of harm has lessened before the intervention can be removed. Winsberg said, "Once you tell people this virus is so dangerous that we need to close schools and you need to stay home from your job, once you tell teachers this is so dangerous that no one should be in school, it's very hard to come back three weeks later and say, 'We're still not sure what's happening, but you should come back to school.'" That hurdle was overcome in Europe (though not without some dissension), where the sociopolitical landscape was not as acrimoniously bifurcated on the issue, and where the media was less sensationalist about risks to children and of school—but in America reopening schools that spring was a nonstarter.

Because of these issues many philosophers don't even acknowledge that the precautionary principle exists. Within philosophy, the precautionary principle is seen as a fallacy known as "question begging." Conventionally, most of us know "begs the question" as an expression meaning "raises the question." But the formal meaning of this phrase traces to an Aristotelian saying meaning *assuming the conclusion*. (The vagaries of translation from ancient Greek to Latin to English over a couple millennia yielded the mismatched wording today.) Philosophers reject question begging because an argument's premise should not be based on an assumption that its conclusion is true instead of supporting it with evidence. This is also known as a circular argument. God's word is infallible because it says so in the Bible, which was written by God.

In a practical and informal sense, the precautionary principle can be sensible. If you have good reason to believe something terrible will happen if you do a certain action, then the precautionary principle would dictate for you to not do that action. If you think your children might get killed or grievously harmed by going to school, then "to be safe" you would keep them home. The problem is there was a wealth of evidence early on that children were not at great risk from the coronavirus, that schools and children were not drivers of the pandemic, and, on the other side of the scale, that being out of school for an extended period would put a great number of children at risk of a multitude of harms. Are we to believe that the public health authorities in Europe—where many cities in the spring of 2020 had comparable case rates to those in American cities, where the schools are not so radically different from ours that transmission dynamics there would alter the epidemiology of the disease in a manner totally divorced from how it would function in schools in the US—were somehow less cautious than their American counterparts? Of course not. They simply did not default to the philosophical and rhetorical fallacy of school closures equating to acting "out of an abundance of caution."

"We ignored a question under the assumption that it was already answered," Winsberg told me. The Europeans, on the other hand, actually asked the question: What, in fact, are the net harms and net benefits of closing schools, and keeping them closed? And by actually asking the question, rather than begging the question, they arrived at a different conclusion than we did.

The fallacy of the precautionary principle and the rhetoric of being "safe" by closing schools was damagingly effective at keeping schools closed because it positioned anyone who questioned this policy as someone who didn't value children's safety. It set opposition as immoral. Everyone agrees *in the abstract* that preventing death is more important than preventing learning loss and other harms of being out of school. But in reality that agreement only extends to a certain point. Is keeping one million children out of school worth preventing one death? If so, for how long? And what evidence is there for us to even conduct these calculations? Why would preventing death above all other considerations be the policy for schools during the pandemic when it's not the policy for schools outside the pandemic? Again, we've always tolerated a certain number of deaths (and other harms) from schools being open in regular times. And this is the case for society in general. We allow for highway speeds of sixty-five miles per hour, knowing that more people will die than if the limit were twenty-five miles per hour. Society and individuals do not value the avoidance of death above all other considerations.

People claimed that they were preventing potential death by keeping schools closed and that this was the moral imperative. But they didn't know how much death they were preventing. In fact, it's possible closing schools did not prevent any deaths at all, or even led to an increase in deaths, since we don't know whether an individual infected in school would have been infected outside of school anyway, or whether school closures increased children's breadth of contacts, especially elderly people

who had to take care of them. Moreover, even if school closures prevented a certain number of deaths and other harms, a certain number of
deaths and harms occurred as a result of the closures as well.

The precautionary principle, in effect, is the opposite of a cost-benefit
calculation. It relies on what Winsberg calls a "duty analysis," in which
instead of a cost-benefit calculation, decisions are simply guided by a
"duty" toward prioritizing a certain interest, in this case attempting to
prevent COVID infections, over other interests.

When there was an absence of information, claiming decisions were
made by following the precautionary principle offered an illusion of
harm reduction. But, in reality, in the absence of information you're just
consulting your own intuition, Winsberg said. And in the US intuition
was valued over empirical evidence.

But the intuitions of citizens, and of the broader public health community, such as regular doctors serving as trusted community members,
or epidemiologists on social media, who weren't intimately familiar with
the data, were distorted. The health authorities, by their own admission,
drummed up fear with the aim of increasing obedience to their guidelines. On March 15, Anthony Fauci said, "If it looks like you're overreacting you're probably doing the right thing." In the UK behavioral scientists
working for the government's emergency advisory group suggested a
series of methods to improve the public's compliance with social distancing guidelines. "Coercion" and "persuasion" were among the techniques
cited. "The perceived level of personal threat needs to be increased among
those who are complacent, using hard-hitting emotional messaging," the
advisers said. The media's tendency to emphasize or exaggerate risk aided
the authorities' mission, like tossing accelerant on a fire. Occasionally the
intention was made explicit. The *Times* published a piece in March titled
"Complacency, Not Panic, Is the Real Danger."

This is part of the problem with making decisions based on intuition
rather than evidence. Our intuitions are heavily skewed by all sorts of
factors, a large portion of which we are not consciously aware of. What
many people perceived to be the potential net harms and net benefits of
school closures were—in part because of the openly admitted objective
of the authorities, often with assistance from the media—the result of a
deliberately manipulative information environment.

Moreover, even without the skew from authorities and the media, there is a superficial logic to thinking school closures would reduce transmission. But—as I have, and will continue to detail—the historical evidence, along with a deeper consideration of how humans operate and interact, disabuses that intuition. As I have shown, and will continue to show, our assumptions are often wrong. That is why we need to rely on evidence and the scientific method, not intuition, for important policy decisions.

To be clear, as the saying goes, absence of evidence is not the same as evidence of absence. It is possible that school closures were going to have some effect, during a certain duration of time, in certain locations. But the authorities did not say that. They did not say, "We don't have strong evidence this is going to work, certainly not once we pass a few weeks, but let's try it anyway; maybe it'll help, and we think that unknown possibility of benefit is worth it." Instead, using the language of certainty, riding on the delusive vehicle of the precautionary principle, people were misled into believing a specificity of potential harm from schools. As Winsberg noted, teachers who were sent the message that being in school could kill them were not inclined to go back.

A core problem with the American policy, both Winsberg and Jeremy Howick, the Oxford philosopher of science, said is that closing schools quickly became the default position. The norm, of course, is for schools to be open. But rather than schools needing to be proven exceptionally dangerous to warrant their closures, teachers unions and others demanded that schools be proven to be safe to be reopened. (The definition of "safe," of course, was left open to interpretation.) The burden of proof had flipped. This is the opposite of what should happen. In medicine and public health intervening is not supposed to be the default—this is the foundation of nonmaleficence in bioethics, often referred to as "first do no harm."

Even interventions that seemingly would only have an upside are not always beneficial, and can be harmful. Take, for example, noninvasive testing of patients who come to the emergency room complaining of chest pain. The American Heart Association guidelines endorse a variety of tests in this scenario, such as stress electrocardiograms and stress echocardiograms. Patients with normal results can be discharged; those with abnormal results get admitted and undergo further, often invasive testing. This makes intuitive sense. Why not use noninvasive tests "just to make sure" there's nothing wrong? Because "there is no evidence that early noninvasive testing benefits patients," wrote researchers in *JAMA Internal Medicine*. Further, they noted, in addition to more than $3 billion in hospital costs each year, this testing protocol may lead to overtreatment, with invasive procedures that increase potential for injury without improved outcomes. The reasons are complex for these findings, and the authors note some patients may benefit from early testing. But the point is interventions that seem obvious and that make intuitive sense often do not achieve the expected result.

Notoriously, abstinence-only programs in high schools are correlated with more teen pregnancies. Administration of medications and public health interventions no doubt are well-intentioned. But evidence-based medicine would say before you intervene—give a new drug or, say, bar children from attending school—that you have to see evidence of benefit *and* a net reduction in harm. EBM does not countenance you intervening first and continuing to intervene until there's confirmation of harm, Howick said. If we do the latter—operating on the precautionary principle, based on assumptions—we wind up unnecessarily harming some patients with chest pain and tragically increasing the number of children with life-altering peanut allergies.

The language itself that is used in public health and in medicine reflects our bias toward action. We are all familiar with the phrase "risk benefit"— it's even used in this book—when talking about interventions. Yet this wording frames our perception and weights the analysis of interventions in a one-sided manner. We think of "benefits" on one side, yet only think of "risks," rather than "harms," on the other side. An analysis of PubMed, a database of medical literature, found that variations of the phrase "benefit risk" appeared 3,977 times. By contrast, variations of "benefit harm" appeared only 156 times, and the more uncertain "potential benefit" and "risk of harm" appeared only 8 times combined.

Unlike medical interventions, which patients or their proxies can refuse, children and their parents did not have a choice in accepting school closures. Because they can take the form of social programs, public health interventions often are imposed on a population whether they like it or not—think of kids and the D.A.R.E. program, or abstinence-only lectures, or the revamping of a cafeteria lunch menu with ostensibly healthier entrees, for example. But school closures were more than just a program. A long-term school closure is uniquely absolute in its impact, almost spherical in its envelopment of a child's life. One would be hard-pressed to cite a public health intervention of this scale and personal imposition that was enacted without evidence of a net benefit (and, later, with evidence to the contrary), for which participation was compulsory. There was no option to attend school for those who wanted to. Conversely, keeping schools open, or reopening them shortly after they closed, as was done in much of Europe, would not have prevented families from keeping their children home from school if they chose to do so. Through the first year or more of the pandemic, once schools in many areas did open fully or partially, the option of staying home was also almost universally available.

"The precautionary principle is a burden of proof claim," Winsberg said. As a society we agree on what the default action is. And if you disagree then, certainly after a brief time, the burden is on you to prove why we need to veer from the default. The answer can't just be your intuition for an indefinite period of time.

Once the empirical evidence emerged from Europe that opening schools did not lead to disaster, and in fact did not lead to any noticeable difference in case rates, it's important to understand that schools did not remain closed in the US out of an abundance of caution. To continue to claim, after the European evidence to the contrary, that school closures were being maintained out of caution is the equivalent of declaring "Because I said so!" Winsberg noted. You can't do that forever in a democracy. Rather, Winsberg said, we need to bring everyone's values to the table and figure out if some people are being harmed more than others.

Saying you're closing schools—or, later, only allowing kids to attend two days a week, or forcing them to wear masks all day or not allowing a five-year-old to put his arm around a friend—"out of an abundance of caution" silenced debate. In a time when much of the public had been whipped into a state of fear, a person who claimed that a decision was made "out of an abundance of caution" was absolved from having to provide evidence, or near any defense at all, and rendered any opposition morally suspect.

Yet caution was never defined. The caution of school closures was different for a wealthy teenager, with his own bedroom, MacBook, tutors, and parents working from home, there to help him if needed, than it was for an underprivileged third grader, with no computer or internet access, taken care of by a single parent who had to work outside the home, than it was for a middle-class kid with an abusive stepfather in the house, than it was for a child with attention deficit disorder whose brain was cognitively incapable of "remote learning" for more than a few minutes. An abundance of caution was experienced very differently by different kids and different families. "Caution" only ran in one direction.

*   *   *

Who decided what is cautious? The public health establishment, politicians, and the journalists and editors of the prestige media. Each of these groups are part of the cultural or political elite in America. (Teachers unions and, to a far lesser extent, parents also had a say in defining "cautious," but their perception of the cost-benefit of closures, and the ability to act on that perception, was largely dictated by the guidance from the public health establishment, the rules passed by the politicians, and the narrative formed by the media.)

And, drilling down, who laid the foundation for the public health establishment's, politicians', and the media's response? The modelers. But the top modelers, who by and large work at eminent universities, are highly educated, make upper-middle-class salaries, and live in comfortable homes in comfortable neighborhoods, not only created the framework of what was considered "cautious." They also served as a reflection of elite society's priorities and blind spots. The models of the pandemic had many flaws, but their final flaw was that the modelers' membership among the elite brought a list of biases that prioritized the values and circumstances of their select segment of society.

This phenomenon is not exclusive to modelers. The people who create the frameworks within which we live can have enormous, even if at times inadvertent, control over the parameters of that frame.

A study of facial recognition technology developed in different regions found that the "Western algorithm recognized Caucasian faces more accurately than East Asian faces and the East Asian algorithm recognized East Asian faces more accurately than Caucasian faces." For generations, the default thermostat setting in corporate offices, which are disproportionately run by men, has been decidedly chilly, in part because that's more comfortable for men. The vast, public infrastructure projects of Robert Moses in New York City during the mid-twentieth century, which prioritized cars and highways over walkable urban spaces, advantaged residents who were wealthier, who could afford their own vehicles for travel.

"The core question is 'In what ways do models incorporate our social and ethical values?'" Stephanie Harvard, a public health economist at the University of British Columbia, and a frequent collaborator with Winsberg, told me. Harvard's focus is on "knowledge translation" (known as KT in the field), how evidence-based research gets incorporated into practice and policy. She studies how to build a better bridge between evidence and policy. Her entire area of scholarship is a refutation of the notion that Cuomo or Fauci or anyone else was "following the science," as they so often claimed: science itself is the pursuit of knowledge and acquisition of evidence; how we choose to conduct society or make laws based on that evidence is a wholly separate process.

The models, or "the science," did not tell us to close schools. Rather, the models purported to forecast what would happen to viral transmission if we closed the schools. (Which, as I extensively detailed, due to catastrophically flawed methodology, they failed to do.) But the possibly bigger problem with the models is not the faulty inputs they relied on. Rather, it's the inputs they left out.

"There's this preconception that models are this scientific device, and you use scientific reasoning to build them," said Harvard. But that is not so. What you choose to model shows what you value. "Nobody denies that if I'm a cancer researcher I think cancer is important," she said. "It's exactly the same, though harder to see, if you build a model in a pandemic on hospitalizations and death. That's what you think is important in a specific way." When we're making highly consequential decisions for society, such as whether schools should close (and remain closed), Harvard said, in part it's about scientific evidence, but it's also a question of *what* we look into. And this very much is an ethical issue. So, the first question is what exactly gets modeled. Then the next question is to what extent do you model externalities.

"Pretty clearly early on the COVID models left out costs," Winsberg told me. "There's nothing in the model about what will happen to hospital systems if healthcare workers' children are forced to stay home. There's nothing in the model about what will happen to the economy if nonessential businesses are forced to close. There's nothing in the model about if you make people socially isolated, especially children and teens, how that may impact drug abuse, depression, eating disorders, and other effects." Models, he said, cannot be morally neutral.

"It's tempting to be overly crude about this, but it's also quite dramatic the extent to which the people who did best during the pandemic, how much they were like the people that built the models," Winsberg said. "To realize that those of us whom you might think of as being in the laptop class, those who do our work at desks on the internet, how much better we fared in the pandemic than people who work in meat packing plants, or deliver our groceries, or live in parts of the world where the internet is not readily available."

* * *

It's understandable that families, even those who would suffer the most hardship from their children being kept out of school, initially would nevertheless want schools closed, considering the fear of death that permeated much of the populace. But, remember, as Branch-Elliman had explained, and as detailed in the playbook, closing schools, among other NPIs, is a temporizing measure, intended to delay transmission until the imminent and predictable arrival of a vaccine or effective treatment (as is typical for the flu). This intervention was never supposed to last as long as it did in many areas. Part of the reason it was able to endure for so long was that the only official government mission, using quantifiable metrics from models, was to mitigate the spread of the virus. This may have made sense for the initial few weeks. But after that time continuing to only model cases, deaths, and hospitalizations related to the virus, and not model second-order effects of the mitigations, placed viral mitigation above all other concerns. To put a fine point on it: The risks of the coronavirus to an eighty-five-year-old were orders of magnitude higher than they were to a child. Similarly, the harms to the family of a corporate attorney who could do her work from a luxurious home without losing a dime in income, and her children who had comfortable places to do their remote learning or had tutors or were in private school, were entirely different from the harms to a small business owner whose finances would be wiped out if no one came to their store for months on end, or children in homes without adequate parental support or physical space or tools to do remote learning. The models, and the resultant policies to close schools or require hybrid schedules for months or in many instances for more than a year, had a completely different cost-benefit for children overall, and less-privileged children in particular, than they did for the elderly or well off. The models only showed the (falsely presumed) upside—reducing viral transmission. No one modeled the downsides, which, with wild disproportionality, were shouldered by children.

10

IGNORING DAYCARES, AND THE CONTINUED REFUSAL OF EVIDENCE

Not modeling and, in turn, not seriously addressing second-order effects of school closures led to a very strange omission of evidence by public health officials. We already knew about schools reopening in Europe, which was ignored. But there was something happening right here in America that, remarkably, was also dismissed. From the onset of the closures, many frontline workers, from doctors and nurses to grocery store clerks and kitchen staff, had sent their young children to special government-run daycares and to YMCAs. In the spring of 2020, the Y cared for up to 40,000 children from ages one to fourteen, at more than 1,000 sites, often in partnership with local and state governments. The New York City Department of Education alone cared for more than 10,000 kids at 170 sites. The YMCA centers grouped kids into "pods" that didn't mix with each other. Yet social distancing and masks were not uniformly observed or used, and if a child was sick they were told to stay home (notably similar circumstances to those in Swedish schools). The Y said while there were a few COVID cases among staff, there were no records of outbreaks at its more than 1,000 sites.

This astonishing circumstance came to the public's attention through a June news piece by NPR reporter Anya Kamenetz. (The above details are quoted from Kamenetz's reporting.) Yet throughout March, April, and May, government officials either knew all of this and ignored it, or should have known it but made no effort to.

While schools, particularly for older kids, are structured differently from daycares, the notion that more than 50,000 children spent each day in person with each other, not to mention without uniform masking or distancing, and no obvious calamity ensued, was a remarkable piece of evidence. Yet on May 1, New York governor Andrew Cuomo announced that schools in his state would not open the rest of the academic year. His policy mirrored that of nearly all forty-nine of his peers. (With a few exceptions in Montana and Wyoming, the entire school system in America remained closed from March through June.) Was Cuomo not aware of the New York City Department of Education program? Ignoring what happened with 50,000 kids in the Y and New York City's program was yet another flight from evidence-based public health, just as it was with ignoring the April 8 CDC report and, later, the May 18 determination by the EU's education ministers.

As Jeremy Howick and Eric Winsberg, the philosophers of science, had explained, the burden of proof of safety and benefit should fall on the intervention, not on the status quo. Ethically speaking, a well-designed study in which outcomes and other variables are systematically tracked and adjusted for was not necessary or appropriate as the only means of adjudicating whether schools should reopen. (Indeed, those types of trials were never conducted to that end. Schools, at different times in different places, simply eventually opened.) This evidence of tens of thousands of kids together for months, right here, in America, and, of specific relevance to Cuomo, in New York City, was pretended away.

And even if officials felt, going against the ethical norm of medicine, that a return to school required more than this strong but informal observational evidence why didn't they systematically monitor case rates and social distancing measures in daycare centers? This was a perfect experimental setup, involving a large number of children in different states, to simulate what could happen in schools. But it was not taken advantage of.

"We had hired McKinsey to crunch numbers," said the source with highly placed insider knowledge of the Cuomo administration. "They'd basically look at the IHME models, and Columbia's and others, showing something like 170,000 people in the hospital. It was crazy. We had something like 50,000 hospital beds. Even if we canceled all elective surgeries, we'd have at most 35,000 beds." But, the source said, "Very quickly we saw that every projection was wrong." Later, "in early April I was paying close attention to the numbers, and I saw growth slowing. That's when I knew we would be fine." Knowing this, and that some 10,000 kids had been in New York City–run daycares without incident, I asked the source what the conversations were like at the time about reopening schools. "I don't remember any discussion in spring 2020 to reopen schools," was the response.

I was astonished. I had eagerly, if naively, looked forward to talking with this source to learn about the behind-the-scenes discussions administration members held in which they reviewed the data on kids and schools and how they came to their conclusion to keep schools closed. Yet the Cuomo administration, and likely most other governors, even after more than a month, and then two months of closures, were not meeting in a war room each day discussing how to get schools open. Schools were simply not on the agenda.

So a circular logic—based on the unethical flipping of burden toward proving the safety of *non*intervention—ensured schools would remain closed. The authorities seemingly required high-level evidence that schools were "safe" in order to reopen them, yet the authorities didn't attempt to acquire any evidence.

* * *

With the government not bothering to track what was happening in daycares, this was one of the first of many instances during the pandemic in which a few outside researchers, often reluctantly, and sometimes with no particular expertise, took the initiative to gather data on their own. An economist at Brown University named Emily Oster was a natural fit for the task. She had published two best-selling books, one on pregnancy, the other on parenting, that took a data-driven approach, using evidence to debunk myths such as expectant moms being told they shouldn't eat sushi, or offering encouragement for new parents about sleep training. Her modus operandi was to cast an economist's analytical eye on certain conventional wisdoms and shibboleths around parenting that tended toward a particular American neuroticism.

Oster saw that schools were closed, daycares were open, and, frustratingly, that "there was this incredible dearth of information." Oster had recently started a newsletter so she began, in May, by asking her readers to ask their daycare centers to sign up with her and provide data.

She was fortunate to also get a company that runs a number of centers to participate. "I asked two basic questions: 'How many kids are there? And how many COVID cases are there?'" Oster told me. She knew this was far from a proper study, but because state and local health agencies, education departments, the CDC, and NIH failed to act, this was better than nothing. Any information at all would be valuable. On June 19 she released a newsletter with her findings. Out of some 14,000 children and 5,000 staff, the infection rate was around 0.1 percent. This result came too late for schools to open that spring, but it echoed Kamenetz's report of the YMCAs and NYC centers. Oster's data were powerful evidence that, even without systematic testing and other methodological protocols, one could surmise that daycare centers were not drivers of transmission. And if daycare centers—where little kids tumble around and pick noses and rub eyes—hardly bastions of hygiene, had this result then it was a reasonable extrapolation that schools would fare similarly.

The general direction of Oster's findings was furthered by a subsequent formal study published by in the journal *Pediatrics*. Walter Gilliam, an expert in early childhood education research at Yale School of Medicine, and coauthors analyzed survey results from more than 57,335 childcare providers from 28 states about their COVID status and other factors during April and May. About half of the respondents were working in person during that time and the other half were home because their programs had closed. This fifty–fifty split "was an essential condition that made the study possible," Gilliam told me. Employing a variety of methods, using matched and unmatched cohorts and controlling for relevant variables, the authors concluded: "Exposure to childcare during the early months of the US pandemic was not associated with an elevated risk for COVID-19 transmission to providers." Also of note is that 88 percent of the respondents who worked in person said their facilities did not have universal masking of the children.

Considering roughly half of the respondents said their facilities were closed during the study period of April and May, it's worth asking: How did those closures affect the families with parents or guardians who couldn't just "stay home to save lives," as public health campaigns ordered? More than 7 million American children under age six are in some form of professionally run childcare every week. Based on Gilliam's survey data, if roughly half the childcare programs were closed in the US during April and May what happened to all of those children? Surely, plenty of these children's parents worked outside the home. So with their childcare facility closed the children would have to be cared for by a relative or neighbor or as part of some other ad hoc arrangement while the parents continued to work, or the parents would have been compelled to stay home. This is the scenario Winsberg lamented—the modelers, and the authorities who ordered social distancing measures that resulted in mass closures of schools, daycares, and businesses based on the modelers' projections, did not factor in the second-order effects to people who were not like them. Did the parents whose jobs required on-site work yet whose childcare facilities were closed have to stay home and lose income or their employment entirely?

The closures of many professional childcare centers, coupled with the requirement for only certain types of workers to appear in person for their jobs, inequitably impacted millions of families. Moreover, as the portion of daycares that remained open showed, regardless of school closures, millions of children (and adults) were still physically interacting. How many of the children who continued to go to daycare had older siblings whose schools were of course closed? Prior to the pandemic more than 6 million children aged five and under were cared for by a relative each week. How many of those children continued that arrangement or were put into different external childcare after the social distancing orders? Beyond a couple weeks it was fantastical to think that a large segment of society—in particular, a portion of the more than 12 million kids under age six who pre-pandemic were in some form of nonparental care arrangement each week, in addition to millions of essential workers—was not going to continue to circulate and mix even with schools remaining closed. Still, it was apparent early on that daycares were not driving transmission; they merely reflected, or had lower transmission rates than what were in the community.

Gilliam's paper wasn't published until October, but one is left wondering why the CDC, other entities under the umbrella of NIH, or state health departments didn't conduct an analysis such as his. The various levels of government certainly had the resources to do so. By mid-May they could have had six weeks' worth of data, and after seeing the benign results in childcare centers governors could have allowed (or ordered) schools to reopen for the final four to six weeks of school. The answer is self-evident: Scientists (and governments) study what they feel is important. Acquiring daycare data, as Oster had done, and analyzing it, as Gilliam had done a short while later, simply wasn't of interest to the powers that be. As the Cuomo administration source indicated, opening schools simply wasn't seen as urgent. Discussing the possibility of opening them wasn't even on the governor's agenda.

* * *

The fiasco of the government's neglect to compile even basic data from daycares, and health officials' willful refusal to reckon with the basic findings Kamenetz and Oster reported, was of a piece with the authorities' overall approach.

For all the error in believing the models initially, it was the continued belief in the models *after* empirical evidence emerged that school closures were not impacting case rates in any significant or noticeable way that represented a true departure from science. There was no evidence that, whatever their differences from ours, open schools in Europe (and, later, in Florida and elsewhere in the US that reopened the following academic year) were different in ways that would yield meaningful differences in outcomes. Claims were repeatedly made about class size, or community rates, or testing, or HVAC systems, but were all based on conjecture. There were zero studies that showed any benefit on transmission of six feet of distancing versus three feet in a classroom, or the effect of using a HEPA filter versus opening a window in a classroom. Conjecture is not unreasonable in the absence of evidence. But it was a striking departure from evidence-based science that conjecture was valued *over* observable evidence to the contrary.

In the US, the burden of proof had inverted. The accepted position was that the daycare evidence and European evidence, when it was acknowledged at all, could casually be dismissed by making any claim one wanted about why that evidence wasn't applicable to US schools. The attitude was that any of these claims about HEPA filters or testing or what have you were true until proven wrong. Yet the government chose not to run any studies to verify whether these claims were true. It was a fait accompli.

To make matters worse, officials and health professionals openly acknowledged that they didn't know the exact benefits of any particular intervention. The public simply had to trust them that the measures, in some unquantifiable manner, were effective. This was the philosophy behind the so-called "Swiss cheese model," based on targeted layered containment cited in the playbooks, in which multiple interventions had to be implemented at once, precisely because it was not known which ones worked, if at all, and to what extent. The media, and in turn much of the public, readily bought in to the Swiss cheese model, with cartoon diagrams—depicting layers of Swiss, with green spiky virions absurdly enlarged to fit one-at-a-time in the holes—circulating online and featured in outlets like the *Times*. Yet there was no evidence this metaphor had any relation to reality. It's possible one slice is nearly solid, doing all of the work, and the rest of the slices are so riddled with holes that they are effectively useless, where even layering them does nothing to stop something—say, a microscopic virus—from sliding through. It's possible *none* of the slices make a difference. This is what happens when there is no burden of systematically identifying the effect, or lack thereof, of each intervention in proper randomized trials.

Ignoring or dismissing real world evidence, and insisting on requiring interventions where the benefit—if there was any at all—was unknown and the government refused to conduct tests to find out—was extremely important for three reasons. First, it kept many schools closed because public health authorities, politicians, and teachers unions—who, in part, based their demands on the claims made by public health authorities—pointed to things like a lack of HEPA filters as a reason schools weren't "safe" to reopen. Second, when schools eventually reopened, in large swaths of the country they only operated on so-called hybrid schedules, in which children could only attend part time in order for schools to comply with distancing guidelines that necessitated sparsely crowded classrooms. Lastly, children's experience in the buildings was profoundly degraded, with mandatory masking all day, plastic barriers placed around them on their desks, rules against any physical contact whatsoever, and even a prohibition against talking during meals. (Yes, many schools had mandatory silent lunches.) To be clear, *none* of these interventions had any high-quality empirical evidence behind them. Some of them may have intuitively seemed to be effective. Some may have had mechanical testing that showed an effect in a laboratory. But, as I've detailed extensively, what we think works, or what shows an effect in a lab, or what makes sense in theory, over and over again has proven to not be the same thing as an effect in the real world.

And it was not just health officials operating by this process but seemingly nearly the entire public health and medical establishment. From a local pediatrician posting on Facebook to an emergency medicine physician, to an epidemiologist with 50,000 Twitter followers who has zero expertise in infectious diseases, they *believed* this was the science because that is what the establishment—the CDC, Fauci, Birx—told them, not because they had read the relevant research themselves. In turn, the public was told over and over—from officials and workaday health professionals—that this was what "the science" said to do.

Believing in the effect of interventions—and imposing them on the citizenry—without scientific validation meant we were following a model of public health that was faith-based, as opposed to evidence-based. This was even more bizarre because with European schools and American daycares, where many or most of these interventions were not in place, we had copious evidence that if they offered any benefit at all, it was not meaningful. Decisions were guided not just by faith in the unknown, but faith against observable reality.

11

TECHNOLOGICAL SOLUTIONISM

Society in the middle of the last century was, of course, far less scientifically advanced than the 2020s. Superficially, then, it may seem strange that during a pandemic at that time the health establishment, in some regards, was far more sensible. But unlike the COVID crisis—when so much empirical and observational evidence was dismissed, and an ethos of unearned certainty around the wisdom of interventions prevailed— officials and administrators sixty-odd years earlier had a better grasp of the limitations of NPIs.

In February 1957, a new influenza strain, known as H2N2, emerged in China. By June of that year it had spread around the world. The 1957–1958 pandemic of Asian influenza ultimately infected approximately 25 percent of the population.

There are several comparisons to draw in relation to schools from the response in 1957–1958 to the COVID pandemic. The first is that in 1957–1958 closing schools and limiting public gatherings were expressly not recommended as strategies to mitigate the pandemic's impact. The Association of State and Territorial Health Officials wrote at the time, "there is no practical advantage in the closing of schools or the curtailment of public gatherings as it relates to the spread of this disease." Similarly, the health commissioner of Nassau County on Long Island, New York, said public schools should stay open even in an epidemic. "Children would get sick just as easily out of school," he said in a 1957 interview.

These official guidelines to keep schools open, of course, stand in stark contrast to what happened in the COVID pandemic. But they're especially salient because, unlike with COVID, children were much more likely to develop symptomatic or severe disease from the Asian flu. By the fall it was estimated that more than 60 percent of students had clinical illness. "The outbreaks were so explosive that the evidence of an epidemic in progress in a county was quickly apparent by school absenteeism," noted a detailed analysis of the public health response to the pandemic by D. A. Henderson, Jennifer Nuzzo, and coauthors, in a 2009 paper.

Reading through several October 1957 *New York Times* articles the numbers of sick children are astounding. In New York City, on October 7, more than 280,000 students were out sick, 29 percent of total enrollment; in Manhattan, the rate reached 43 percent. On October 1, in Passaic High School in New Jersey, 536 out of 1,300 total students were out sick. A few miles east, across the Passaic River, in Garfield High School, 415 students out of 1,695, were absent. In Dobbs Ferry, New York, in Westchester County, about twenty miles north of Midtown Manhattan, 98 cases were reported, out of 300 total students in a residential school.

Yet the schools remained open.

In fact, the only time schools were closed was when there were too many teachers absent for the school to run properly. Similarly, high school football games were only canceled if there were too many sick players.

Compare this to COVID and children—around 40 percent of those infected had no symptoms at all, and, with rare exception, the remainder of kids who were infected had mild illness. During the COVID pandemic—when confronted with a virus that was so benign to almost all kids that nearly half of them didn't even know when they were infected (were it not for a test)—many schools were preemptively closed, and athletics seasons canceled, *for more than a year,* in part to "protect" children.

All of this illustrates a fundamental difference in how we view risk and conduct society today versus six decades ago. There used to be an acceptance that part of life entails coming down with a flu-like illness periodically, and that, other than perhaps for a brief window of time, closing schools wasn't going to affect that one way or the other. (This isn't a call to blindly harken back to the past and all of its unsafe practices. We're better off with seatbelt laws, among countless other changes. But it's instructive to compare how society back then versus today was far more measured in how it handled a risk to children from a virus that was known to be unpleasant but, in all likelihood, not dangerous.)

*   *   *

Despite the lockdown example from China, despite the models, the media, and the retreat from evidence, there was one overarching determinant, more than any other, that allowed for and encouraged the closures. And, in part, this determinant, which was absent years ago, explains why 1957 played out as it did, in contrast to 2020 and 2021.

On May 5, 2020, while children across the country were grinding through the end of their second month of remote learning (and millions of children in Europe had been returning to class), New York governor Andrew Cuomo gave a press conference, as he had done every day since the beginning of the pandemic—much to the delight of the legacy media and professional class. He wore a dark navy suit with a crimson tie and crisp white shirt. He sat erect. His tie had a perfect knot, and hung perfectly centered. The lines of his jacket's lapels formed a tight V down his torso and angled at the top to shoulder pads that jutted stiffly outward like the wing serifs in the Van Halen logo. Backdropped by the flags of the United States and New York on either side of him, Cuomo's figure and the video's frame were a cinematic display of geometry and symmetry. With his usual Powerpoint slides accompanying him, Cuomo cited cases and hospitalizations and deaths in his usual no-nonsense tone. This daily performance earned him an Emmy Award for his "masterful use of television to inform and calm people around the world."

A little past eight minutes into the briefing, Cuomo shifted from his general comments to focus on education. It was here where he laid out his vision for the future. The presentation also explains why my source within the administration said reopening schools that spring was never considered. The words "Reimagine Education" appeared on a slide as he delivered his remarks: "The old model of everybody goes and sits in a classroom and the teacher is in front of that classroom and teaches that class and you do that all across the city, all across the state, all these buildings, all these physical classrooms. Why? With all the technology you have?"

Here was America's governor, the Emmy Award winner, the man who had steadied the ship, now telling the country, the world even, that remote learning, the scourge of millions of children and embittered parents, was actually quite excellent. So excellent that actual classrooms with people? That was old-timey school. Remote learning—this was the vanguard.

"It's not just about reopening schools, let's open a better school," Cuomo said. He announced that the state would be working with the Bill and Melinda Gates Foundation on the project. Cuomo called Bill Gates a visionary and said Gates's ideas and thoughts on technology and education had been spoken about for years. "We have a moment in history where we can advance those ideas. When does change come to a society? You get moments in history where people say 'I'm ready for change.' This is one of those moments. Let's start talking about revolutionizing education."

The next day, Cuomo upped the ante and announced that Eric Schmidt, Google's former CEO and executive chairman, would lead a fifteen-member commission to improve New York's use of "advanced technological tools." Naturally, Schmidt included remote learning among his first priorities. The journalist and activist Naomi Klein referred to the plans as the "screen new deal," in which the months of isolation, she wrote derisively, were "a living laboratory for a permanent—and highly profitable—no-touch future."

None of this should have been a surprise. The critical part about the laptop class comprising the people who designed the models, crafted the pandemic guidance, and backed the policies to enforce interventions, including school closures, is that they had . . . laptops. The communications technologies that allowed white collar professionals to work from home were sold to the public by those same professionals as an acceptable substitute for school.

It is a counterfactual—but one supported by the last hundred years of evidence, given that past epidemics did not lead to societal shutdowns or school closures on the order seen in the COVID pandemic—that if the pandemic had struck just ten or fifteen years earlier, if there were closures at all, in short order most professionals would have resumed going to work and children would have resumed school because there would have been no capability for anything resembling the remote work and remote school that instantly took over in 2020. In short, nearly the entire COVID pandemic response only happened because technology enabled it to happen.

As late as 2010, a mere decade before the start of the pandemic, just 60 percent of American adults even had broadband in their homes. In 2005, it was only 29 percent. Without broadband there's no Zoom, Google Meet, Microsoft Teams, and the rest of the video conferencing apps. Nor was there sufficient adoption of smartphones or the infrastructure to handle mass use of live video on the cellular network. And connectivity aside, there weren't any mainstream video conferencing apps at the time that would have worked for the masses. For example, though Skype began in 2003, it originally was only for voice calls over the internet, and when video was introduced later it was primitive.

While some remote schooling can be conducted by a teacher assigning work via email, "synchronous" learning, a euphemism for live instruction, which was the foundation of many remote learning programs, relied on video conferencing. And the school districts that only offered asynchronous instruction—where there was no real-time interaction between students and their teacher—still were largely dependent on platforms like Google Classroom, which began in a rudimentary form in 2014, to organize work by subjects, allow teachers to share assignments, and allow students to submit completed work. In just a few short years, though, the tools advanced rapidly.

The state of technology in spring of 2020 gave politicians and public health officials a society-altering lever. They put their hands on it, squeezed tight, and pulled.

In some ways, the health officials, so eager to take advantage of these new technologies to enable the imposition of wide-scale interventions, were simply the inadvertent accomplices to a bigger project that predated them. While the lockdowns and subsequent work- and school-from-home were a vast experiment, the ground had been laid for remote learning, and, more broadly, injecting of technological tools into American schooling for a long time. In some ways the school closures were simply the culmination of plans that were in the works for decades. It was as if, in the eyes of some, the pandemic had allowed the school system to actualize itself to its ideal form.

Toward the end of March, the official social distancing plans so nascent that society was still enduring its initial fifteen days to slow the spread, Schmidt published an editorial in the *Wall Street Journal* in which he outlined his aspirations for America. We should be thinking not just about how to use technology during the pandemic, he wrote, but how we'd use it once the crisis had passed. This included accelerating "the trend toward remote learning." In this bright future, there would be "no requirement of proximity." Schmidt advocated for making network connectivity more affordable and widely available, surely an admirable aim toward equity. What Cuomo, Gates, Schmidt, and the rest took as a given was that in the post-pandemic world more technology in the schools—or instead of schools—was an inherent good.

In my late twenties, I was having a football catch one day. As I threw a beautiful, arcing twenty-yard pass I felt a lightning bolt run through my arm. In the days after, any time I extended my arm quickly a knife tried to debone my triceps. I saw a top orthopedist, a clinician trained in the latest surgical techniques who treated players on the New York Jets, among other professional athletes, and he ordered an MRI. When we discussed the results he said I had a labral tear, and that if I wanted improvement I would need surgery, which he could perform. "You can see Maria at the front desk to get started on scheduling and paperwork," he said blithely while walking out of the exam room. I decided to wait a few months and did nothing. The injury—whatever it was—eventually went away on its own.

If you have back pain a surgeon is inclined to tell you an operation will solve your problem, a chiropractor will say you need an adjustment, an acupuncturist will suggest acupuncture, and an herbalist will prescribe herbs. When you bring in technologists—in particular those who became billionaires selling technological products—to oversee your state's education plans, you can predict that their blueprint is going to include more technology.

Schmidt said remote learning was a "massive experiment," and that with data acquired from the experiment we could build better distance-learning tools. That likely is true. And yet it missed a larger lesson that the Marshall McLuhan adage captures well—the medium is the message. With a sore back—or in my case, arm—instead of an advanced surgical procedure the best treatment was some ibuprofen and taking it easy for a few months. Maybe making better distance-learning tools was beside the point. Perhaps the remedy to the deficits of remote learning was not more sophisticated remote learning, but teachers in person with their students.

The championing of what's known as edutech of course is not limited to remote connectivity. In many districts it permeates nearly every aspect of a public school student's experience. Reminiscent of the study I referred to earlier on pediatric screen use, which found that even after school closures had largely ended screen use remained elevated, the schools that began using all sorts of apps and software programs in remote learning have retained much of these tools as part of their regular instruction. I know in my own children's district this certainly has been the case. Amazed at the amount of edutech programs the kids were using on a regular basis, a fellow parent in town joked to me that it was only a matter of time before the high school football team would be playing at Zearn Math Field and students would be dining in the Google Classroom Café.

Schmidt and Gates and Cuomo did not seem to entertain the idea that perhaps *less* technology in schools might be preferable. Their view was not unusual, however. It matched a long-term fetishization of injecting technology into American schools. And this widely held ethos not just validated but actively cheered the notion that closing schools and sending sixty million children and adolescents into remote learning was an amazing opportunity. Sure, lip service was paid to the importance of in-person schooling, but remote learning was positioned as a fully viable and acceptable long-term plan.

How did we get to a point where, among politicians and many citizens, there was an unquestioning embrace of remote learning?

One place to start, according to Katie Day Good, a communications scholar at Miami University whose research focuses on technology use in education, is the Cold War. In 1957 the Soviet Union launched Sputnik, and American lawmakers panicked, Good told me. Until that moment, Americans had felt superior technologically. Now our legislators worried we were behind the Russians, and the only way to catch and surpass them was to produce more scientists and engineers. The National Defense Education Act passed, and a mass program of federal student loans, primarily aimed at promoting the study of science and math, began. But this represented more of an anxiety about a lack of tech-minded education.

To see the origins of the infusion of electronic tech in education we need to take a longer view, and look back to the 1910s and 1920s. At the time, Good explained, there was a push for students to be prepared to enter the newly technologized work environment. The school system was swelling and becoming bureaucratized. Schools, formerly one-room schoolhouses, were becoming huge buildings, which were seen as the crown jewel of progressive infrastructure, she said. A national competitiveness began to take hold, and bringing the right materials into the classroom was seen as a way to gain an edge.

Americans tend to care about the industries and products that are made in the US. It's part of the national psyche. In the early part of the twentieth century, Good explained, captains of industry, especially from the media and communications technology industries like radio, television, books, and magazines, began to make overtures to education leaders, who were eager to listen. The motion picture business had tried to get schools to buy projectors in the first decade or so of the 1900s, an effort that was largely rebuffed. But after World War I, the power of this new medium was undeniable. In generations past, the offspring of the wealthy had a rite of passage known as the Grand Tour, during which they traveled around Europe and educated themselves about the outside world. Now, there was the idea that, for the first time, you could bring the world to an average student, Good said. With technology as the vehicle, this was how you made a child aware of what was happening outside our borders and brought them information that was formerly only accessible in great libraries or institutions.

Enter Thomas Edison, who was seen as a towering figure of American culture, and science and business, the man at the vanguard to lead the country into the future—and he was deeply invested in how our education system should operate. In 1922 Edison said, "I believe that the motion picture is destined to revolutionize our educational system." The following year he said the movie screen would replace the blackboard and the motion picture film would take the place of textbooks. Film, he said, made it possible to touch every branch of human knowledge. If Americans wanted to succeed, if individual schools and the students within them wanted to succeed, this new technology was the path to get there.

Then something interesting happened. A man named Harry Arthur Wise was skeptical of Edison's claims. "Like many new educative devices," Wise wrote, in a critical 1939 book, "the motion picture was received into the school with a confidence and an enthusiasm not well founded." Wise wasn't simply pontificating. He had reviewed the results of seven studies on teaching with film, and conducted his own study. Wise warned teachers to not abandon their normal routines in an effort to cater to this high-tech device, Todd Oppenheimer recounted in his 2004 book, *The Flickering Mind*, on the failure of technology to improve our schools.

In the next decade, there was a new technology to get excited about and, yet again, for confident claims to be made about its use in education. Oppenheimer introduces us to William Levenson, the director of the Cleveland public schools' radio station, who said "the time may come when a portable radio receiver will be as common in the classroom as is the blackboard." He said radio instruction would be fully integrated into school life as a new educational medium.

And, predictably, a couple decades later in the 1960s, yet another technology was touted as necessary for an effective education. This time, Oppenheimer wrote, it was television, and it was championed by the president, Lyndon Johnson. In 1964, a project in American Samoa, at the time still using one-room schoolhouses, was undertaken to teach the children there through televised instruction. A decade later it was deemed a bust. No matter. By the early 1970s more than 100 million dollars from the federal government and private philanthropy, including the Ford Foundation, were funneled into televised learning.

The pattern reliably keeps repeating. Oppenheimer's history recounts when, in the 1990s, Bill Clinton said that the bridge to the twenty-first century would be one where "computers are as much a part of the classroom as blackboards." In 2002, the director of education under George W. Bush talked about the forthcoming advantages of computers personalizing education. And so on. Each time promises were made, each time we were told more money was needed. And the promises rarely panned out.

Echoes of Edison's and the others' pronouncements over the decades, of course, can be heard in the bluster from the tech titans of today assuring us they have the magic answer for improving education.

The cycle of the tech industry always promising something anew for schools, and education leaders and politicians as the eager marks, is an important pattern to recognize. It shows us that the pitch for remote learning, and its welcome reception by so many people, was but the latest chapter in a predictable story. For a century, industry pioneers, politicians, and some willing education leaders in the US have marketed the idea of technology as a substitute for experience. This was the way poor children could travel the world—through film or other media.

Yet the notion of "experience" mediated through technology has always been at odds with the educational doctrine of the importance of firsthand experience. "Something that worries me," Katie Day Good, the scholar of communications technology in schools, said, "is that teachers have long been the most skeptical of tech, and defenders of first-hand learning." You can go back to John Dewey when thinking about this. "But during the pandemic," she said, "well, well, well, teachers sang a different tune. There was all this talk about how kids could thrive with remote learning."

One final, critical point is that the word technology generally has the connotation today of a device or service that's electronic. Yet any tool is a technology. A pencil is a technology. And, according to Good, the public school building itself is the most important educational technology. It is publicly owned and operated. Silicon Valley products are not. Remote learning, the latest manifestation in a long line of ever-newer electronic technologies, was valued over the foundational technology of school as a physical place—the former sets us apart, the latter brings us together.

The policy makers and others advocating for remote learning should have known that a screen was never going to actually substitute for the academic and, perhaps more importantly, human connection that happens when students are together, in person.

The evidence base for any benefits at all from digital tools before the pandemic was "equivocal at best," wrote Natalie Wexler, in the *MIT Technology Review*. A study of millions of high school students in the thirty-six member countries of the Organization for Economic Co-operation and Development (OECD) found that those who used computers heavily at school "do a lot worse in most learning outcomes, even after accounting for social background and student demographics." Further, the OECD found that "technology is of little help in bridging the skills divide between advantaged and disadvantaged students." Studies have shown that students who use digital devices in class do worse on exams. Wexler also reported on a study that found that eighth graders who took Algebra I online did much worse than those who took the course in person. And on and on.

What exactly did the education community think was going to happen with the "pivot to remote," as it was often termed? And what exactly did

Cuomo, Gates, and Schmidt think was going to happen with their attempt to integrate yet more digital tools into education following the pandemic?

Lest anyone think this is a partisan affliction, Jeb Bush, the former Republican governor of Florida, penned a *Washington Post* opinion piece in May 2020, just a few days before Cuomo's press conference, titled "It's Time to Embrace Distance Learning—and Not Just Because of the Coronavirus." Bush said longer term "all K–12 schools need to adapt to distance learning." Why? "The $200-billion-plus market for corporate learning is exploding with content libraries, assessment tools, workflow learning and 'micro-learning.' Learning is no longer modeled on the traditional classroom," he wrote, "but has become digital, individualized and delivered on smartphones or laptops." Bush said some might push back against this but the "benefits are clear." Are they? And benefits to whom? Bush is now the chairman of Excel*in*Ed, a nonprofit that supports "transforming" education.

Throughout our history there seems to be a never-ending attraction to new technological tools in education. Education professionals and politicians seem to be particularly vulnerable to their siren song. The promise of the *new* exotic thing is somehow always enticing, despite the garbage heap of evidence that the promise is usually a lie.

Immediately, in the spring of 2020, the evidence of what was or should have been expected was readily, painfully apparent. Even preliminary research from the spring showed severe learning gaps. A remarkable study of the effect of the spring closures in the Netherlands is alarming in its clarity. "The Netherlands," the authors of the study, which was published in the *Proceedings of the National Academy of Sciences* journal, wrote, "is interesting as a 'best-case' scenario, with a short lockdown, equitable school funding, and world-leading rates of broadband access." Despite all of these favorable conditions remote learning there was a total bust.

The authors looked at data from 350,000 students and used the fact that national examinations took place before and after lockdown, then compared progress during this period to the same period in the three previous years. The authors found that the learning loss was equivalent to the exact amount of time that schools were closed. The kids learned nothing.

Granted, this was just one study. And most kids over the long haul of remote schooling did learn at least some material. But, as I will show later in the book, directionally, its bracing results are not an anomaly.

Beyond hard data were the endless anecdotal and personal experiences that made obvious to parents and kids all they needed to know. For an enormous number of students, "distance learning" had proven to be a farcical misnomer. Blunt headlines, such as "The Results Are In for Remote Learning: It Didn't Work," from the *Wall Street Journal*, topped articles laden with anecdotes of frustrated children, and quotes from psychologists and education experts attesting to the varied ills of trying to learn through a computer.

In a Sunday *New York Times* piece at the end of April 2020 called "Why Zoom Is Terrible," the writer Kate Murphy quoted an information technology professor who said, "In-person communication resembles video conferencing about as much as a real blueberry muffin resembles a packaged blueberry muffin that contains not a single blueberry but artificial flavors, textures and preservatives." Murphy wrote about the peculiar fatigue that many people were reporting they experienced after spending long hours on video conferences. "The problem is that the way the video images are digitally encoded and decoded, altered and adjusted, patched and synthesized introduces all kinds of artifacts: blocking, freezing, blurring, jerkiness and out-of-sync audio," Murphy wrote. "These disruptions, some below our conscious awareness, confound perception and scramble subtle social cues. Our brains strain to fill in the gaps and make sense of the disorder, which makes us feel vaguely disturbed, uneasy and tired without quite knowing why."

Humans are superbly skilled at detecting the most minute body language and facial muscle changes. Those granular details get lost in the digital compression that occurs over the internet, not to mention the noticeable glitches, buffering, and pixelation. The audio quality, similarly, often leads participants to miss intonations in people's voices that convey something important beyond the words being said. To use another food metaphor, video conferencing, at limited times, can give you the basic information you need in the way a protein powder can give you the amino acids you need. But without real food—the spices and fiber and natural sugars and compounds and textures—you don't get the all the nutrition you need or the basic pleasure from eating we crave. As realistic as video is, it is merely a simulacrum of physical connection. It should go without saying, and without the need for any studies or data, that being in physical space with other humans is superior to connecting through some form of media. It's an empirical, experienced reality of all people, except the rare few recluses who genuinely are averse to human interaction.

This lack of nutrition and pleasure was equally as bad, if not worse, with so-called asynchronous instruction for kids, where there was no live interaction with another human at all, and instead lessons were delivered via prerecorded videos, animated apps, and solitary assignments.

In the summer of 2020, a meme surfaced on Reddit that captured what was obvious to millions of parents. A child, who looks like she just rolled out of bed, with tousled hair, her small head just barely above the desk, has a look somewhere between blankness and confusion and sadness as she stares at a screen.

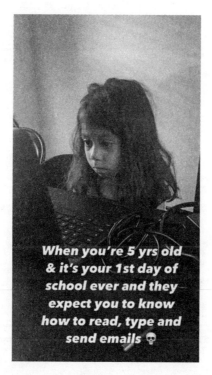

Social media meme of little girl bewildered by remote learning. Source: Reddit.

TRIBALISM, PUBLIC HEALTH, THE ELITE, AND THE MEDIA
JUNE THROUGH AUGUST 2020

12

IF TRUMP IS FOR IT, THEN WE'RE AGAINST IT

On June 24, in the second piece I wrote for *Wired*, on the proposed in-school mitigations, I cited the meeting of the EU education ministers as the lede. It was more than a month after the meeting had occurred, but, dismayingly, it was still a scoop. (The ministers met again, near the end of June, some two months after many schools had reopened there, and announced the same conclusion as they did in May. Presiding over both meetings, Blaženka Divjak, a Croatian mathematics professor, who served as the rotating chair of the council, in lightly accented English caveated that many countries had predominantly opened only their primary grades to varying degrees. Still, she said there was "no indication that reopening furthered the spread of COVID-19.") The conclusions from neither the first nor second meeting were covered in the *New York Times*, the *Washington Post*, NBC, CBS, ABC, CNN, the *New Yorker*, the *Atlantic*, or anywhere else in the US media as far as I could tell. Dismissing Sweden's schools as an outlier, while not necessarily an epidemiologically sound argument, was one thing. But this was twenty-two countries.

It's hard to convey the sense of unreality I felt at the time, witnessing this blackout on what was beyond question extremely relevant information. I was a freelancer, a bit of a generalist but with a focus on science, culture, and psychology. I had never covered the education beat, and, like nearly everyone else, I had never covered a pandemic. Surely staff writers at major media outlets, with the resources of a newsroom and multiple tiers of editors, could have dug for the videos of the meetings and emailed with a press officer at the EU as I had. Few journalists seemed to know or care about the statements from the EU. This made no sense since school closures, and the heated discussion about schools' supposed lack of safety and children as viral vectors, was one of the most important stories in the country (or at least should have been).

The conclusions in both the May and June meetings were easy to miss in the videos. There were no trumpets blaring. There wasn't a Powerpoint slide with graphics or bullet points. The statements were mentioned alongside various other comments about trying to improve remote learning, and obligatory remarks about turning a crisis into an opportunity. The statements weren't quite buried, but the absence of emphasis seemed to imply that the observations about schools not raising case rates were simply accepted as a noncontroversial matter of fact.

I noticed after my second *Wired* piece that, while the general tide was still against its premise warning of excessive measures imposed on children that lacked evidence and carried costs, it gained a few more mainstream voices of support relative to my first piece. Immediately after it was published, for example, I noticed that some prominent editorial writers and journalists at major news outlets began following me on Twitter. Then, five days after publication Michelle Goldberg, a widely read opinion writer for the *Times*, published a piece titled "Remote School Is a Nightmare. Few in Power Care." Goldberg focused on the frustrations of parents, who at that point had no information about whether and under what conditions schools would open in the fall, though it was all but certain for much of the country that if they opened it would be in a hybrid model. Goldberg cited my *Wired* piece and its evidence about European schools, and Kamenetz's NPR piece on the YMCAs. But other than that, the column did not question the narrative about schools being unsafe. Rather, via an interview with Randi Weingarten, the head of the American Federation of Teachers, the second-largest teachers union in the country, it took it as a given that, as Weingarten warned, if schools didn't get $100 billion to open "safely," schools might not open at all. The incongruity between printing Weingarten's claim and citing evidence from Europe and daycares, where no such infusion of money happened, was not addressed. Still, an influential voice at the most influential media outlet in the country was openly talking about downsides of school closures (even if assumptions about the necessity and wisdom of proposed safety measures went unchallenged).

A few days after Goldberg's piece, Jennifer Nuzzo and Dr. Joshua Sharf-stein, a pediatrician, coauthored an editorial in the *Times* in which they were critical of states that had opened many aspects of society, from bars to gyms to restaurants, while schools remained closed. They ticked off a number of harms from the spring school closures, including an inter-ruption of in-school meal programs, increased child abuse, widening of racial and economic divides, and learning loss, and they cited Austria, Germany, Denmark, and Norway as successful examples of countries where schools reopened, with various mitigations in place. Nuzzo and Sharfstein's piece popularized the meme #schoolsbeforebars, succinctly highlighting the corrosive fatuity of the situation. "Deciding whether to reopen schools is not only a question of benefits versus risks," they wrote, "but also a matter of priorities."

If we as a society were so concerned about the spread of SARS-CoV-2, why were bars and restaurants open? It didn't make sense epidemiologi-cally for schools to be closed while these other aspects of society, patron-ized by people at far higher risk than children, were open. And since epidemiologically it didn't make sense, that raised the question of our cultural values. I had asked my source with knowledge of the Cuomo administration a series of questions about how they weighed the evi-dence about the risks associated with opening schools—what metrics did they use, how did they arrive at the benchmarks, what data were they gathering, and so forth. But the person's answer, that opening schools simply wasn't on the agenda at all that spring, showed I shouldn't have been asking a series of questions of "how," but, rather, I merely should have asked one question: *if* they discussed opening schools, period.

Around the same time as my *Wired* piece, and Nuzzo and Goldberg's editorials, the American Academy of Pediatrics released guidance that argued forcefully and unambiguously for opening schools. "All policy considerations for the coming school year should start with a goal of having students physically present in school," the guidance stated. "The importance of in-person learning is well-documented, and there is already evidence of the negative impacts on children because of school closures in the spring of 2020," the guidance continued, saying that school clo-sures made it harder to identify and address sexual abuse, physical abuse, substance abuse, and depression. Beyond the educational and social impacts, the academy wrote, the spring closures impacted food insecurity and negatively affected children's physical activity. Notably, the guidance highlighted the particular harms of school closures on children with special needs and those from underprivileged backgrounds. People were asked to reflect on the impacts to "different races, ethnic and vulnerable populations."

The AAP guidance parted ways from the CDC's in that it said being as close as three feet was acceptable, as opposed to the CDC's six-foot recommendation. In an interview shortly after the guidance was released, Dr. Sean O'Leary, one of the AAP authors, elaborated: "The downsides of having kids at home versus in school are outweighed by the small incremental gain you would get from having kids six feet apart as opposed to five, four or three." The CDC's guidance didn't quite say students *couldn't* be closer than six feet; rather, it said students should distance six feet "when feasible." This type of language, using vague phrases like "when feasible," was a hallmark of the CDC guidelines throughout the pandemic. The wording left state health departments, which were issuing policy, and school districts, which were tasked with following state or CDC guidance, uncertain about interpretation of this language and uncertain about implementation. What is or is not "feasible," is, of course, highly subjective. The AAP's clarity was a welcome relief. However, as a private organization, its guidance did not carry the political weight of the CDC's, which was the default.

The academy also suggested that temperature checks were likely an ineffective screening tool, and O'Leary said MIS-C was rare and that nearly all children who developed the syndrome recovered. "So much of our world relies on kids being in school and parents being able to work," O'Leary said as a summation. The AAP's guidance, and subsequent related interviews and news coverage, threw a bit of cold water on the panic about schools and children, and its flexible approach to metrics, such as distancing requirements, made plain the priority was getting kids into school.

The prevailing narrative still emphasized risks to children and the notion of kids as viral vectors endangering society, implying that open schools were a menace. Schools throughout the country had been shut down for months, a radically ahistorical event. Yet until then questioning the presumed net benefit of school closures on reducing transmission was virtually nonexistent in mainstream media outlets and the public conversation. The AAP's guidance and columns like Goldberg's indicated a new appetite for allowing that, whatever the presumed benefits, closures carried harms, too, which should be considered. More than three months after schools had closed, and nearly two months after my first *Wired* piece was largely ignored, an actual discussion in the public arena, of the kind that Winsberg, Harvard, and others suggested should have occurred far earlier, perhaps at the base level of the models themselves, was beginning to take place. Unlike during the spring, it was ever so slightly becoming acceptable for a closed school to no longer be seen exclusively as a precautionary act.

Then, on July 6, President Trump tweeted the following: "SCHOOLS MUST OPEN IN THE FALL!!!" The president's view on keeping as much of society running as possible, including schools, was no secret. But once overall lockdowns became a foregone conclusion he was initially loosely supportive, tweeting on March 17 that we "MUST #FlattenTheCurve of the spread of coronavirus. Social distancing, closing schools, limiting non-essential businesses. . . ." Prior to his declaration on July 6, Trump tweeted only one other time about schools after the March tweet. On May 24, he wrote: "Schools in our country should be opened ASAP. Very good information now available." The lone tweet about opening schools in the three and a half months following the "flatten the curve" tweet is significant because Trump cranked out an astonishing 3,784 tweets during that time frame. So July 6, with its all caps and triple exclamation points, hit like a thunderclap. From then until the end of August the storm raged, with Trump tweeting about opening schools seventeen more times. On July 8: "In Germany, Denmark, Norway, Sweden and many other countries, SCHOOLS ARE OPEN WITH NO PROBLEMS. The Dems think it would be bad for them politically if U.S. schools open before the November Election, but is important for the children & families. May cut off funding if not open!" On July 10: "Now that we have witnessed it on a large scale basis, and firsthand, Virtual Learning has proven to be TERRIBLE compared to In School, or On Campus, Learning. Not even close! Schools must be open in the Fall. If not open, why would the Federal Government give Funding? It won't!!!" He goaded at-the-time candidate Biden by name in several of the tweets, saying he and Democrats didn't want to open schools in the fall for political reasons. He mentioned that "top pediatricians" and scientific evidence supported the opening of schools, and that teachers unions were an obstacle. For good measure, on August 3, Trump reprised the tweet that launched the offensive: "OPEN THE SCHOOLS!!!" The official White House Twitter account also contained a series of pro–open schools messages, including multiple video clips of an event with Betsy DeVos, Trump's education secretary, and a clip of Dr. Scott Atlas, an adviser on the Coronavirus Task Force, saying the "president's priority is to open the schools." Both Atlas and DeVos were widely reviled by Left.

Anyone involved in decision making around schools was now, to no small extent, going to be seen through the binary lens of either with Trump or against Trump that had already been fixed on much of public and political life in America for the past three and a half years. Whatever momentum that began to build from the op-eds and experts arguing for kids to be back in school immediately met an indomitable headwind. The notion of opening schools was now seen as explicitly part of Trump's "open everything up" campaign, and in the process became radioactive to many liberals and much of the intelligentsia. This was a demonstrably obvious fact of the political and social reality of the Trump presidency, which was hated and feared with such breadth and intensity that the day after his inauguration it spawned what was reported to be the largest single-day protest in American history. The Left and much of the cosmopolitan elite in America saw Trump as so clownish, ignorant, malignant, and harmful to society that, with rare exception, it was anathema for a Democratic politician or official, or journalist or news organization (other than conservative outlets), to ever be seen as agreeing with him on anything. This dynamic was no less ingrained in much of the professional and influencer classes in publishing, technology, entertainment, medicine, academia, and polite society in blue state America.

His brief endorsement of flattening the curve notwithstanding, Trump's initial denials about the dangers of the virus, and his constant calls for the economy to reopen framed the debate about the pandemic response in many people's eyes in moralistic terms, as one between those who cared about money versus those who cared about people's well-being. (Sample headlines: "Trump Cares More About the Stock Market Than Humans,"

Washington Post, March 23; "Trump Mostly Focuses on Economy, Rather Than Health," CNN, May 21; "Trump's Choice: The Economy or Human Lives," *US News*, March 24. And so on. This narrative extended to Republicans in general: "Georgia's Experiment in Human Sacrifice," read the title of an *Atlantic* article from April 29, 2020, as the state was relaxing some restrictions, warning readers, that "the state is about to find out how many people need to lose their lives to shore up the economy.") It was an absurd false binary. Yes, it could be argued that demanding the right to a haircut in March of 2020 was a morally obtuse position. But much of the objections to enforced NPIs were rooted in legitimate fears over very real harms. As Winsberg and many others explained, shutting down vast sectors of society carried wildly divergent costs for different people. The ability to stay home without incurring significant repercussions—a loss of income or, worse, the shuttering of one's business; a child with special needs incapable of functioning alone on a computer all day—which, in short order, for many folks could easily prove worse than the virus itself, was largely limited to a certain class of people. Nevertheless, much of the pandemic policies were seen by liberals and portrayed by the media through this cleft frame—open, closed; risky, cautious; bad, virtuous.

In part because of Trump's boorishness, delusional statements (e.g., his repeated claim that the virus would just "go away"), and frequent infidelity to facts many on the Left, along with plenty of political centrists, seemingly were compelled to feel, and demonstrate, that every single idea, even ones they otherwise might favor, that emanated from the president must be resisted. In 2018, for example, when Trump announced plans to withdraw troops from Syria and Afghanistan, many Democrats, including Nancy Pelosi, the House minority leader at the time, among other prominent Congress members, and the *Times* editorial board, criticized the decision, even though before Trump's announcement they had long expressed misgivings about keeping American troops in the region before Trump took office. When the COVID vaccine development was fast-tracked under Trump as Operation Warp Speed numerous high-profile Democrats, including then–vice presidential candidate Kamala Harris, cast doubt on whether they would take it after it was approved. Once Biden came into office, however, Democrats immediately began championing the very same forthcoming vaccines.

Hypocrisy among politicians from both parties of course is nothing new, and these are complex issues with granular details to be debated. But Trump's combativeness and lack of nuance was monumental, and typically elicited not only a reactive posture by Democratic politicians, but an automatic recoil from liberals in general, no matter the topic or message. It was Newtonian physics played out in a psychosocial context: any stance taken by Trump was going to be met with an equal and opposite stance. Thus, it was inevitable that Trump's position on schools would be opposed, vigorously.

Even those on the Right recognized the problem. "I thought it was really good and useful to have someone with a big megaphone make those arguments," about opening schools, said Rick Hess, the director of education policy at the American Enterprise Institute, a conservative think tank, in an August interview with the *Times*. "But," Hess added, "he made them in such a five-thumbed, unserious, reckless way. If you had told me that Trump was doing this as a favor to the schools-must-not-open crowd, I'd believe you."

A survey of Chicago Teachers Union members saw a jump from around 50 percent to 80 percent, from June to August, of those who were "extremely uncomfortable" returning to the classroom. A survey of members of the American Federation of Teachers, the second-largest teachers union in the country, echoed the Chicago results. The change in attitudes reflected in the surveys cannot definitively nor should it exclusively be attributed to Trump, but comments by the president of the Chicago Teachers Union, Jesse Sharkey, are telling. Sharkey was quoted in the same *Times* piece saying that Trump's advocacy for opening schools, and his referencing of open schools in Scandinavia, where Sharkey said case rates were lower than in the US, undermined the credibility of a safe reopening of schools. He said it was against the science, and that "it didn't help" that Trump was the messenger. As the union president, Sharkey's view both mirrored and influenced those of many of his members. (A 2017 survey found that 68 percent of teachers said their unions represented some or a lot of their views.)

The California State Assembly's education committee chair similarly noted that Trump's advocacy for opening schools "changed the political calculus" in his state, according to the *Times*. "It's a political hot potato now," he said. In a July interview shortly after Trump's tweet, Randi Wein-garten, the head of the American Federation of Teachers, said Trump's "defiance of science has made it impossible to do what he wanted to do." The day after the "open the schools" tweet, Lily Eskelsen García, at the time the president of the National Education Association, the country's largest teachers union, said, "The reality is no one should listen to Donald Trump or Betsy DeVos when it comes to what is best for students." Then she added the obligatory closer: "Our number one priority is that we keep our students safe." In a separate interview she said, "He is saying, 'Sac-rifice your children, sacrifice their teachers, sacrifice their families that they could infect, because I need something to sell in November.'" Seth Meyers, the host of NBC's late night talk show, a format where many Americans get their news, posted a segment on July 13 titled, "Donald Trump Is the Last Person We Can Trust to Safely Reopen Schools." Cabi-net members also served as a proxy for Trump. Neera Tanden, at the time the president of the Center for American Progress, an influential liberal think tank, and later White House staff secretary under Biden, tweeted to her hundreds of thousands of followers numerous times that summer saying it was Trump's fault that kids were in remote learning. And in a tweet against Trump's secretary of education, on July 12 she wrote: "Who are the parents who actually believe Betsy DeVos is actually focused on the best interests of their children's health? Honestly, she makes me think we shouldn't send kids to school."

In short, Trump's advocacy for schools to open, ironically, made them less likely to open, simply because he was the one advocating for it. For Democratic politicians, members of the medical and public health fields, and those in the professional classes in general, regardless of their views on the matter, just the appearance of agreeing with Trump was enough to deter them from doing so.

*   *   *

But more often it wasn't optics, or at least not optics alone, that guided the opposition. Rather, as politicians, union bosses, and media coverage sampled above made explicit, the message was axiomatic: Trump want-ing schools to open meant that opening them was a bad idea. This was a man with a history of poor decisions and abhorrent behavior on related and unrelated matters; assuredly, he was wrong on schools, too. Of course Seth Meyers said Trump was the last person to trust on opening schools. Trump was the last person to trust on everything. Vague and unfalsifiable claims that Trump wasn't following "the science" on schools served not as their own argument, but as a justification for the axiom.

The problem with this type of reasoning is that it *feels* right, even though it's often wrong.

Deductive reasoning is a hallmark of human logic. Life presents us with certain information, and based on this information we can infer a conclusion. With deductive reasoning, as long as the original information is factual, it is impossible for the conclusion to not be true. All dogs are descended from wolves. A husky is a type of dog. Therefore, huskies are descended from wolves.

The type of reasoning applied to Trump, however, was not deductive. It was inductive. Unlike deduction, in which the conclusion is certain, with induction the conclusion is only probable. It's an assumption based on a pattern. In my childhood in suburban New Jersey all the squirrels I saw were gray. If someone had asked me what color all squirrels are, I would have answered, "All squirrels are gray." Except this is false. There is a sizable number of black squirrels, which I've seen as an adult, in New York State. (There are also red squirrels and plenty of variations between these colors.) Unlike deductive reasoning, conclusions from inductive reasoning are only probable, not certain, and can lead to false conclusions like a childhood assumption about all squirrels being gray.

David Hume, the influential eighteenth-century Scottish philosopher, warned about the inductive reasoning fallacy. Like two of our other heroes—John Locke, the seventeenth-century Enlightenment philosopher who counseled us to not rely merely on the opinions of experts but to seek evidence for ourselves, and James Lind, the Royal Navy physician who ran the proto-randomized trial for scurvy treatments—Hume was an empiricist. And a resolute one at that. He was fundamentally against assuming anything. Hume basically wrote the first draft of the modern financial services disclaimer, "Past performance does not guarantee future results." (Taken to an extreme, Hume's argument means you can never trust any amount of evidence for drawing a conclusion about the future, since you never know for certain if an observed pattern will change. Hume's induction problem has been discussed by philosophers in complex ways, but we need not get into that here. The core of Hume's empiricist philosophy, valuing experience and observation over speculation, serves as a lodestar against assumptions. The practice of evidence-based medicine, which launched in part from Hume's viewpoint, resolves his inductive reasoning problem to a large degree, though not entirely, with randomized trials, where if they are large enough and conducted well can give strong confidence in a statistical probability of future results.)

The politicians', union leaders' and others' inductive fallacy was: Trump is bad, therefore all of Trump's positions are bad, therefore his position on schools must be bad. The error of this thinking could be summed up as "Even a broken clock is right twice a day." While some, like the union leaders and others, openly argued that Trump had been wrong on many things before, therefore we could not trust him to be right on this, more people simply intuited this thought process and then post facto found or contrived an explanation to support this assumption. As quoted earlier, this often took the form of the false statement "The countries in Europe that Trump referenced could open their schools because, unlike us, they controlled the virus." This tendency is known as "confirmation bias," the seeking out and interpreting of evidence so that it supports one's prior beliefs.

The claim about European countries controlling the virus, and therefore having earned the privilege to open their schools, was fallacious for several reasons. First, there is no universal benchmark that defines "controlling the virus" as it relates to schools being able to open. Second, as I will detail later, innumerable American cities and towns had similar case rates to counterparts in Europe where schools opened. These details, however, *disconfirmed* people's bias, and so were ignored or dismissed.

13

POLITICS AND TRIBALISM

Just four days after Trump's thunderous tweet, the American Academy of Pediatrics (AAP) released a statement that was an about-face on the guidance it had issued only eleven days earlier. Now, instead of serving as an opposition to the CDC's highly restrictive guidance on schools that, if followed, would compel most of them to remain closed or only partially open, the Academy was in step with the CDC and the broader public health establishment's narrative. The AAP's guidance still expressed the "goal of children returning safely to school" and the value of being "physically present in the classroom." But its new statement seemed to contradict that goal by now adding instead that "science and community circumstances" should determine whether kids would return to school. Of course, "science and community circumstances" can mean anything that anyone wants it to mean. In effect, the new guidance allowed for any criteria named in the service of being "safe" to prevent schools from opening. The reversal was perceived as so overt that, among other outlets, NPR covered the story, titling its piece "Nation's Pediatricians Walk Back Support for In-Person School."

Without mentioning Trump, the AAP's new guidance statement seemed intended to directly address his tweets. The release said that "evidence, not politics" should drive decision-making, and that we should leave it up to the "experts" to tell us when to open schools. (In a strange bit of internal inconsistency, the statement also read that parents, educators and school leaders "must be at the center of decisions" on when to reopen. Were parents, school leaders, and educators now deemed "experts" on the "science"?) In another apparent nod to Trump, it read that "withholding funding" from schools that didn't open full-time would be a misguided approach. Instead—unlike the original document, which made no mention of money or lawmakers—the new AAP statement declared that reopening schools would "clearly require substantial new investments," and called for Congress and the White House to provide resources to schools so they could educate children safely. Its final paragraph noted that "educators are invaluable in children's lives."

The most dramatic parting of ways from the original AAP guidance, though, was not just the new text itself, but its authorship. The new guidance was released as a joint statement from the AAP with the American Federation of Teachers and the National Education Association, the two largest teachers unions in the country, and the School Superintendents Association. One need not resort to conspiracy theories or rely on an informant for insight into what led to the changes. The statement's coauthors were listed publicly.

From that point forward the messaging from the AAP and CDC, along with the American Medical Association, American Academy of Family Physicians, and a long list of other American public health and medical organizations remained in relative lockstep on schools, masks, and pediatric vaccines, despite the fact that each of these issues were being handled very differently by public health agencies in much of Europe. (More on this in endnotes.)

Against this backdrop a strange phenomenon had been occurring for me. Starting with my first *Wired* piece, my inbox began receiving a steady beat of emails from doctors—a pediatric immunologist at an Ivy League university hospital, the editor in chief of a leading pediatric medical journal, the head of pediatrics at a major hospital chain, among many rank and file physicians—and nonmedical people as well. Nearly all of them included some variation of: "I read your recent article. Thank you so much for writing about this. I'm a liberal but . . ." or "I didn't vote for Trump but . . ." and then would go on to say they were dismayed by the lack of critical thinking and discussion regarding NPIs, in particular mitigations imposed on children, most importantly school closures. They were worried about what they referred to as "groupthink" among those in their field. The same conversations took place when I spoke with health professionals whom I contacted after seeing a scholarly paper they had authored that suggested even a modicum of skepticism about the evidence behind NPIs or the wisdom of implementing them on children.

On a call with a pediatrician who had reached out to me, and who worked at a major university hospital, after a long discussion about the lack of evidence behind NPIs I asked, "What do your colleagues say about your thoughts on this?" And he replied, "I don't talk about this at work. Total third rail."

A small but ever-growing "underground" formed of dissenting doctors and health professionals (including former CDC employees), from New York, Boston, San Francisco, and a list of locales in between. Dovetailing with the "I didn't vote for Trump" preamble that started so many conversations and relationships among us was the insistence by most of them that they remain anonymous or that our communications remain fully off the record. If they wouldn't go on the record, why did they want to speak with me? Because our conversations and text groups and email chains, in what over the months and years turned into a loose whisper network across the country, made each of the members feel less alone. Most everyone struggled with the alienation that came with being a heretic—they from their medical colleagues, I from the legacy media.

This isn't to say everyone who was deemed a "contrarian" fit this mold. A number of them were quite public with their views. And not every dissenting medical professional was an alienated Democrat or Independent. But most were. And something was deeply wrong that physicians—many of whom, such as pediatricians, immunologists, and infectious diseases specialists, had expertise of specific relevance to the pandemic—were afraid to speak out.

I was frustrated and troubled by this. But I was also sympathetic. If you worked at a large hospital, there were severe professional repercussions for speaking against the CDC, or the views of your colleagues, your bosses, or "the narrative." This wasn't just in their minds. Multiple experts I interviewed had been reprimanded by superiors for publicly questioning, either on social media or via interviews with the press, the restrictions on children and school closures, or for pointing out inconvenient data. One doctor who worked in the pediatric intensive care unit of a university hospital gave an interview to a medical news site in which she said that in the few weeks right after teens were first eligible for second doses of the COVID vaccine her PICU had more patients with vaccine-related myocarditis than they had teen patients with COVID in almost an entire year. She was not a COVID denier, or a Republican operative. She simply told the truth. The next day she was dressed down by the head of her department. She didn't speak about it again.

Most didn't reach the point of reprimand, however, because they simply chose not to say anything publicly to begin with based on the obvious professional and social climate.

Physicians in general overrepresent as liberal. And infectious diseases and pediatrics are ranked number one and number three most liberal, respectively, of all medical specialties. (Just 23 percent of ID docs were registered Republicans, 2016 data showed.) And university hospitals—where it's more common to find prominent and influential physicians, who are cited in the media and looked up to by peers—were likely even more ideologically imbalanced. The academy itself is extremely liberal leaning. One study found just 12 percent of faculty identified as conservative. And university hospitals are often in urban centers or, by default, in college towns, both of which also lean heavily Democratic. Indeed, research by Stanford political scientist Adam Bonica found that, not surprisingly, Democratic physicians tend to practice in Democratic areas, and Republican physicians in Republican areas. The political tilt is even more pronounced with epidemiologists (who, with some exception, are not also medical doctors). Data from 2018 showed that just 4.4 percent of epidemiologists identify as conservative or right leaning. The political divide in America during the pandemic meant that for a medical or public health professional to publicly agree with anything said by Trump—and, in turn, to go against Anthony Fauci, the AAP, or other leaders and organizations perceived as bulwarks against Trump—was to condemn oneself to the out-group. Public skepticism and criticism, therefore, was largely left to conservative mavericks like Rand Paul.

Even if professional repercussions were not a specific concern, most (though not all) humans do not well tolerate being seen as contrarian to their group, or even thinking contrary to their group. This is obvious through all of history, with a rich literature on in-group-/out-group bias, social identity theory, peer pressure, and groupthink among peoples in nations, religions, and professions. This human tendency is exaggerated within medicine, a field that strongly self-selects for rule followers, not iconoclasts. To get into medical school you typically need to have excellent grades, which requires a temperament suited to buckling down and doing what you're told; once in medical school, a large portion of success hinges on mass amounts of memorization and thinking through pre-established decision trees for diagnoses and treatments; and in practice residents must function within a strict hierarchy, with attending physicians at the top, whose opinions are not typically encouraged to be seriously challenged. Values like discipline and a discouragement of rogue behavior often serve medicine well. But during the pandemic we were left with a circumstance in which the professionals who were looked to most often by the media and the public for direction were in highly politically homogeneous specialties, within an already left-leaning field, in a vocation largely built on conformity.

Many days my phone would ping constantly with texts coming in from sources—most of whom were highly placed experts at esteemed institutions—complaining about the latest guidance, or announcement from Cuomo, Newsom, Fauci, or *New York Times* article that they felt misrepresented risks to children or incorrectly summarized a recent study. The result of all of this, for me, was to have a private awareness that the public perception of uniformity within the public health establishment was misplaced. Not every expert was persuaded that school closures met an evidentiary burden of benefit to outweigh their known costs, or that there was sufficient evidence behind the distancing recommendations or mask mandates, or that children were in great danger, or that they should be seen primarily as viral vectors putting teachers and society at risk. Some of the experts were public on some of these points, but a much, much larger number stayed silent. From my years of interviewing and developing relationships with many dozens of these people, I believe it was still a small minority of public health professionals who dissented. But, critically, it was not nearly as small as people thought.

* * *

Arguing for open schools and for fewer mitigations imposed on children not only would mean health professionals going against colleagues, but it also would mean being out of step with their political tribe. Within the medical field the lack of public dissent regarding schools and kids should be seen within a broader context of an existing ethos of "safetyism" that defined the in-group of the Left.

While people of all political persuasions have their irrational fears, during the pandemic the Left's fears were expressly focused on COVID, in particular around schools, and children in general. And the public acknowledgment—or performance—of that fear was very much a signal of one's membership in the Left.

In part, as I've discussed, this exaggerated perception of risk was a result of gross misrepresentations of danger by public health authorities, along with the media. Numerous polls show that Americans in general, but especially Democrats, wildly overestimated the likelihood of hospitalization or deaths from COVID for every age group except for the elderly (where the probability was dramatically underestimated). A Gallup poll in 2020 showed Democrats thought the share of COVID deaths for people under age twenty-five was *eighty-seven times* higher than the actual proportion.

This degree of innumeracy and ignorance both reflected and reinforced a mindset that exalted safety, or at least the perception of it, above all other concerns—a mindset that already defined the political Left in the decade leading up to the pandemic. Psychologist Jonathan Haidt and his coauthor Greg Lukianoff popularized the term "safetyism" in *Coddling of the American Mind*, a 2018 book in which they describe the phenomenon as one that elevates safety to a "sacred value," and people become unwilling to make trade-offs demanded by other practical and moral concerns.

Much of *Coddling* documents the shift in culture on college campuses, where the authors detail the rise of safe spaces, trigger warnings, and the general notion that students are treated as fragile and that they will incur harm by being exposed to ideas they may find challenging or upsetting. But the foundations for the college years, of course, form in childhood and adolescence. Long relegated to sepia-toned nostalgia is the ethos of the 1950s, when kids would disappear for hours after school, returning home at dark for dinner. Even through the 1980s and early 1990s, in my own childhood, in a world before the norm of cell phones, I'd ride bikes with my best friend, or oftentimes alone, many long afternoons, getting into various kinds of minor trouble, out of reach of parents or anyone for that matter.

As is well covered, much of childhood today is steeped in the culture of "helicopter parents" (or the newer version—bulldozer parents, who don't just hover over their kids but push all obstacles out of their way), who are in constant contact with or surveillance of their kids. Depending how much faith one has in social science data, kids today apparently are more anxious than they used to be, which Haidt and Lukianoff see as directly related to growing up where so much of daily life is seen as a threat, and where parents supervise and schedule nearly every granular aspect of their children's lives.

While safetyism, particularly regarding child rearing, can be seen as an American phenomenon, it's far more entrenched on the progressive Left, perhaps especially among the more well-to-do, as its roots are embedded in a modern leftist ideology. In this culture young people are perceived—and perceive themselves—to be not only at risk of harm from physical threats, but even unintentional insults are intolerable, wrote the sociologists Bradley Campbell and Jason Manning in an influential 2014 paper on the topic. Campbell and Manning explicate what they call a "victimhood culture," in which one's moral status gets raised by being a victim. This is distinct from earlier cultures, when it was generally embarrassing and a diminishment to be seen as a victim.

Against this backdrop of perceiving danger and harm lurking in every aspect of life it is no wonder that Democrats had a dramatically exaggerated sense of the risk that COVID posed to most of the population, especially so to young people. Moreover, publicly communicating—through words or actions—fear of the virus was a form of in-group signaling against Trump and Republicans. The more fear, the more "seriously" you took COVID, the more virtuous you were and the more you raised your status among other progressives or Democrats. The phrase "we're a very COVID-safe family" was spoken proudly to me many times by some friends and neighbors in my town to explain some aggressively "safe" behavior or viewpoint of theirs. (On playdates at a friend's house—obligatorily outdoors-only—my eleven-year-old daughter was denied use of their bathroom. "We take COVID seriously," was the reason given.) Opposing the opening of schools—and when schools were open, advocating for maximum interventions—was a natural fit within this milieu. It was a social class marker.

As part of a culture of safetyism, the insistence that schools were unsafe was accepted as virtuous, and positioned as being for children's benefit. But in actuality—consciously or not—this argument was made to serve certain adults, and largely was to children's detriment.

It is a long-held truism within medicine, psychology, and sociology that excessive efforts to be "safe," and specifically to overprotect children against one or a number of specific threats, increases other harms in any number of predictable and unpredictable ways. Often, this safetyism is reflective of what Joan Tronto, the feminist scholar, calls "protective care."

Good care happens when everyone involved thinks about the situation from the standpoint of the one who needs care. With protective care, however, the views and needs of the *caregivers* "often shape, distort, and reimagine, the needs" of the care receivers. Providing "protection" when it is unnecessary ultimately makes the dependents weak, and lends itself all too well to paternalism, Tronto told me.

"Frightened by the complexity of the virus, persuaded by the adults in the school system, and living in a world deeply shaped by partisan expectations," Tronto summed it up, "leaders even in progressive places opted for safety over equity."

The constant yet selective application of the terms "equity" and "safety" by those who wanted schools closed, as if merely saying the words justified any position they held—and ignoring the fact that achieving equity and safety in one arena often results in inequity and harm in another—ultimately neutered and, in an Orwellian sense, even countered their meanings.

14

THE MEDIA, PART II

Publicly, nearly the entire medical establishment was against Trump, and therefore against schools opening full time. Some of the arguments were overt, but most were simply in effect against opening (and against Trump) without saying so explicitly. Declaring that children should be in school but then advocating for mitigations such as six feet of distancing—which meant that, at most, kids could only attend school part time—or calling for unreachable benchmarks of community case rates to make it "safe" for schools to open, was, in actuality, the same as saying they should be closed.

This stance might have been questioned more by regular citizens if the media had not unquestioningly reported the claims health officials and politicians made, and repeatedly framed stories for maximum fear. With official claims unchallenged and uninvestigated, news reports and Democratic politicians' statements coalesced into an orchestrated performance of the wrongness of Trump's view on schools and the moral correctness of opposing it.

For example:

On July 14, Reuters ran a story titled "Trump Calls COVID School Closures a 'Terrible Decision' as Cases and Deaths Rise." To make sure the insinuation didn't get lost on readers, at the top of the article was a photo of a person on a stretcher, feet visible halfway out of the back of an ambulance, with a hearse in the background for good measure. The week before, the *LA Times* ran a piece that said Trump exhibited "magical thinking" by going against CDC guidance that said kids needed to be distanced and wear masks, among other measures.

In a July interview with the *Atlantic*, Arne Duncan, education secretary under Obama, said he was infuriated that the country lacked the will and discipline to "do the right thing" so that schools could open. The right thing being extensive mitigation measures. The piece's viewpoint was that opening schools was of paramount importance but, echoing Neera Tanden, the influential Democratic insider, it was Trump's failures that prevented them from doing so. Austin Beutner, the superintendent of the Los Angeles Unified School District, was quoted in the piece saying that for his district to open there needed to be a system of testing and contact tracing in place, which every level of government had proved incapable of providing. Opening schools, he said, was "not practical" and "not safe." Schools should be open but, Duncan said, administrators were given "no choice" other than for them to remain closed.

On July 8, a CNBC article on Trump's push to open schools said parents and educators were "growing increasingly anxious about whether there is any way to make in-person school safe enough." That same day the *Washington Post* ran a story that quoted Senator Patty Murray from Washington, the top Democrat on the Senate Education Committee, saying Trump was "trying to bully schools into reopening, no matter the risk." Representative Robert Scott, Democrat from Virginia, and chair of the House Education Committee, said Trump's move to open schools was "not only irresponsible, it is dangerous."

"President Donald Trump's new push to open schools shows he's learned nothing from calamities sparked by his demands for premature state openings" began a CNN piece, also on July 8. The piece, by Stephen Collinson, a CNN White House reporter, cited Trump's tweet about schools having opened in Germany, Denmark, and Sweden without problems, but, similar to comments by Jesse Sharkey, of the Chicago Teachers Union, he said, "All those countries have suppressed the virus in one way or the other."

Opening schools in the fall "could be dangerous to students, parents, and teachers," began still another piece on July 8, in *Vanity Fair*. "The trouble is," the article continued, in the vein of Collinson and Sharkey, "most of the countries returning to some semblance of normalcy got the virus more or less under control *before* taking cautious steps toward reopening, unlike the U.S." And results in Sweden, one of the countries

Trump cited for opening schools successfully, the article claimed, had been "catastrophic."

On July 7, Lily Eskelsen Garcia, the NEA president, promoted the "child as viral vector" narrative during a *CBS News* interview. Speaking of Trump, she said, "I dare him to sit at the back of a classroom and breathe the air of those little kids." The following month the NEA published an article stating that too many schools are in older buildings with dysfunctional HVAC systems, and therefore were unsafe to open. "All schools should be shut down throughout the country. Just too risky. I fear for my children's safety," the piece quoted an unnamed parent. A *Washington Post* article, citing a Government Accountability Office report, said 40 percent of schools were estimated to need updates or replacements to HVAC systems, and that this raised issues for schools planning to reopen in the fall.

A *Politico* piece on July 10 questioned the "rush" to open schools in the fall. The article, like many other pieces, highlighted Trump's threat to withhold federal funds from schools that didn't open. Many lawmakers questioned whether Trump even had the authority to make good on that threat, so Trump's posture and the reactionary umbrage with it were both in no small part theatrical. Regardless, Trump's "rampage," the article said, had created a backlash, even among some Republicans, and that schools needed funding to reopen "safely."

A *New Yorker* piece a few weeks later that centered on teachers' fears of going back to school was titled, "Teachers across the Country Worry about a Rush to Reopen Schools." A lengthy opinion piece, complete with detailed graphics, in the *Times* that weekend quoted a Harvard professor who said there was a "rush" to open schools in the South, where it wasn't safe to do so because there were too many cases. A July piece in the online magazine *Vox* quoted the president of the Massachusetts Teachers Association: "We cannot rush into opening schools just because the calendar says we have to return to school by August or September."

On July 17, California governor Gavin Newsom, mirroring the talking point of Cuomo, Fauci, and others, tweeted that in his state "science will determine when a school can be physically open." And that when they open students should maintain six feet of distance when possible, and that "all staff and students 3rd grade and above must wear masks," a policy presumably also determined by "science." (The CDC advised that all children beginning at age two should wear masks. Yet third grade is composed of eight- and nine-year-olds. How could "the science" be off by seven years, and whose science was correct, the CDC's or Newsom's? Coverage of Newsom's policies, in the *Times* and *ABC News*, among other outlets, did not comment on or investigate the difference between the CDC's and California's age cutoffs for the mask requirements or how those cutoffs were arrived at, nor was there discussion of the evidence behind Newsom's six feet of distancing policy. Much of this was moot, though, in the summer of 2020, since millions of children in California didn't set foot in a school for more than a year anyway.)

On July 11, the *New York Times* ran a triple-byline 2,200-word feature titled "How to Reopen Schools: What Science and Other Countries Teach Us." The article reads as the pièce de résistance of the July media onslaught on Trump and schools. It began by saying there was "enormous pressure to bring students back—from parents, from pediatricians and child development specialists, and from President Trump," followed by a quote from a school nurse saying that going back to school felt like playing Russian roulette with kids and staff. No nation has attempted to bring children back to school with the virus "raging at levels like America's," the article, by Apoorva Mandavilli, Benedict Carey, a *Times* science reporter for 16 years, and Pam Belluck, a Pulitzer Prize–winning science writer, stated. "Experience abroad has shown that measures such as physical distancing and wearing masks in schools can make a difference," the authors wrote, and that controlling community spread was critical to enabling schools to open. They noted children were at low risk but reminded readers that the risk was "not zero," and then mentioned that a small number of children needed intensive care and suffered from a related inflammatory syndrome (remember, this is the condition, MIS-C, that the head of the Royal Academy of Pediatrics explicitly had said was so rare, and treatable, that it was irrelevant to any discussion about schools).

The larger concern, the authors wrote, was kids spreading the virus to family members and teachers. They noted that evidence suggested children were less likely to spread the virus, but that it was inconclusive. And, they wrote, this evidence was collected in countries practicing social distancing and with inadequate pediatric testing. A biologist quoted in the article said the risk of opening would depend on containing transmission through masks and limiting capacity. Even if children don't spread the virus easily "all it would take is one or two to seed" an outbreak, the authors wrote. Dr. Megan Ranney, an emergency medicine physician with no expertise in infectious diseases or the effectiveness of mitigations, was quoted saying that schools should randomly test students.

The articles cited above are just a sample of the broader mediascape. I could have easily included five times as many examples from major news outlets with similar claims and framing. Collectively, this was the narrative on schools the media drilled into the American public: Trump is not only wrong, but recklessly so; schools present unique dangers to kids and society; it is morally incumbent to oppose Trump's position; "the science" and "experts" tell us schools should not open, or if and when they do open a series of specific benchmarks need to be met and specific mitigations need to be in place for schools to be "safe."

Hume and Locke would be displeased. Evidence matters. Every single claim or implication I referenced from the *Times* flagship feature on schools was either false, an unverified assumption, or misleading. And many of the claims in the other news articles I referenced suffer similarly.

I'm going to address each of the major claims in the *Times* piece and the other articles above because these claims were made time and again in the media, and they profoundly misled the public about the risks of open schools, and exaggerated or outright fabricated the hurdles that needed to be overcome for schools to open.

First, let's start with the notion that the objective to open schools in the fall was a "rush," as the *Politico* piece and many others referred to it. Schools in Europe had already reopened months earlier. Between the spring closures and the summer break, American kids would have been out of school for almost half a year come that fall. It was only by flipping the burden of proof onto the status quo (open schools), while removing it from the intervention (closed schools)—a reversal of the ethical standard of how medicine and public health are intended to be practiced—and ignoring evidence from Europe, where tens of millions of children had already been back in class without notable effect, that allowing American kids to attend school after six months would be considered a rush.

Next, even with granting some literary license, likening attending school to playing Russian roulette, as was quoted in the *Times* article, was so hyperbolic and divorced from the statistical reality of risk as to be nothing other than histrionic and grossly misleading to readers. The notion of pointing a revolver with a loaded chamber to a child's head and pulling the trigger, as the *Times* saw fit to print, dovetailed nicely with the Reuters hearse. The same pediatric data from China in February, and the host of studies and governmental reports in March and beyond had not changed. Children were at extraordinarily low risk of serious harm, well below a long list of typical threats—from motor vehicles to drownings—they faced in any given year.

What about the purported danger to teachers implied or explicitly noted in many of the articles, which presented kids as human sprinklers spraying viral particles in infectious mists all over their classrooms, putting adults at home and in school at unique risk? First, we have the findings of the two EU education ministers' meetings to contend with. The conclusions drawn were broad; the Croatian minister's statements were not referencing a study on teachers in schools. And there was no pretense or expectation that there was zero transmission in schools. But if schools were overt superspreaders the effect would have been unmissable.

As compelling as the observational evidence cited by the education ministers was, it could be seen as an illuminating yet diffuse light. Yet at the end of June we had a laser: a concise, eleven-page report from the Swedish government that should have made headlines. Featuring several tables and a minimalist bar graph, the report detailed the incidence rate of COVID cases among different professions. The data showed that primary school teachers in Sweden, who had been working uninterrupted throughout the pandemic, teaching hundreds of thousands of students in person, were at no higher risk of infection than average compared with other professions. (Taxi drivers and pizza bakers, for example, were at nearly five times higher risk of infection than teachers.) This was a fireworks moment. One of the key concerns health officials, teachers unions, and politicians expressed was the possible risk that children posed to school staff. These data directly addressed those concerns.

This was one report from one country, and data analysis of this nature has many variables. Still, the sample size was massive, and because lower schools hadn't closed, instead of relying on modeling or conjecture, as authorities were doing in the States, the researchers were able to look at real world, empirical evidence of infection incidence of teachers actually working in schools. This was the evidence, ostensibly, we all were waiting for. And yet, instead of highlighting this groundbreaking report, the *Times* published a steady stream of articles around that time portraying Sweden as either the climax or denouement in a disaster film. Sweden was the "world's cautionary tale," one headline warned ominously. It was a "pariah," read another. "Sweden Took Its Own Path. Now It Is Paying the Price," read a third, among many others. The dire coverage left one to envision either a scene of utter chaos, air raid sirens screaming, people running for the hills, or near silence, a toddler walking alone amid a wasteland portrayed in washed-out colors, a filthy doll abandoned on an empty playground.

A second Swedish report, released in July, conducted jointly with Finland, where schools had shut down from March 18 to May 13, concluded that there was no difference in cases in children between the two countries. Whether schools were open or not "had no measurable direct impact," the report concluded. And out of more than one million Swedish children in school there were zero deaths.

These were inconvenient data for a narrative about undue risks to teachers and the overall danger of schools. And so, they were largely ignored by authorities and the media.

As for the suggestion from Dr. Ranney, the emergency medicine physician, for random testing, without specifics on the percentage of students tested and at what frequency, there was (and still is) no evidence that this practice yields a meaningful reduction in in-school transmission. This is especially so if there is a low community rate because the fewer cases there are overall the lower the likelihood of finding a positive individual among a small random sample. In areas with very high community rates, if a large enough sample of students is tested often enough it might be beneficial, but this differentiation went unsaid by Ranney or at least it wasn't included in the article. Like many interventions, the devil is in the details as to whether there is benefit at all, and if so to what extent. Blanket statements like "masks work" and that there should be "random testing" can easily lead to net costs since they can wind up being implemented in a manner that is not effective. As Dr. Monica Gandhi, an infectious diseases specialist at University of California, San Francisco, along with two coauthors later argued in a *Washington Post* editorial, there are numerous downsides to systematic testing for students, including, most importantly, the possibility of false positives wrongly keeping uninfected kids out of school. Gandhi outlined a scenario in which a case rate of 15 per 10,000 people per week could translate to more than 90 percent of positive test results being incorrect. Gandhi and her coauthors calculated that with a positivity rate of 0.4 percent, which was the rate in New York City schools that fall when more than 234,000 asymptomatic students and staff were tested, 40,000 tests would need to be performed to prevent one in-school transmission. "Overall," they wrote, this kind of testing "fails a cost-benefit analysis." My own district tried to implement a voluntary program of testing 5 percent of the student body each week, but not enough parents signed up, so it never was implemented.

Finally, the claim, made in nearly every piece, that the countries in Europe that reopened their schools only could do so because they had "controlled" the virus, was misleading on multiple levels:

First, it was simply untrue, when viewing many city-by-city comparisons. For example, multiple major cities in Germany, including Berlin and Hamburg, that had opened their lower schools at the beginning of May had higher cases rates than those in many large American cities, including Los Angeles and San Francisco. (The German cities had an average of around 11 cases per 100,000 daily over 7 days, versus 8 per 100,000 in Los Angeles, and 3 per 100,000 in San Francisco.) Other European population centers, such as Copenhagen, Oslo, and Helsinki, where schools began opening at the end of April and into May, had rates on par with or above those in Seattle and Portland the first week of May (6, 2.5, and 1.8 per 100,000, respectively, versus 4.4 and 2.0 per 100,000). In Paris, where schools had begun opening at the end of May, the rate in the first week of June was an average of 8.15 per 100,000, daily over 7 days, on par with New York City's, at 8.6, and well above San Francisco, Seattle, Portland, and a long list of smaller cities and towns around the US.

Second, relatedly, in regard to school closures, viewing cases through a national lens, rather than regionally or locally, goes against pre-pandemic guidelines, and logic, which is why regional or city comparisons, as I illustrated above, are more appropriate. European countries have, respectively, millions or tens of millions of citizens, and the US has hundreds of millions of citizens, spread over millions of square miles. Why should opening schools in Berkeley be based on the case rate in Baton Rouge? The idea that, as the *Times* reported it, no country had opened schools with the virus "raging" as it was in the US was to spuriously view America's massive geographic area and population as one entity, which made no more sense epidemiologically than viewing all of Europe as one entity, rather than as separate countries with differing circumstances. The case rate in New York, for example, on the day the *Times* piece was published was the second-lowest case rate during the entire pandemic through the summer of 2022.

Discussing the coronavirus cases at a national level, and suggesting that schools should be closed everywhere is like a doctor suggesting a full body cast when you have a broken left ankle and a contusion on your hip.

Third, rarely did officials or journalists define and defend what "controlling the virus" actually meant. What metrics meant a virus was sufficiently under control for a school to open? And how were those metrics arrived at? Were they based on models that were based on assumptions? Were they based on pediatric influenza transmission patterns, which, early on, differed dramatically from those of the coronavirus? Further, the assumption that a high community rate, however it was defined, meant that schools should stay closed because that would reduce transmission

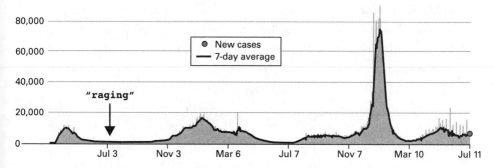

Seven-day average, new cases in New York. *New York Times*, with "raging" added by David Zweig.

was not borne out by any quality evidence. The notion that children all stayed isolated at home while schools were closed, especially once closures continued beyond a few weeks, was never evidence-based. Recall Robert Barro's analysis, and the absence of impact of school closures over the long term. Recall the implementation science concept of voltage drop, the gap between the ideal and the actual, and that people's adherence to measures diminishes over time. Recall that even from day one plenty of families were incapable of isolating themselves because, unlike most modelers, the parents had to leave their homes to work, and as a result their children often had to interact with people outside the home, either neighbors or relatives looking after them or in daycare centers. Retrospective studies looking at cell phone mobility data, which showed people's adherence to staying home waned over time, support what the observational data from Europe had already shown: closing schools was not correlated with meaningfully lowering the impact of COVID. Though some people—who had both the financial and vocational ability, as well as the inclination—could seal themselves off at home, that was not the norm, especially as more time elapsed. Moreover, other observational studies, including one published in the CDC's journal *MMWR*, found that even in communities with extremely high rates of infection, open schools had a lower prevalence of cases than the surrounding community and only a tiny portion of those cases was determined to result from in-school transmission.

There is perhaps no more perfect evidence that the society-wide mitigation measures were doomed to fail than the authors and directors of this guidance themselves. Neil Ferguson, the famed Imperial College modeler, argued vigorously for the necessity of society-wide social distancing. Yet he got busted for trysts with a married woman who left her family to visit him at least twice during British lockdowns in March and April 2020. He resigned from his government advisory role after the scandal broke. On the day after Thanksgiving 2020, Deborah Birx traveled to one of her vacation homes, where she congregated with three generations of her family from two different households. That month Birx had warned that the US was entering the deadliest phase of the pandemic, and urged the public in countless media appearances to not gather with extended family for the holidays.

The public rightfully was infuriated at Birx's and Ferguson's hypocrisy. But the bigger point is that their own behavior simply proved that the models, and the guidance based on them, were never going to work as expected. There is a reason why the mitigations they so adamantly championed are, at best, temporizing measures. The architects of the lockdowns themselves couldn't adhere to them. Ferguson didn't even make it past March before breaking the rules. Humans, in real life, do not operate according to models. They get bored, they get frustrated, they get lonely. We are social creatures. Unless people are welded inside their homes, eventually most of them are going to come out.

The hypocrisy was not just a moral failing of Birx and Ferguson, but rather an intellectual failing, to not understand—or at least be honest about—human nature, even within themselves. But the media, which had so credulously and scoldingly amplified the supposed morality and effectiveness of lockdowns, did not take the Ferguson and Birx episodes as opportunities to examine the veracity of their reporting. Instead, incurious stenographic reporting on modeled reductions of cases and deaths from social distancing, and claims by officials, like Anthony Fauci, and health professionals about the value of closures, mask mandates, and so on, continued apace.

*   *   *

It's also worth looking at a brief case study to further explicate how the media relied on "expert" opinion, rather than evidence. And how doing so was deceiving in several ways.

In June, the *Times* ran a piece: "How 132 Epidemiologists Are Deciding When to Send Their Children to School." The subtitle quoted one saying this was "the dreaded question." More than a dozen participants said they would wait to send kids back until there was a vaccine, which they acknowledged could be a year or more. While some opinions expressing concern about keeping kids out of school were included, the tenor and framing of the article was made clear in the subtitle, which said experts were "struggling to weigh virus risks and uncertainty against family well-being." The entire premise falsely positioned school as a place that raised the risk of harm.

But the salient point about the *Times* piece is not the views it shared, but rather that it contained no discussion of evidence. It contained no mention of the European schoolchildren who had been back in school for more than a month. It contained no mention of how wildly off the models, which had specific predictions about the impact of school closures, had been. What exactly were these epidemiologists basing their opinions on? We don't know, because the article simply consisted of a list of quotes.

The article's introduction read:

The comments below give a sense of how experts are considering this difficult question in their lives.

This exemplified what is known as an appeal to authority, a logical fallacy, in which instead of providing evidence behind a claim, one merely points to the authority of the person saying it, suggesting that that alone makes the claim true. Philosophers consider this an invalid form of argument. The article—of a piece with much of the pandemic reporting in the *Times*—epitomized how the media helped enable the flight from evidence-based public health to the retrograde reliance on "expert opinion" for decision-making.

It gets worse, though. What the *Times* didn't reveal is that many of these epidemiologists' expertise had absolutely nothing to do with infectious diseases. One "expert" quoted in the piece—who said "it would be really stupid to reopen schools in September"—was a consultant for smokeless tobacco companies. Other "experts" quoted didn't have children, even though the title of the article was how epidemiologists were deciding when to send "their" kids to school. Still other "experts" in the article included someone whose research focused on substance abuse, a PhD student whose research was on exposure to heavy metals, a professor who specialized in disparities in maternal health, and cancer researchers. I only learned of the "experts'" actual expertise because I looked them up. (Only names and affiliations were given, not area of focus or experience.) Readers were told "epidemiologist" meant "expert" on this topic. But it did not. Epidemiology is a broad field, in which only a specific subset of practitioners specializes in infectious diseases. And even those people are credentialed for understanding the spread of diseases, which is totally different from an expertise in weighing costs and benefits of a family's child being kept out of school. Why should readers care that a childless grad student, who studies the health effects of cigarettes, has "reservations" about sending kids back to school?

In short, not only did the article suffer from the appeal to authority fallacy, the "authorities" surveyed in the article weren't even experts in the subject on which they were giving their opinion.

Seen through the media lens that amplified opinions more than reporting facts, it is not surprising that, despite all of the empirical evidence—from the tens of thousands of American children in daycare; from Sweden, which never closed its lower schools; from a score of countries in Europe that had reopened their schools and said it went fine—the child-and-school-as-superspreader narrative continued to prevail in America.

Further, evidence suggests that the epidemiologists who made the models, advised the politicians, and gave interviews to the media not only were more likely to be of a class that *could* seal themselves or their families at home, but also may have been more likely to possess a certain psychology to *want* to seal themselves or their families at home compared to the general public. It's not irrelevant that in a survey nearly three-quarters of epidemiologists described themselves as risk averse.

Eli Perencevich, a physician and infectious diseases epidemiologist at the University of Iowa, who was a prominent voice and fierce advocate for school closures and maximizing other mitigations, makes for a compelling example. Back in 2013, Perencevich wrote a strange and detailed post in which he boasted of, among other actions, locking his kindergarten-aged child in the bathroom for twenty-four hours to avoid contracting norovirus from him. He ended the post by saying "most of these steps are easily reproducible in any household."

Eleanor Murray, an epidemiologist at Boston University, with more than a hundred thousand Twitter followers and whose opinions frequently appeared in the *New York Times*, *Washington Post*, and other media outlets, and advised health departments, was perhaps the public health professional most notorious for anxiety and what, to many critics, came across as pedophobia and misopedia. Murray was extremely vocal, bordering on militant in her advocacy for school closures, masking children, and other mitigations, often directed at the young. She also repeatedly tweeted about her personal struggles with an anxiety disorder, but this was not mentioned when she was quoted in news articles sharing her opinion on the necessity and wisdom of COVID mitigations. "I am so so worried for all the young children in my life," she tweeted in August of 2021, more than a year after the pandemic began and it was irrefutably established that kids, by and large, were fine. That same month she also tweeted: "Genuine q for ppl more concerned about schools being closed than covid: are you aware mandatory schooling is barely a century old in this country?" In June of 2022, long after the CDC rescinded its mask recommendation for schools, she urged people to call their local health departments to keep kids masked until summer.

I cite Murray and Perencevich because they had high profiles. But they were not outliers among their peers, given the survey results and tenor of comments by innumerable epidemiologists in the press and on social media. Also, it's important to see epidemiologists' perception of risk aversion through the frame of health practitioners' bias toward action, a belief that measures should be implemented, even in the absence of evidence of benefit, or even when there is evidence of harm.

The media relentlessly cited these professionals' opinions on schools and mitigations for children, which were based not on evidence but on personal values and fears that were not necessarily aligned with those of much of the public.

DEEP DIVE: IT'S "BASIC PHYSICS"— MITIGATION MISINFORMATION, AND THE CASE OF HEPA FILTERS

Unfortunately, when journalists weren't focusing their articles on expert opinion, they often broadcast "expert" views that veered toward rank misinformation.

More than three months after the initial closures, and, by the fall, nearly six months after them, pegging the opening of schools to an arbitrary community rate, as many officials had done with the blessing of health authorities, was not only epidemiologically unsound but also ethically dubious. Recall the #SchoolsBeforeBars philosophy. Even with higher community rates politicians could have compelled other aspects of society to remain shut down while schools stayed open. That's exactly what happened in England, France, and Germany. Despite what Americans were told, keeping schools closed was not a science-based policy. It was a values-based policy. And in the US, particularly blue state America, the value was on businesses staying open, where adults—who, with few exceptions, were at substantially higher risk from the virus than children—could congregate, while schools—which could have been filled with children, who with rare exception were at a statistical zero of risk of serious harm—stayed closed.

Aside from the deceiving claims about Europe "controlling" the virus, relative to the US, there was a list of claims, regularly cited by the media, about what mitigations within schools were necessary. The claims that American schools, especially those in cities, suffered from specific disadvantages relative to European counterparts, and that because of these supposed disadvantages schools shouldn't open, were also unfounded.

Masks were repeatedly cited as an essential component of the "Swiss cheese" approach of mitigation in schools. This matched the CDC's recommendation for all children, including those as young as age two, to wear masks for the duration of every school day. Yet in Germany there was no mask mandate for children in primary school. In France no kids under age twelve were required to wear masks. Similar pediatric masking guidelines were in place throughout Europe in part because, in contrast to the CDC, the World Health Organization said no children under age six should wear masks at all, and those aged six to eleven should only wear them under certain circumstances. The European Centre for Disease Prevention and Control did not recommend masks for any child in primary school.

The CDC never produced any data that masking toddlers and kindergarteners yielded any benefit to justify its more aggressive guidance compared to that of the World Health Organization and the ECDC. Moreover, as I detailed earlier, meta-analyses, and even a systematic review from the CDC itself, of masking trials before the pandemic did not find that community mask mandates conferred any clinically meaningful benefit. Claims about mask mandates being necessary and beneficial for schools in particular were even further divorced from any evidence base. A full year later, in the summer of 2021, the CDC published what it said was the first comparative study of mask mandates in schools, covering some 90,000 students. The result found a nonstatistically significant effect of student masking. In other words, even with 90,000 students the effect size was so small that researchers could not say if there was any benefit.

Distancing in many of the European schools, including those in big cities, was either one meter (roughly three feet) from the outset, or began at two meters and dropped to one meter shortly after, as happened in Denmark, or there was no specific distancing requirement at all, such as in Sweden. The six feet of distancing rule for schools that was in place in much of the US remained not only untethered from any evidence base before the pandemic, but, worse, was also divorced from the real-world evidence of millions of European children in school without that requirement. This distancing rule is one of the reasons the hybrid schedule— which came about largely because schools had to operate at lower density to comply with six feet of distancing—became the dominant model in school districts in much of the US, particularly in the Northeast and mid-Atlantic regions, for close to an entire school year, but was largely absent in Europe. Mostly, the schools there were either open or closed. And there was no evidence before the pandemic that distancing in schools reduced overall rates of infection that somehow would have overridden this new evidence from Europe to the contrary.

Testing was not uniformly being conducted in widespread fashion throughout these cities and regions of Europe which had opened their schools, even though testing was often cited as a necessary intervention for schools to open "safely" in the US. Moreover, there was no evidence prior to the pandemic that random testing worked, particularly for a highly contagious respiratory virus that had already spread among the population.

With rare exception, the schools in European countries were not equipped with forced-air HVAC systems or outfitted with HEPA filters. Guidelines in some of these countries suggested opening windows; often national health authorities did not suggest specific ventilation requirements for schools at all. The claim that schools throughout America required massive infusions of money to purchase HEPA filters and the like for them to be "safe" to open was belied by the fact that these types of filtration systems were almost entirely absent from schools in Europe. (This isn't to imply that, outside the context of the pandemic, ventilation and clean air aren't important, and that some portion of American schools with aging infrastructures aren't in desperate need of repairs and replacements to HVAC systems, among a long list of other renovations. But as evidenced by the European schools, and contrary to the claims by American experts and media, the need for those upgrades was unrelated to making schools safe in relation to the coronavirus.) Schools in Europe relied almost exclusively on opening windows or doors (or in some cases no specific ventilation intervention at all), and there was no observed effect on transmission. What's more, simple, inexpensive enhancements, such as putting a fan in a window, had been shown to increase ventilation. In addition to the observational evidence from Europe showing a lack of ill effects of not having sophisticated HVAC systems in place in classrooms, there was no evidence showing a decrease in school transmission when using HEPA filters versus fans in windows or even just open doors. Nor was there any real-world evidence before the pandemic that HEPA filters reduced viral transmission in this type of environment.

HEPA filters may indeed confer some benefit on reducing coronavirus transmission in schools, but no one knew then or knows now, more than three years later, what amount that benefit was, if any. Considering the evidence from Europe, where open schools were not found to have contributed to overall case rates and where heightened (or any) filtration was not the norm, it's hard to imagine how this intervention would have a clinically meaningful effect. To claim that HEPA filters and expensive HVAC upgrades were required for schools to be safe when its effect, if any, on reducing transmission could not be quantified, rendered a cost-benefit analysis impossible, just as was the case with school closures. (Some infectious diseases specialists who were extremely vocal advocates for HEPA filters in schools admitted privately to colleagues—in messages that were shared confidentially with me—that there was no real-world evidence of their benefit on transmission and that randomized trials were needed.)

Kimberly Prather, an atmospheric chemist who was very prominent on Twitter and in the media during the pandemic, with more than 70,000 followers on the social media platform and numerous interviews given to the *Washington Post*, *Time*, the *Boston Globe*, the *New York Times* and the *San Francisco Chronicle*, among other outlets, repeatedly tweeted that NPIs such as masks and air filtration "worked" because it was "basic physics." She wrote that asking for trials to determine the effect of these interventions on transmission was "ludicrous." She sometimes accompanied these claims with the statement, "Science is not a belief system."

Remember Alfred Korzybski's adage. Prather is not wrong about basic physics. She was wrong because she mistook the map for the territory, artificially bridging the distance between the theoretical and the actual.

Prather, and the many others who shared her view, did not understand that two things can be true at the same time: HEPA filters clean indoor air *and* they may not have a meaningful effect on students' or a community's overall case rates. No one should have claimed, especially not with certitude, that HEPA filters and most of the HVAC upgrades were necessary to open schools "safely." In fact, more than four years after the start of the pandemic, in the summer of 2024, as I type this sentence, there still are no published studies that show that this intervention in

schools reduces coronavirus transmission. There are only two comparative studies of the effect of HEPA filters in schools on the incidence of
COVID infection. One, on German kindergartens, was published in *BMJ
Open* in 2023. Of 2,360 children in 32 kindergartens, some with HEPA
filters, others without, the study concluded that HEPA filters did "not
lead to reduced COVID-19 prevalence." The authors had hypothesized—
as so many health professionals asserted—that HEPA filters would have
a preventative effect. But "this hypothesis was rejected," they wrote. (In
fact, COVID prevalence was higher in the kindergartens with HEPA filters.) The other study, published by the CDC in its journal *MMWR*, in
May 2021, did not find a statistically significant benefit on transmission
reduction in schools with HEPA filters versus those without HEPA filters.
This result doesn't mean there is no benefit, but that the study, despite
including more than 30,000 students in the comparative groups, failed
to demonstrate that HEPA filters reduced infections more than doing
nothing at all. Prather's condescending dismissal of the need for trials
to find out how much, if any, effect there is on actual transmission was
woefully misguided.

In early 2020, when physicians were scrambling to figure out effective
therapies for patients who were seriously ill from COVID, transfusing "convalescent plasma (CP)"—antibody-rich plasma from a COVID-recovered
person—into the patient surfaced as a promising treatment. The general
idea had been around for more than a century. Although it lacked proper
controlled trials, there was some observational evidence the practice had
worked for other viruses, and it made intuitive sense. Some physician
researchers believed so strongly in its likely ability to help critically ill
COVID patients that they refused to conduct trials that included a proper
control group, i.e. participants who would be getting a placebo or, in this
instance, plasma from regular people who hadn't had COVID, because
physicians felt it would be unethical to hold back this powerful treatment
from patients. When proper trials were finally conducted and published
later that summer and in the fall, convalescent plasma failed to yield any
benefits for those with moderate disease, failed to prevent progression of
disease in high-risk outpatients, and failed to reduce mortality. Moreover,
the treatment carried risks of blood clotting and other dangerous side
effects. Much later CP was found to possibly help a narrow subgroup of

patients, an encouraging finding, though it was a far cry from the anticipated benefit initially.

Dr. H. Clifford Lane, a clinical director at the National Institute of
Allergy and Infectious Diseases, conducted a CP randomized trial on
influenza patients in 2019, which found no significant benefit. "Everything that's going on right now in terms of trying to find an effective
treatment for COVID-19 is driven by fear and this strong desire to do
something for patients," he said in an April 2020 *JAMA* interview. Yet,
he said, "Many of the things that are so promising in theory fall apart
when really studied rigorously." Notice the theme, once again, of the
desire to *do something* despite no known benefit. In this instance even
trial evidence showed no significant benefit and the possibility for harm.
There appears to be a perennial, and not ill-intended, need among clinicians and health experts to feel useful, and to show the public they have
some control.

Just as with a long list of other treatments, a few more of which I will
detail later, including radical mastectomies, doctors' intuition about what
would work was wrong. This is fine on its own, except for the fact that too
often treatments based on intuition were proposed with such hubris that
a trial was deemed unethical. In schools, the demand for HEPA filters,
masks, distancing, and, most importantly, partial and full closures were
all based on intuitions but no real-world data. Each of these interventions
carried with it significant costs to children, particularly over the long
term. (Even requiring seemingly benign interventions like HEPA filters or
HVAC upgrades in many instances produced harms, since their absence
was cited as a reason to keep schools closed, and their implementation
diverted money from other areas.) Yet because these interventions made
intuitive sense to health authorities and many regular people alike, suggestions that we needed actual high-quality data on their benefit were
dismissed, and those who questioned their benefit were often maligned
as fools or for not caring about the welfare of children or the community.
Prather's claims not only showed a misunderstanding of the disconnect
between lab results and the real world, but also demonstrated yet another
instance in a long history of a humility deficit among health professionals that proved to be unearned.

Dr. Vinay Prasad, an oncologist and professor in the Department of Epidemiology at the University of California, San Francisco, has written extensively about evidence-based medicine, and during the pandemic he became an evangelist for the need for randomized trials for NPIs. "No one knows which interventions slow spread, and which do not," he wrote in early 2022. The way to figure this out is "cluster RCTs [randomized controlled trials], but we ran zero in the USA." Prasad argued that the government should be given a grace period to implement various NPIs, but after that grace period—he suggested three months—they need to have produced solid evidence of benefit, via RCTs, or lose the ability to mandate the intervention. In cluster RCTs groups, as opposed to individuals, are randomly allocated to the treatment or control arms. Randomized trials, while not perfect, typically generate a more robust form of evidence than observational data, which is subject to all sorts of biases. And, considering RCTs are looking at outcomes in people or the world, in this instance reduction in virus transmission, they generate evidence of relevance that is multiple levels above that from lab studies or models. Running proper RCTs is expensive and can be complex. But when taking into account the untold billions of dollars spent on NPIs, and the costs of lost school time for students in districts that were unable to open because they didn't employ interventions (such as HVAC upgrades) that teachers unions demanded or authorities required, whatever the RCT cost it would have been worth it to find out which of these interventions actually worked, and, if so, to what extent.

Some clinicians and researchers, such as Branch-Elliman, have suggested that running an RCT on masks or some of the other NPIs for schools may have been too infeasible to conduct properly, since, in part, it would rely on parents and children accepting whatever arm the child was assigned to. (For example, it's perhaps unlikely that a parent who is opposed to mask mandates would agree to their child being forced to mask for months as part of a trial.) And EBM is not only about RCTs or bust. It's also about making choices based on the best available evidence. But the best available evidence regarding all of these NPIs, from a vast natural experiment in schools throughout Europe, showed that their absence had no noticeable impact.

* * *

Speaking of HEPA filters, I want to take us on a brief tangent to discuss not school ventilation per se, but the broader messaging around it and a case study of sorts of the dubious influence of the expert class and its disconnect from evidence-based public health. Don't worry, I'm not going to get into the minutia of HVAC systems and aerosols.

It was often claimed, in news articles, by teachers unions, and others, that many schools, particularly those in inner cities, had classrooms with windows that didn't open or no windows at all, which made the schools unsafe to operate without sufficient HVAC upgrades. And it was asserted that this rendered comparisons to Europe (where it was inferred, incorrectly, that all classrooms had their windows open all the time) inappropriate. I was also sometimes given this response personally when I discussed opening schools with regular people or with education professionals: "That's *Europe*. Things are different there. We have overcrowded schools with windows that don't open." Often the statements were nonspecific; for example, an NPR report on schools in Philadelphia that said, "In some buildings windows can't open or can open only a little bit." In interviews in the summer of 2020, Michael Mulgrew, the head of the United Federation of Teachers, New York City's main teachers union, mentioned classrooms without windows as a concern. On multiple occasions Randi Weingarten, head of the AFT union, publicly mentioned concerns about classrooms without windows or windows that couldn't open. A letter sent by BASIC (a coalition of education and civic groups, including the American Federation of Teachers, two school principal associations, the National Wildlife Federation, and around forty other organizations) in July 2020 asked Congress for $10 billion for emergency repairs for 14,000 schools as part of a COVID relief package. Among the issues listed by the coalition was "windows can't open to increase fresh air in classrooms."

The claims about windows intrigued me for a few reasons. First, state and local laws typically require some form of ventilation in classrooms. In New York City, for example, if a classroom does not have windows that can open, it must have an exhaust fan or an intake fan or an HVAC unit that circulates and filters air. In New York City, as of September 6, 2020,

96 percent of its classrooms passed ventilation inspection, which meant they had at least one operational method of ventilation. Out of 62,000 classrooms, 200 did not meet the criteria, and a DOE official told me that those rooms were not going to be used until or unless that was remedied. It's possible, of course, or in the case of New York City, definitive, that some classrooms were not in compliance with guidelines, and some classrooms didn't have operable windows and had dysfunctional ventilation systems. But those classrooms, at least in New York City, were not going to be used. Many newer school buildings were designed to not have operable windows and instead to rely on HVAC systems. Merely having a classroom without windows that open did not mean there wasn't ventilation. Also remember that opening windows was not a requirement or even explicitly recommended for many European schools, and in general they did not have forced-air HVAC systems either. And once fall and winter arrived many classes, particularly in colder northern European areas, kept their windows closed.

Setting aside that American classrooms that have inoperable windows typically have another form of ventilation, and setting aside that many European classrooms didn't open their windows or have mechanical ventilation, this claim about schools with windows that don't open, which was regularly repeated as a reason for American schools to stay closed, vexed me for almost two years. How many classrooms in American schools actually had windows that didn't open? And, more saliently, of those classrooms how many also did not have a functional HVAC system? The answers to these questions were vital because the windows narrative blocked kids from attending school. I contacted numerous districts but got no answers. I contacted the National Council on School Facilities, an organization that deals in all matters related to school buildings, and with which I had previously corresponded about distancing guidelines, but did not receive a reply. I sent BASIC an email asking for data on schools with classrooms without operable windows and no other ventilation—since this was one of the reasons listed in their letter asking for $10 billion for schools—and did not get a response from them either.

After months of thinking about the issue, and researching it off and on, and then more or less giving up, I came across a May 2021 Johns Hopkins School Ventilation Report. It contained this line: "Windows cannot be opened in many schools." Finally, I was going to get to the bottom of this. The forty-six-page document was written by scholars at the Bloomberg School of Public Health and the Center for Health Security, both at Johns Hopkins University, an elite institution. It had seven coauthors and listed eight "expert reviewers." To produce the report and its recommendations, thirty-two experts in air quality, engineering, and education policy were interviewed, and the relevant peer-reviewed literature and engineering best practices were examined.

Finally, I hit it big. It can take a while but sometimes you get lucky with research, and the right experts and the right documents surface. An extensive report devoted to school ventilation would obviously contain a detailed account of this infrastructure problem of windows that cannot be opened, with localized statistics.

Yet as I scanned the document I began to get worried. No matter how closely I read it, I could not find any additional information about windows beyond that one sentence. I then saw that at the end of the sentence about windows that cannot open there was a footnote citing a Government Accountability Office report. *This* is where I'd find the information I sought. As comprehensive as the Hopkins report was, these types of statistics on windows were too granular to include, and I should not have been surprised to need to dig another layer deeper.

I found and then carefully reviewed the ninety-four-page GAO report. Yet, strangely, there was nothing in it either about inoperable windows. I figured I must have been missing something, so I emailed the GAO report's author. He told me that I was correct; there was nothing in his report about windows not being able to open.

To recap: the Johns Hopkins report made a claim about inoperable windows. It cited another report as the source of that claim, yet the source did not contain any information related to the claim. I reached out to two authors of the Hopkins report raising this issue, along with a few others. After five emails back and forth, Paula Olsiewski, one of the authors, suggested we arrange a call.

Olsiewski, a senior scholar at the Johns Hopkins Center for Health Security, and a leader in the field of the microbiology and chemistry of indoor environments, was warm, animated, and generous with her time and knowledge, offering lots of details about ventilation science. Yet, no matter how many times I gently prodded, during our hour-long call she did not answer my question about how many schools had windows that didn't open, let alone windows that didn't open and no other source of ventilation.

I'm thankful scientists like Olsiewski exist and that they have devoted their professional lives to trying to improve conditions for the rest of us. Not that I needed to be persuaded, but Olsiewski made a detailed case for why clean air in schools is an unmitigated good. (And there is no doubt that filters help take particulates out of the air.) The question is not whether Olsiewski and her colleagues' work over the years toward improving indoor air quality is a noble goal. The question is whether claims about windows, and, more broadly, demands for HEPA filters and the like were valid reasons to keep schools closed during the pandemic.

How did the authors of the Hopkins report know that there were "many schools" with windows that didn't open if they couldn't tell me a number? What was "many"? One percent? Five percent? Twenty percent? And of those schools was it every classroom in the building that didn't have windows that opened or just a portion of classrooms? And of those classrooms without windows that opened how many did not have functional mechanical ventilation? The answers to these questions matter. Without quantifying the scope of the purported problem or being able to quantify the benefit of the proposed solution we're left with mere guesswork and opinions.

The Hopkins report had other claims I was concerned about. Numerous times it recommended the use of HEPA filters to "help reduce the potential for SARS-CoV-2 transmission." But, as I've detailed, lab tests showing reductions of virus in the air from HEPA filters is different from knowing how much, if any, reduction in transmission of the coronavirus they lead to in a classroom. The only real-world data on this at the time, as noted earlier, from the *MMWR* paper, was not promising.

According to a systematic review of studies on air filtration and circulation in hospitals before the pandemic, there were zero randomized trials, which is considered the highest level of evidence, on HEPA filters regarding transmission reduction. Of the remaining lower levels of evidence none indicates how whatever benefit some of these systems may have shown in hospitals would translate to a school. While HEPA filters may provide transmission reduction in a medical setting, it's possible that in a school, an environment that obviously has a lower percentage of sick people than a hospital, the benefit may be negligible. For example, imagine if a study showed that HEPA filters reduced transmission by 50 percent in a hospital. That sounds like a big deal! Now imagine they do the same in schools, except a school had two cases out of 1,000 students before HEPA filters; after their installation a 50 percent reduction would be one fewer case out of a thousand. This is the difference between relative reductions, which is the percentage, and absolute reductions, which is the actual number. Beyond that, the systems in hospitals that showed benefit may be far more robust than what was capable of being installed in most schools.

Indeed, even ventilation, i.e. bringing in fresh air (as opposed to filtration, which cleans the air), which has generally been considered the single-most or perhaps second-most important mitigation in schools, has very limited real-world evidence to support it having a significant impact on SARS-CoV-2 transmission in schools. The *MMWR* study I mentioned earlier found that schools that employed ventilation techniques (opening windows or doors or use of fans) had 2.94 cases per 500 students versus 4.19 cases per 500 students in schools without ventilation over a span of four weeks. So ventilation was associated with 1.25 fewer cases out of 500 students over an entire month. Moreover, 2.94 and 4.19 are "point estimates," essentially best-guess extrapolations. As is typical, the authors had given a range of possible outcomes, called a "confidence interval" in statistical language, with cases in schools employing ventilation techniques ranging as high as 3.5 and cases in the no-ventilation schools ranging as low as 3.63. Therefore, it's possible there was basically no difference at all. Similarly, a study in the journal the *Lancet*, preliminarily published in fall of 2022, could not find a consistent effect of ventilation on the number of cases in Dutch schools. Two-and-a-half years into the pandemic, by all accounts, these were the only two comparative studies on ventilation in schools. The results did not suggest there was a meaningful effect.

The Hopkins report also stated: "School systems should use . . . ultraviolet germicidal irradiation." The citation given for this claim was a CDC/NIOSH report on UVGI used for tuberculosis in healthcare facilities. My query to the authors about how UVGI use in a healthcare facility for a bacterial infection could be extrapolated to the efficacy and safety of using this intervention on SARS-CoV-2 in schools went unanswered. And the report stated: "If schools only have natural ventilation, HVAC systems should be installed." My query about what empirical or real-world evidence there is that schools using natural ventilation would benefit from installing HVAC systems for reducing the spread of SARS-CoV-2 also went unanswered. The *MMWR* study referenced earlier is the only one of relevance I am aware of on this point. It did look at HEPA filters and open windows *together* as an intervention but the outcomes were only compared to doing nothing at all, versus being compared to only opening windows.

White papers like the Hopkins report are often important and influential because they form the foundation of scientific knowledge on a particular topic that researchers cite for years to come and, ultimately, filter up to policy makers. Major scholarly reports like this are not always cited by the media or known to the public, but they influence policy makers and professionals within the field, who in turn speak to the media, consult for school districts and teachers unions, and communicate directly with large audiences on social media. The academics who write these reports also use their authorship as a credential demonstrating expertise to consult to lawmakers and others. And it is extremely unlikely that state or local officials fact-check claims in scholarly papers, as I've done here. Several infectious diseases experts told me that no officials for whom they consulted ever questioned the citations or methodologies in their papers.

Experts were welcome to *infer* that there would be a reduction in transmission from HEPA filters, but, as I've detailed extensively, inferences without direct data in medicine and public health are wrong with great frequency. It seemed obvious to allergists that to "play it safe" infants shouldn't be given any peanut-derived food. It seemed obvious that convalescent plasma would help COVID patients. It seemed obvious that adults at risk of cardiovascular adverse events should take a daily low-dose aspirin. That is until evidence showed adults over sixty initiating this practice did not prevent fatal heart attacks or strokes, and increased the risk of internal bleeding. This isn't to suggest that HEPA filters would cause direct harm, but without any evidence of a quantifiable benefit the most that experts should have said was, "It appears this intervention works in healthcare environments, we think that benefit might translate to schools, but we don't know whether it will or to what extent."

HEPA filters, insofar as the money for them wasn't diverted from other important repairs or services for schools or children, even without quantifiable evidence of transmission reduction are most likely a net good. Who wouldn't want clean air? But in all but the rarest circumstances, resources are always finite, and when money and attention are committed to one endeavor they are diverted from something else. So having robust data on the effectiveness of an intervention is critical. Perhaps the money spent on HEPA filters and the like could have been put to more effective use elsewhere. More problematically, unverified, unquantifiable claims about windows, and more broadly about the necessity of ventilation upgrades that unions, politicians and others made—which also happened to go against what was seen in Europe—were used to prevent schools from opening. Evidence matters.

I focused on this one report because its numerous claims without evidence are emblematic of a larger phenomenon I witnessed over and over as I did research during the pandemic. It's distressingly similar to the Russian doll experience of citations in the epidemiological models. This happened in scholarly reports such as the Hopkins one, studies in the CDC journal *MMWR*, and in peer-reviewed papers in other journals. It's hard to overstate how pervasive this practice is, and for someone not in the academy it's a phenomenon by which I am still shocked and disappointed.

But when I asked a number of my sources—infectious diseases doctors, epidemiologists, a statistician, an oncologist, who all regularly publish research—about the practice of making claims without evidence I was met with a mix of bemused shrugs and resigned disgust. But what about peer review? "Reviewers don't click on citations," a source told me with a laugh. Indeed, there is a wealth of disquieting research that shows, for a variety of reasons—from clubbiness in certain specialties in which it's often likely for reviewers to have a bias toward agreeing with the findings of the paper they're reviewing, to the fact that review is generally unpaid and laborious and, as such, reviewers simply are unlikely to invest the time necessary to inspect every claim and citation—though peer review can perform an important function, it often does not deserve the imprimatur of "quality" that much of the public associates with it. Multiple experiments have even shown that a large portion of peer reviewers did not catch purposefully inserted overt falsities in scholarly papers.

The Hopkins report epitomizes a system of how credentialed experts can make claims without evidence yet not be called out for them. These unsupported claims, made in scholarly reports and in papers published in scientific journals, formed the foundation of "truth" upon which, at least in part, policies on NPIs for schools came to be suggested, required, and implemented.

And, as the Kim Prather tweets show—and her comments were far from an anomaly among public health professionals—to question the transmission reduction benefit of a HEPA filter or other interventions in schools was to risk being demonized as a "science denier." Journalists like me, and scientists or researchers from other disciplines, like the economist Emily Oster, were told to "stay in your lane," and not question the experts.

*   *   *

For each intervention cited—HEPA filters, masks, barriers, six feet of distancing, or closures—the fallacy was two-layered: first there was no direct or quantifiable evidence to begin with that it would be advantageous. Swiss cheese is not EBM. You don't do a whole bunch of stuff, not know which thing works, and keep saying month after month that we must continue doing it all. A doctor doesn't give a patient a medicine cabinet's worth of pills and say, "I don't know which of these will help you, but for the next year just keep taking all of them. Oh, and I know they each have a cost and side effects but, trust me, it's worth it." Second, we had real-world evidence from Europe that showed the *absence* of these interventions did not lead to any clinically significant rise in transmission. Yet all of these measures were still insisted upon. Worse, claims about Europe controlling the virus as the reason it earned the privilege to open schools were baldly untrue, as a simple comparison of case rates in different cities and regions in Europe and the US at the same time, as I did earlier in the book, makes clear.

In summary, the long list of claims, the filibuster of excuses about why schools could not open that were made repeatedly by politicians, union leaders, influencers, the media, and health authorities—and others in the medical field who had no expertise on viral transmission or mitigation, but whom journalists treated as experts anyway—was a systematic fiction.

Even more than two years later, in the fall of 2022, after the reckoning of abysmal academic outcomes from school closures became an acceptable admission in polite society, many epidemiologists, other public health professionals, and pundits simply framed this as the unfortunate consequence of a wrenching decision between saving lives from COVID or harming kids by keeping them out of school. But this damned if you do, damned if you don't narrative was a false binary, representing a fundamental misunderstanding about the lack of benefit of school closures. Much of Europe, and many areas in the US where schools were kept open the longest in aggregate, suffered no greater numbers of cases, or subsequent morbidity and mortality, than areas where schools were closed the longest.

15

GROUPTHINK

There certainly is a wide range of school and community conditions throughout the US and Europe. And different researchers are going to run analyses of varying pandemic data on schools and children and transmission for years, possibly even decades to come, and they will find endless different results, since any retrospective study will be designed, purposefully or not, to tease out different effects. What is clear, though, is that it was observable in real time that the schools in Europe did not drive transmission in their countries. Nothing overt happened, despite tens of millions of children being in school. And, as I detailed earlier, the schools there were not so different from those in the US in any meaningful epidemiological way. For a new drug or an intervention—in this case, school closures—to be implemented the effect size needs to be sufficiently large as to clearly offset whatever costs might be incurred. With the observational data from Europe it was clear that the intervention of school closures failed that test. The question is why—after it was clear the intervention was a failure, after it was clear that open schools did not lead to calamity, indeed after it was clear that primary schools in Sweden, with more than a million students who attended without interruption, with a population density and community case rates in Stockholm on par with or higher than in much of the US, did not lead to an elevated rate of infection among teachers versus other professionals, and, through the middle of June, out of 1.8 million children under the age of sixteen, there were zero deaths and a total of eight children who went to the ICU with COVID—the obvious evidence regarding children and schools was ignored, waved away, and pretended into non-existence, and not just by journalists who were too biased or incompetent or by politicians who were too partisan, but by the experts, namely the academics, the scholars, the scientists.

The seventeenth-century artist Johannes Vermeer is one of the most celebrated painters of the Dutch Golden Age. Most readers are likely familiar with *Girl with a Pearl Earring*, his most famous work and considered his masterpiece, although all of his paintings are extraordinarily valuable, hanging in the world's top museums, studied by art professionals, and selling in private hands for many millions of dollars. In the 1930s and 1940s a number of new Vermeers surfaced, selling for around $30 million in today's money. In 1937, an eminent Dutch art historian proclaimed one of the newfound works, *The Supper at Emmaus*, to be the artist's greatest painting. Dutch art experts, along with critics and admirers around the world, swooned. *Emmaus* and some of the other new works were special. Unlike most of Vermeer's works, which tended to be small and depicting middle class life, enlivened with bright colors and flooded with light, the newly discovered works were often huge and had a darker quality and religious subject matter. In 1945 the truth came out: *Emmaus* was a fake, as were all the other "new" Vermeers. This was revealed not because the art world figured it out, but only because the forger confessed to the crime so he wouldn't be punished for treason for having sold a prized "Vermeer" to Hermann Goering, the infamous Nazi official. (The forger claimed he was a hero for ripping off Goering.) For eight years, paintings that even people who were not aficionados could plainly see looked nothing like the oeuvre of Vermeer were nonetheless lauded by experts, and in turn much of society, as creations of the Dutch master.

Dr. Robert McNutt is an internal medicine physician, oncologist, a National Library of Medicine fellow with a focus on decision analysis, a director of several programs for the Society of Medical Decision Making, an instructor of evidence-based medicine, and was an associate editor at *JAMA*, the *Journal of the American Medical Association*, for nearly twenty years. I got connected with McNutt and a small group of EBM experts via Dr. Rita Redberg, the editor in chief of *JAMA Internal Medicine*, when I inquired with her about the "Less Is More" series in the journal, which exposes the harms of implementing medical practices that lack sufficient evidence of benefit. I wanted to gain insights into how so many American medical and public health professionals not just went along with but vigorously advocated for an intervention—school closures, and, more broadly, the Swiss cheese of other NPIs on children—when there was no quality evidence of benefit, there was known evidence of harm, and there was real-world evidence of no effect (from Europe). "One of the reasons I wrote back to you is I was worried you are going down a path without knowing the past decision making that's occurred," McNutt said to me during a several-hours-long interview. The phenomenon you are describing about schools, he said, "we've been doing forever." The surprise isn't that this happened, he explained, it's that it doesn't happen even more often. Part of my error was that I approached what happened with American schools and children with a sense of surreality, an assumption that the dynamic at play, whether more broadly or just through the lens of public health, was a terrible fluke, an anomaly.

"Look, Dave, this isn't new," he continued. "For more than seventy-five years we did radical mastectomies on women out of theory. I lived with the experience of many patients, taking off breasts, muscle, fascia, lymph nodes—we did it without a shred of evidence." Many women were so damaged after the surgery they even had trouble moving their arms because of all the chest muscle that was cut out. For the better part of a century this act of ravage, perpetrated with the best of intentions, continued until a surgeon named Dr. Bernard Fisher questioned the practice; he had seen how cancer spread throughout the body early in the course of the disease, which indicated that removing so much tissue near the tumor was not likely bringing any benefit in exchange for the horrible disfigurement it caused. A large number of surgeons at the time thought Fisher's idea was so wrong that it was unethical, and that to do anything less than a radical mastectomy was malpractice. Fisher forged ahead and ran a randomized trial, which showed that, indeed, women who underwent the comparatively minor "simple" mastectomy, which was far less invasive, lived just as long as those who had undergone radical mastectomies. The result was so clear that the trial shut down after two years. "And yet it still took ten years after Fisher's trial for the practice to entirely wind down." McNutt said that the medical and public health community do things "all the time" without evidence, and that that doesn't stop the experts from insisting the practices are correct and repudiating anyone who disagrees. McNutt regaled and horrified me with a long list of

examples of consensus standards of care, from estrogen therapy to pros-
tate cancer treatments, in which even observing the great harm these
interventions caused, the mere suggestion that more robust evidence was
needed for them to continue was met with scorn, only for the practice to
ultimately change after proper evidence was accrued.

Unlike art critics or surgical oncologists, where the groupthink divorced
from evidence was relatively confined to the experts, for school closures
and the various mitigations imposed on kids the groupthink would need
to extend far beyond. Preventing fifty million children from attending
school, some of them for an entire year, and when they finally were in
the buildings mandating compliance with any number of unproven measures that didn't allow a child to put an arm around a friend's shoulder or
seeing one another's faces, would require more than just the experts. This
was a societal phenomenon that needed buy-in from the media and the
cultural elite. There was one key dynamic that allowed this to happen in
the US: the ideological homogeneity among public health professionals,
media professionals, and much of the influencer class.

Positions on radical mastectomies and peanut allergies are not associated with a political viewpoint. But views on school closures and mitigations were tightly aligned with either Republicans or Democrats, and
that matters significantly when deconstructing the decisions behind the
policies. It is important to note that there was nothing inherently progressive about pushing for school closures and maximizing mitigations
imposed on children. With arguable exceptions, almost all of western
and northern Europe, even the countries with conservative parties in
power at a given time, are far more politically progressive than the US,
and yet, by and large, they opened schools earlier, longer, and with far
fewer restrictions than did the US. Conversely, the conservative party in
Sweden pushed for more restrictions in that country. Israel, which was
led for the first year of the pandemic by Benjamin Netanyahu, a right-
leaning politician, had fairly strict social distancing rules in comparison
to those in much of the US. Australia, which was governed through spring
2022 by Scott Morrison, the head of his country's center-right political
party, famously was perhaps the most tightly locked-down democracy
in the world. Seen through this international lens, the US progressives'
adamance and near uniformity in backing school closures and harsher

mitigation measures takes on an unmistakable tribal hue rather than an ideological one.

In our hyper-partisan domestic climate, shared political beliefs fueled a sort of exclusionary esprit de corps, predisposing the members of powerful factions of society—media and public health professionals and left-leaning influencers—to see and then position the NPIs, in particular as they related to schools, as oppositional to Trump and Republicans. In so doing the overall cohesion of the group, and individually one's in-group identity and status, were reinforced. The public health establishment was like a company selling a product it believed was excellent, even though it wasn't, and the media and cultural elite ran the most expensive public relations campaign in history for it for free.

Through the fallacy of inductive reasoning, and through groupthink, seemingly most of these people *believed* in the righteousness of their position, data be damned. Collective delusions are as old as time, in part because they foster social cohesion. The nineteenth-century French sociologist Émile Durkheim wrote of this phenomenon in his examination of the origins of religion. One's commitment to a group's outlandish beliefs affirms their membership in the group.

Further, to maintain that belief, and strengthen bonds and enthusiasm within the group, there must be an out-group to blame and vilify. There is a dense literature, from historians to wildlife researchers, observing the effect on in-group cohesion by members uniting against a common enemy. This practice is so deeply embedded in the basic functions of primate society that it's even seen outside of humans, in chimpanzees.

Jonathan Haidt, the social psychologist, has said about tribalism that it's an "us against them mindset. We evolved for war," he explained, "and as soon as the war is declared there can be no nuance." Haidt gave the anecdote of George Orwell in the 1930s in the lead up to World War II. Paraphrasing Orwell, he said, "If you write about problems of British slums suddenly you're giving fuel to the Nazis."

Many times after one of my articles that was critical of mitigations or, later, pediatric vaccine mandates, published I would get an alarmed reaction from certain friends or journalists: "But this is going to give fuel to the Trumpers!" or "What about the anti-vaxxers?!" Conspicuously, they didn't say that the evidence I presented was incorrect.

In short, between rampant tribalism, and the motivated and inductive reasoning that coupled with it, many people seemed emotionally and intellectually incapable of tolerating agreeing with people they found to be odious. To do so would mean to suffer a sort of moral injury, an internally directed guilt by association that threatened people's very identities and sense of self.

* * *

While legacy media outlets, in particular the *Times*, carried enormous influence on the narrative around schools and risks toward children, social media, and its use by the influencer class, played a critical role as well. Over and over, when prominent conservatives made statements about schools and children, they were often viewed and portrayed in the most uncharitable and often baldly misleading light. (Dishonorable behavior of course is not exclusive to one side. But the Left dominates the public health establishment, prestige media, and professional class. Acting in concert—as a tribe, if you will—and aided by social media, these powerful factions exerted considerable control over school policy and the public narrative around it, in part by distorting statements from and demonizing the opposition.) An episode early in the pandemic, in April of 2020, was one of the first examples of this phenomenon, setting the template for untold iterations to come over the following two years.

Dr. Mehmet Oz, the cardiothoracic surgeon and celebrity TV doctor with a penchant for hawking "miracle" pills like those made from green coffee bean extract, had already long been mocked and disliked by the liberal elite. But near the onset of the pandemic he had also become more of a conservative darling as he expressed optimism about hydroxychloroquine as a COVID treatment, and was reportedly a source of pandemic guidance for Trump. Then, during an April 15 interview on FOX, he apparently said something monstrous.

As was widely quoted, Oz said we should open schools because only 2 to 3 percent of kids would die. Predictably, social media exploded in a spasm of horrified indignation. "I am wondering if Dr Oz would say this if it was his own kids were part of the 2–3%. . . . How morally outrageous of someone who says he is a doctor," tweeted Randi Weingarten, the head of the AFT. Joe Scarborough, the cable TV news host, said on his show before playing the clip, "Here's Dr Oz saying 'yeah, kids are going to die.'" Then after the clip ran Scarborough said, "Two to three percent mortality *for our children*? My God." Soledad O'Brien, another television newsperson, called the comments "insane." And so on.

Except Oz did not say 2 to 3 percent of children would die from opening school. This is what Oz said: "We need our mojo back. Let's start with things that are really critical to the nation, where we think we might be able to open without getting into a lot of trouble. Schools are a very appetizing opportunity. I just saw a nice piece in the *Lancet* arguing that opening schools may only cost us 2 to 3 percent in terms of total mortality . . . to get every child back into a school where they are safely being educated, being fed, with a theoretical risk on the backside, might be a tradeoff some folks might consider."

It needs to be said that Oz did an absolutely terrible job of relaying the findings from the *Lancet* paper. The relevant text in the paper, which itself was referring to a model, suggested that school closures as an isolated measure, with no other NPIs, would only reduce overall COVID mortality by 2 to 4 percent. This of course is different from saying opening schools would "cost" us 2 to 3 percent in total mortality. Regardless, Oz never said anything about opening schools leading to the deaths of 2 to 3 percent of children. (Fun side note: the model referenced in the *Lancet* paper was none other than Report 9 from Imperial College London, which, as you surely recall, was built on some dubious assumptions.) Oz's broader point about thinking about trade-offs got lost in the wash of umbrage. So Oz's initial statement—based on a paper referring to a model—was wrong, and then Weingarten, Scarborough (who has an audience in the millions), other influencers, and many tens of thousands of people on Twitter, falsely attributed a totally different statement to him, with performative condemnation, all the while amplifying the falsehood that 2 to 3 percent of children would die if schools opened. It didn't matter that Oz released a mea culpa shortly after the blowup. Influential voices had already projected the lie, and it circulated among the rest of the populace with far more reach and indelibility than Oz's subsequent apology and explanations. The mental model about opening schools leading to deaths had done its damage.

Countless other examples followed, but let's fast forward to the summer, back to the context of Trump's infamous "open the schools" tweet and subsequent news stories on schools. On July 11, a random, nonfamous person tweeted, "So, Betsy DeVos today said 'only' .02% of kids are likely to die when they go back to school. That's 14,740 children." The tweet was liked 234,000 times, and retweeted 67,000 times, eliciting endless comments of incandescent rage. Other people tweeted similar posts, racking up hundreds of thousands of likes and retweets as well. An Olympic athlete, an NFL quarterback (to his 500,000 followers), a New York state assembly member, a Connecticut Congresswoman, the novelist Anne Lamott, the journalist Kurt Eichenwald (to his 489,000 followers) were all among the retweeters. Collectively, more than one million people saw these tweets and others related to the DeVos quote. At the time, I searched and searched for the source for this statement but could not find it. I emailed the person who wrote what, as far as I could gather, was the original tweet, asking where she got the quote, but she never replied. (She deleted the tweet sometime after my email.) While DeVos certainly had advocated vigorously for schools to be open, like Oz, an incendiary statement that she never made was attributed to her.

An internet fact-checking website called truthorfiction.com pieced together what may have been the source—a thread on Reddit that misattributed a quote from Deborah Birx to DeVos. Further, the Birx quote was, "We know the mortality rate in [people] under 25 from the CDC data is less than .1 percent." Neither Birx nor DeVos said anything remotely resembling the statement that "only .02 percent of kids" were likely to die if they went back to school. As it was with the Oz debacle, the frenzy around the fabrication led to two results: it vilified the enemy, helping to further cement in-group cohesion, and it circulated a falsehood that hyperbolized the danger of opening schools.

Perhaps inevitably, this telephone game with a one-way distortion also had a two-participant version, from New York to Washington. The same week that the DeVos meme blanketed Twitter, the *Times* published a piece titled "As Trump Demanded Schools Reopen, His Experts Warned of 'Highest Risk.'" What the title didn't explain was that Trump wasn't quite warned by "his experts"; the highest risk "warning" was already known in publicly available CDC documents. Further, the CDC had created categories of risk—lowest, more, highest—with the last one meaning opening schools with no mitigations at all. It did not mean, as the headline implied, that the mere act of opening schools was the "highest risk" action relative to opening other aspects of society. Two days after the *Times* piece, Speaker of the House Nancy Pelosi said on CNN that going back to school presented "the biggest risk for the spread of the coronavirus." It's possible Pelosi just made this up or had some other absurdly erroneous source, but its similarity to the *Times* headline was uncanny. Either way, the *Times* headline and Pelosi both perpetuated the same falsehood.

When a group is primed to believe the worst of its perceived enemy, and motivated to diminish them, the easy spread of false and damning information about them is inevitable. Unfortunately for American kids, this meant often benign and reasonable statements about schools from influential figures on the Right were—purposefully or not—distorted by the media and the cultural elite on the Left to fit their accepted yet untrue narrative that opening schools put children and others in grave danger.

Beyond the framing by legacy news outlets and within social media, attacking Trump's stance to open schools became a visible touchstone of Democrats' election strategy. The Biden campaign ran numerous ads with ominous music in the background warning that Trump made "our kids not safe in school" but that he was forcing the schools to open anyway, "risking teachers' and parents' lives." This was not March 2020. This was after tens of millions of children had already been back in school in Europe without any meaningful effect.

A highly partisan and influential left-wing political action committee called Meidas Touch, with more than 1 million Twitter followers and an ad budget that exceeded $1 million, started a campaign with the hashtag #ProtectOurKids. An ad from the group begins with slow-motion scenes of children entering schools. *If Trump gets his way what will happen to our kids?* appears on screen. The video then smash cuts to thunderous music and chaotic scenes of people in the back of ambulances and patients on stretchers, with IV bags astride, being wheeled urgently down hospital halls by teams of worried medical professionals. The music and scenes flicker in rapid-fire succession with a swelling cacophony of beeping medical machines and sirens, until the video cuts to black and the words

"We must protect our children" appear on-screen while the sustained *eeeeee* of a flatlined EKG takes over the soundtrack.

Political advertisements of course are not known for subtlety or honesty. But the absurd and manipulative exaggeration of risks around schools and children in these ads was weaponized to a degree that even for health professionals with just a modicum of knowledge would have been hard to countenance. Yet health officials did not, nor did the medical establishment, nor did the legacy media, come out forcefully to debunk this narrative from Democrats.

16

THE MEDIA, PART III

Many of the claims that journalists, politicians, union leaders, influencers, and public health authorities had been making about schools were statements of conjecture. They were alarmed predictions about what would purportedly happen if schools opened without the necessary conditions for it to be "safe." But by the end of July there was an important shift: no longer was the public only hearing about hypothetical horrors that would occur if kids were allowed to congregate and schools opened. Now they were being fed reported horrors of actual events. There were three pivotal news stories that summer that, to be crass for a moment, scared the shit out of parents around the country, created an instant association in their minds of schools being dangerous, and offered talking points to anyone who wanted to argue that schools weren't safe at all, or weren't safe without some layers of Swiss cheese.

Yet in each of the three news stories, it should come as no surprise now, there were egregious errors and faulty framing, and they all went in one direction: more fear, more risk to children, more impending harm related to schools. Each exemplifies how, through basic errors in looking at evidence and how it was depicted, deeply misleading narratives were formed. Worse still, those false and scary narratives quickly ossified in the minds of the public, helping to prevent schools from opening.

On July 18 the *Times* ran a feature titled "Older Children Spread the Coronavirus Just as Much as Adults, Large Study Finds," with the subheading, "The Study of Nearly 65,000 People in South Korea Suggests That School Reopenings Will Trigger More Outbreaks." Needless to say, without even reading the main text the message was clear. The article, by Apoorva Mandavilli, said the study found that children "between the ages of 10 and 19 can spread the virus at least as well as adults do." She went on to warn that once schools reopened communities could expect to see clusters of infections take root. Dr. Ashish Jha, at the time at Harvard, and later Biden's coronavirus response coordinator, was quoted as saying the study was very carefully done. Middle and high schoolers were more likely to infect others than adults, the article stated. Predictably, the article said schools needed to implement physical distancing and masks. It ended by presenting the opening of schools as a dichotomy— children shouldn't miss out on education and socialization but districts had the "unenviable task" of choosing between the kids' needs or lower transmission.

The article rocketed around Twitter and Facebook. This was the evidence proving what so many people had suspected and feared—opening schools was going to be a disaster. TV doctors, like Leana Wen, a former head of Planned Parenthood turned COVID pundit, who made frequent appearances on CNN before ultimately becoming an analyst for the network, tweeted the article. Randi Weingarten, expectedly, tweeted the article, saying that we could not afford for leaders to act as if schoolchildren "cannot be super spreaders." High-profile Democrats, such as Nikki Fried, who later would run for governor of Florida, tweeted the article and wrote that "Forcing schools to reopen is dangerous and puts our kids, parents, and teachers at risk." Journalists, celebrities like Mia Farrow, and others spread the article. At least one school district, Charlotte-Mecklenburg, North Carolina, the seventeenth-largest in the nation, with 140,000 students, had approved some in-person schooling for the start of the school year but switched the plan to full remote learning, citing the *Times* article specifically as part of the reason for the change. There were reports of other school districts as well canceling in-person schooling because of coverage of the South Korea study.

Yet the study came under immediate criticism from a number of specialists from around the globe, including Dr. Alasdair Munro, a prominent pediatric infectious diseases physician in the UK, who had publicly called out Mandavilli before when she touted dubious findings from the unpublished article about viral loads in children. On its face the data didn't make sense; it showed that kids through age nine had the lowest infectiousness, then ten- to nineteen-year-olds had the highest, then it dropped back down in the twenty to twenty-nine age group. There was no logical explanation for the rate of infectiousness to jump from lowest to highest in one age bracket. A finding like this usually suggests what's known as "confounding"—extraneous variables that distort outcomes because they were not controlled for in the study. As Munro explained in a Twitter thread, there were only a very small number of children as the index case, which could allow an anomaly to skew the results. And nearly every secondary case (the person who ostensibly got infected by the child index case) shared the initial exposure. It's just that the children developed symptoms first so they were assumed to be the spreader. Joseph Allen, a professor at Harvard's school of public health, also took issue with the conclusion. He pointed out that the study's data showed that ten- to nineteen-year-olds were *half as likely* to transmit as adults outside the home, which was the relevant statistic, not in-home transmission, if you're worried about schools.

Zeynep Tufekci, a sociologist and frequent writer for the *Times* herself, later tweeted that it was unfortunate the South Korea story got such "widespread coverage that I'm aware of parents ready to keep their 10-year old under literal house arrest for the next year, simply because of that. This is extremely damaging to children, especially since the 10–19 age group wasn't informative." In a separate thread, Dr. Muge Cevik, an infectious diseases and virology specialist at the University of St. Andrews, in Scotland, tweeted: "This nyt article sadly created a lot of social media traction but it was clear from the start this study was never designed to answer the infectiousness question." And Tufekci added, "This study, and the rushed, sensational reporting around it, more than almost any other, single-handedly caused so many schools who were equipped and ready to shut down and parents to keep kids home, in my observation. Correction will reach almost nobody and damage is done." Tufekci also cautioned against journalists publishing articles on studies immediately after they were released. Had Mandavilli and other journalists waited briefly before writing their articles, and seen the critiques that came out very quickly after the study's publication, or if they had more critically read the study themselves, they (hopefully) would have written about the study differently, or not at all. As it was, Mandavilli's article, and similar uncritical coverage of this manifestly flawed study, directly led to children being prevented from attending school.

But the story doesn't end here. The authors of the Korean study released a second paper in August that essentially walked back the findings from the first study, drawing a conclusion similar to what Munro had written about. To Mandavilli's credit, she wrote about the follow-up study. Unfortunately, as is the nature of news, corrections and retractions and follow-up pieces rarely have the impact of the initial story. The headlines are rarely as enticing. Beyond that, there also is little doubt that the South Korea news, which was the first major story on pediatric transmission, and in particular explicitly tied to the prospect of opening schools, triggered a phenomenon called the "primacy effect." This is a well-documented cognitive bias that shows people have a tendency to remember the first piece of information they receive more than subsequent information. And the primacy effect dovetails with what's known as an "anchoring bias," in which people's decision-making is overly influenced—or "anchored"—by the first piece of information they learn, even to the point of overriding newer, conflicting information. (This is why first impressions are so important. In general it's very hard for us to change our minds.) The initial article, and the false message about kids being superspreaders, were what stuck in people's minds. The school board in North Carolina did not reverse its decision. The damage was done.

The Korea study fiasco is merely an example of the overarching primacy effect and anchoring bias that launched with the pandemic. In January and February, Americans saw images of dead bodies lying in the streets of Wuhan. Then they heard terrifying news about hospitals in Italy, and then in New York City being overrun, or close to it. To a large degree, subsequent statistics about children's low risk didn't matter. The early images and stories anchored people's *feelings* about COVID. Also, recall the Philadelphia versus St. Louis meme. It incorrectly portrayed the effectiveness of NPIs, and specifically school closures, over the long term. But the simplistic lesson, complete with the visualization of the cities' differing epidemiological trajectories, anchored itself in the minds of many Americans. Despite copious evidence seen in real time that, on average, areas with open schools did not have higher case rates than areas with closed schools, many people continued to argue and *believe* that the Philly versus St. Louis "lesson" still held.

Two other stories, both relating to "outbreaks," finish off the trilogy of extremely influential, yet wildly misleading and incendiary news narratives that summer that further inflamed fears about schools.

On July 31 news of an outbreak at a Georgia summer camp, detailed in a CDC report, burst into the public consciousness. It was covered by every major print and web outlet in the country, from the *Times* to *People* magazine, every network TV news broadcast, the morning news shows, and it blanketed social media. The thrust of the story was that hundreds of campers were infected, and that, in part, not wearing masks was to blame. The virus "blazed" through the camp, as the *Times* put it, infecting nearly half the campers and staffers. The *Times* quoted the chief health officer at the University of Michigan describing the outbreak as a "cautionary tale." A piece in the *Washington Post* on the camp story quoted Andrew Noymer, an epidemiologist at the University of California at Irvine: "To me, this is a significant weight added to the side of the scale that says close the schools." On MSNBC, an emergency medicine doctor named Uché Blackstock, after referring to the Georgia camp, told viewers, "Right now, going to school shouldn't be an option." A CNN report said the outbreak could have implications for schools reopening. Chris Lu, a former Obama cabinet member, who would become a member of Biden's transition team that fall, tweeted a link to an article on the outbreak and wrote, "This is an ominous sign for schools in the fall." And so on.

My kids, along with millions of others, had been at camp for more than a month. They played with other children from early morning until late afternoon. They never wore masks. After months of isolation and endless hours of screen time, they could be kids again, and they finally started to seem like their old selves. Other than the counselors, who all wore masks, and the fact that parents had to drop off and pick up their kids since the usual bus service was canceled out of fears of COVID transmission, their days were pretty close to normal. I was so happy to see them revived, and knowing they were running around and socializing with peers, I even found myself singing along to the Taylor Swift songs we blasted on the drive to camp each morning. This was just day camp, but I also knew of kids at sleep-away camp. And summer had gone without issue for all of them as well.

This brought into focus the deep illogic and injury of the Georgia camp story, which can be summarized with a phrase that became popular among myself and some critics of the media's coverage of the pandemic, in particular as it related to kids: It was a "case of the missing denominator." The Georgia camp outbreak was presented as a terror-inducing omen. People who had been fixated on children as drivers of transmission had their "See, we knew it!" moment. What the Georgia story actually showed was that, by and large, camps were operating just fine. Could there be an outbreak at a camp or school? Of course! There likely were others besides the one in Georgia that were smaller and weren't noticed due to a lack of testing and asymptomatic cases. This made the news because it was unusual. We had a tiny numerator with a magnifying glass on it, and an absolutely massive denominator—millions of children in camp without issue—that was ignored.

And here Emily Oster, the Brown economist who collected data on daycares, returns to our story. Unlike the federal government, which reported on an anecdote of one camp, Oster compiled data on many camps. Again, like the daycare data, these data had limitations, and were better considered as information gathering than a proper representative sample. Nevertheless, the data were sizable and useful to get a general idea of what was going on. If there was a large effect size, it would show up in a sample this big. What did Oster's data show? The number of participating camps shifted over time, but during July, when there were the most participants, out of a peak of 8,645 campers and 2,857 staff, there was a total of 4 cases of COVID among campers, and 10 cases among staff over the entire month. Oster's data supported what I saw with my own kids and knew anecdotally from friends. Camps, regardless of mask policies, were not typically sources of outbreaks. As a case study, the CDC paper on the Georgia camp was interesting, but it wasn't informative about camps overall, or about the effect of mitigations. Oster's data suggested that kids being together all day, outside, without masks was a low risk of transmission activity. There was nothing about the Georgia camp outbreak that could be seen as predictive of what would happen in schools in general.

But what about data specifically on schools? This brings us to our third example of deeply misleading—and damaging—narratives. In late spring, a spate of articles began to flood the media describing the "disaster" that took place in Israel when that country reopened all of its schools in late May. The trend of these articles reached its zenith on August 4, when the *Times* ran a major piece titled, "When COVID Subsided, Israel Reopened Its Schools. It Didn't Go Well." To hammer home the message, the subtitle was "As Countries Consider Back-to-School Strategies for the Fall, a Coronavirus Outbreak at a Jerusalem High School Offers a Cautionary Tale." The article, based on a study that had been released two weeks earlier, was coauthored by a Jerusalem correspondent and Pam Belluck, one of the authors of the July 11 piece on "what other countries can teach us" about opening schools. The *Times* Israel article, tweeted by politicians, a torrent of journalists, and, naturally, Randi Weingarten ("Israel opened schools the way Trump wants. It failed"), begins:

As the United States and other countries anxiously consider how to reopen schools, Israel, one of the first countries to do so, illustrates the dangers of moving too precipitously.

The article went on to describe an outbreak at a Jerusalem high school that infected 154 students and 26 staff members. Because of a heat wave the government had exempted schoolchildren from wearing face masks, which was a decision that "proved disastrous," the article said, turning the school into "a petri dish for COVID-19."

But, like the Georgia camp outbreak, the lesson to be learned was the opposite of what the public health officials and the media had portrayed. If not wearing masks was so "disastrous," if this intervention was so critical for controlling transmission in schools, why weren't there large outbreaks at schools all over Israel, which has more than 3 million children under the age of eighteen? Or at least a few dozen outbreaks, or even ten similar to the one at the Jerusalem high school? There were, of course, other cases among children in the country. The *Wall Street Journal* reported on June 3 that at least 261 students and faculty were infected in Israel. But these were not explosive numbers considering the population size.

Again, as with the Georgia school narrative, all the attention was on the numerator (the outlier event) and not on the denominator (the 3 million children). Out of that many schoolchildren it would be bizarre if there weren't an outbreak. The fact that there weren't twenty or a hundred outbreaks similar to the Jerusalem school was the real story. An alternate title to the *Times* piece could have been: "Israel Reopened Its Schools. It Was a Success. Out of More Than 3 Million Children, Just One Known Large Outbreak."

There is an even bigger problem with the framing of the Israeli school outbreak and the broader news coverage that had pinned a rise in Israeli cases to schools. The framing neglected to contextualize that Israel relaxed restrictions across the entire country at the same time it opened schools. Malls, markets, restaurants, bars, and beauty parlors all opened. The *Times* piece mentioned that these other aspects of society had been released from the lockdown, and that Netanyahu told Israelis to grab a beer and "go out and have a good time." But other than that brief passage the piece was centered on the school outbreak.

A *Wall Street Journal* piece from July had a title that warned "Israelis Fear Schools Reopened Too Soon." The piece quoted an Israeli government adviser who said that since many things opened at once it was "difficult to disentangle the effect of each separately." But this detail, like the brief section in the *Times* article, was clearly positioned tangentially. The thrust of the media coverage, as seen in the headlines of dozens of stories, was about how schools were the source of the rise in cases in Israel. This would be like opening ten floodgates in a dam, then pointing to only one of those ten gates and saying, "This gate is causing the water to rise." Moreover, it was possible, even likely, that that gate had less water passing through it than some of the other gates. The crystallization of this bias can be seen in a tweet by Nobel laureate and *New York Times* opinion writer Paul Krugman, shared with his several million followers. On August 1, 2020, Krugman tweeted: "One of the defining features of the US COVID debacle has been refusal to learn from other countries. Now, as much of the country prepares to open schools, we should—but won't—look at what happened in Israel."

He then included the following graph:

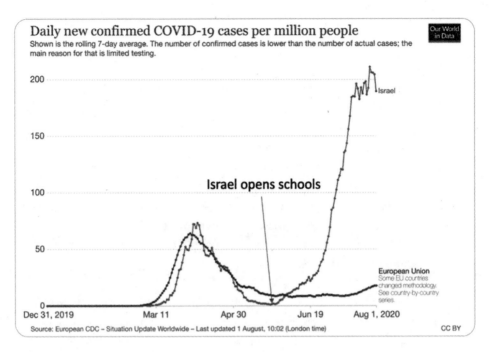

Graph from Paul Krugman's tweet.

It would have been more honest if Krugman had tweeted this instead:

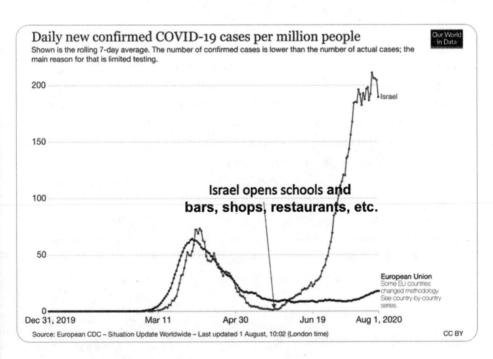

Revised image by David Zweig.

Here is a headline from the *Times of Israel* on May 28, 2020: "Tel Aviv Restaurants, Bars Packed on First Night Open Since Virus Shutdown." The situation couldn't have been clearer. Yet in the months that followed, Krugman, along with the media, and comments from many public health officials, made a strangely selective causal inference related to one specific part of society—schools—that reopened while disregarding all of the other parts of society that reopened. The narrative about Israeli schools was blatantly specious, yet it was so alluring that it was amplified by influencers like Krugman and media outlets from the *Times* on down. And it functioned as a story for people to channel an incredulous indignation at the US's foolishness for not learning this purportedly obvious lesson.

Beyond that, even my revised graph, which includes many aspects of society that had reopened, is misleading. It merely shows an association between the reopening and an increase in cases, not a causation. If you were to look at a graph with the same dates as the Krugman graph, that showed cases in Florida, where, like the rest of America, schools were closed in May, June, and July, you would see that it followed a similar trajectory to Israel, staying low through the end of May and then peaking in mid- to late July. California, the most restricted state in the country, with maximum mask compliance and the most closures, generally followed this trajectory as well, with cases peaking in late July. In summary: there were any number of different countries and different states, each operating under very different circumstances, yet they nevertheless all followed roughly the same epi curve of cases during these months. That correlation does not equal causation is a banal truism. Yet the media, and even celebrated public intellectuals, fell prey to equating the two.

The Israeli schools narrative was simplistic, seductive, and wrong. At the time, a number of professionals, from economists to physicians, pointed out Krugman's faulty reasoning, but he never replied or updated the tweet.

There are two more factors in the *Times* piece on the Israeli school outbreak that are worth highlighting briefly because they exemplify larger phenomena. First, in the piece, Pam Belluck, as she had done in her previous reporting, referred to unnamed "experts" who said schools needed mask mandates, desks six feet apart, smaller class sizes, and ventilation, and that these interventions were "likely to be crucial," for a safe opening.

She said the experts "coalesced around a set of guidelines." Yet she provided no evidence behind the experts' claims. The country, and much of the world, had reverted to "expert opinion"—the lowest form of evidence possible—and journalists, such as Belluck, though she was far from alone, and politicians often presented the opinions as evidentiary fact.

Second, not only was no evidence provided behind the expert claims in Belluck's article, but readers were implicitly being told to value opinion from an "authority" over actual evidence from the real world to the contrary—millions of European kids, many without masks or six feet of distancing, who had attended school that spring without noticeable consequences. It was an egregious example of the "appeal to authority" fallacy, also known as an "argument from authority," which I described earlier. This brings us back to the wisdom of John Locke. In his treatise, *An Essay Concerning Human Understanding*, Locke discussed several types of argument, including what he called, in Latin, *ad verecundiam*. This translates directly as "to modesty," and it is considered the antecedent to the argument from authority because Locke meant the receiver of the argument was too modest in not challenging the authority. Locke described *ad verecundiam* as regular people being overly deferential to the opinions of those with more status. He wrote that it was considered a "breach of modesty" and even seen as insolent for a man to hold his own opinion "against that of some learned doctor, or otherwise approved writer." Locke did not mean we should never value the opinion of an expert, but he implied that credentials alone are not sufficient for making an argument valid.

To be clear, there are plenty of circumstances where expert opinion or rough consensus should guide policy or action. But if something is merely an opinion without high-quality evidence supporting it, it should be presented as such to the public. If it was made clear that some of the policy prescriptions around schools were based on conjecture, rather than solid evidence, that would have led to a very different dynamic, inviting more open questioning of the cost-benefit of the interventions.

Since much of the public relies on the media for information about policies and practices, journalists have an epistemic duty to investigate on their own or to press the experts they are quoting for the evidence behind their claims. As I've detailed, in many circumstances neither of these functions was performed. Succinctly: there was an astonishing lack of curiosity by professionals whose job is to be curious.

Which raises the question: Why is it that journalists, and the broader educated elite traditionally, or at least ideally, bring great skepticism to the claims made by and the motives of every major institution in society, from religion to big business to government, yet when it came to the pandemic policies espoused by Fauci, the CDC, and the public health establishment—especially on schools and children—in so many instances their skepticism all but vanished? At least some part of this could be explained by tribalism. Like Orwell had observed in World War II, for journalists at prestigious outlets, the majority of whom are politically aligned with those in the public health establishment, investigating or critiquing the policies espoused by the people on their team was tantamount to helping the enemy.

Many in public health shared with their peers in the media this instinct against tolerating any public dissent with the tribe. I directly experienced this phenomenon several times after articles I had written that challenged some of the dogma related to school closures, mitigations, and, later, data on the pediatric vaccines. On two separate occasions, once by a pediatrician, and once by an infectious diseases physician, I was told privately that by my calling attention to the lack of evidence or conflicting evidence for a particular policy I was causing harm by allowing Trumpers to question the CDC. I wasn't wrong, but I was helping the wrong people.

* * *

The second week of August brought a reprise of Georgia as the vilified failure, in this instance in Cherokee County schools, where nearly 1,200 students and staff were quarantined at the start of the district's academic year. The *Times* ran with a (presumably) rhetorical headline following the quarantine statistic: "Is This a Successful Reopening?" Like the camp story, the Georgia school quarantines and cases were national news. Covered not only in the *Times*, but the *Wall Street Journal*, the *Washington Post*, NPR, CNN, CBS, NBC, ABC, *USA Today*, *People*, and so on. Much of the coverage framed the Georgia school openings, which were without mask mandates, as foolish and dangerous, risking lives. Innumerable social media posts shared this view, though with more colorful language. The *Times* article linked to photos and videos taken by students, posted online days earlier, of hallways filled with maskless students, which had gone viral, garnering ire.

The *Times* article began by revealing that the first quarantine letter went out just one day after kids had returned to class, and that in other schools in the district students and teachers "immediately" tested positive. This of course meant that the cases originated *outside* of school, since there typically was an incubation period of at least several days from infection to testing positive.

Amazingly, the article even pointed out that cases in Cherokee County mirrored the recent rise in cases in the state overall, where other counties, including Fulton, where Atlanta is located, had not opened schools.

Let's recap for a moment: The public was told that Cherokee County school openings (in particular with unmasked students and the buildings at full attendance) triggered a transmission disaster. Yet the *Times* article, mirroring most of the coverage, *gave details that disproved its thesis*. The cases originated outside of school. And cases in other parts of the state *where schools were closed* had also risen. Despite these facts in plain sight, the story that journalists wanted to tell, and that much of the public wanted to believe, prevailed. The scenario was akin to a prosecutor so gifted at litigating and oration that even though he divulged exculpatory particulars in his closing argument the jury was still persuaded of the defendant's guilt.

But things get even more interesting: Cases in Cherokee county peaked a week after schools opened there and then proceeded to *fall* for the next two months—while schools were open and without mask mandates. On September 9, around one month after Cherokee County schools had opened in full, out of 42,200 students there were 42 cases; out of 4,800 staff, there were 20 cases: 0.09 percent and 0.4 percent, respectively.

This was extremely relevant. If open schools jammed with maskless students were truly the cause of the initial outbreak—and the driver of viral spread in a community—how could cases in the district be near a statistical zero a month later? Looking for followup stories at the time, and unable to find any, I had dug up these data myself. I tweeted about the minuscule Cherokee County schools case rates at the beginning of

September, but, as far as I am aware, not one major news outlet did a follow-up piece reporting this news.

Not only was the denominator (the total number of students and staff) missing in the initial reports that only mentioned the numerator (the number of cases), but because the media failed to do any follow-up coverage, the denominator *as an effect of time* (the total number of students multiplied by roughly thirty school days) was also missing. Like so many other news stories on kids and schools during the pandemic, a provocative anecdote was decontextualized, wildly distorting the public's perception of risks and harms from open schools.

In summary: There was no correlation between opening schools in Cherokee County and an increase in cases. During July, all of Georgia, including counties with closed schools, saw rises in cases. And by the end of August through September, when cases had fallen in Georgia overall, they had also fallen in Cherokee County, with its open and maskless, crowded schools. With the media not reporting any of this context, it's no wonder that the average person, who, understandably, didn't follow the data closely, would have come away with the mistaken impression that Georgia schools opening, especially without masks, was a disaster, and an immoral one at that.

The lack of follow-up reporting on Georgia wasn't exclusive to the Cherokee County schools story. Recall the *Atlantic* article from April 29, 2020, "Georgia's Experiment in Human Sacrifice," which warned of calamitous mortality after Governor Kemp eased restrictions. Something interesting and important happened in the month that followed the article: cases in Georgia remained flat.

The dire predictions made with such confidence and moral disgust were unfounded. Yet the journalist, Amanda Mull, did not publish a mea culpa sequel sharing the good news. She did not, as far as I know, issue a statement acknowledging that she had made a mistake. The article was not appended with a correction or update.

Instead, in August, Mull doubled down with another piece decrying Georgia's foolish and grave errors. She wrote that cases were up again and that Governor Brian Kemp "refused to learn a thing." As evidence of his failings, Mull cited Kemp's rejection of a statewide mask mandate and his opening of bars, restaurants, and gyms, which, she wrote, had "spiked" cases for the beginning of the school year. And yet . . . cases in Georgia fell in August. They continued to fall though all of September, and didn't begin to rise until the beginning of October. Mull did not write another piece about Georgia at the end of August, or in September, or in October.

*   *   *

There is a more fundamental lesson, still, about the media coverage of Georgia and Israel, and, more broadly, of the public health establishment's policies and prescriptions for trying to mitigate cases in schools.

In 1979, a psychologist at Northwestern University named Donald Campbell published an explanation of a phenomenon he observed that became so influential it is now referred to as Campbell's Law. Campbell explained that using a simple measurement to represent a complex goal leads to the measurement itself becoming the goal, replacing the thing it was supposed to represent. For example, a police department may have a set goal of solving a certain percentage of crimes. But research has shown that setting this particular goal can lead to police departments simply recording fewer crimes—the *benchmark* of success becomes the goal, over actual success. Another example is what is known as "teaching to the test." The purpose of a test is to assess someone's knowledge. But if a teacher focuses exclusively on test prep, rather than the genuine education of his or her students, then the test score itself becomes the goal, rather than educating students to increase their knowledge. Focusing on a test score, rather than knowledge, also incentivizes cheating rather than learning.

Campbell detailed that inevitably we work toward improving the metric in any number of ways, even though those ways may be at odds with improving what we actually should care about.

Perhaps nowhere is the problem that Campbell's Law depicts more consequential than in public health. In clinical trials for drugs or other interventions "surrogate markers" (often lab results of a particular biological number) are commonly used to represent the clinical outcome that we care about (extended life or improved well-being). Trials often aim for achieving a particular surrogate "endpoint," which is used to represent a clinical end point. For example, progressive HIV/AIDS is associated with a reduced count of CD4 cells (a type of white blood cell). Therefore, to treat HIV patients, drugs were developed that improved CD4 counts, as a surrogate end point for survival. Unfortunately, trials found that some of the drugs that improved CD4 counts did not decrease death rates.

It is extremely common for interventions to be employed based on surrogates even though in many instances surrogate end points do "not provide compelling or definitive evidence about the treatment's effect on clinical efficacy measures," as the biostatistician Thomas Fleming wrote in a paper on surrogate end points. So why do we continue to not only use surrogates, but to conflate them with what they are supposed to represent? Quite simply, because life is complicated and it's easier to work toward affecting an outcome that's relatively easy to measure.

This brings us back to the news coverage of the school outbreaks. The media narrative about the Georgia schools story was about cases—the surrogate end point. But the reporting failed to mention the primary end point—which is what we really care about—how many kids became very sick or died as a result of getting infected in school, and, more generally, how many adults developed severe disease or died as a result of the schools opening. The stories didn't cover this because no one knew the answer. And yet this is all that really matters.

Here's what Georgia Department of Health data show: COVID hospitalizations for all ages in Georgia *fell* by more than 40 percent from the first day of school on August 3, to a month later. And they continued to fall the month after that, with COVID hospitalizations by October 3 less than half of what they were when schools opened.

The Israeli school outbreak was portrayed as a disaster and a grim omen for what would happen in the US if we let kids back in school. Here is a crucial fact that was not widely reported: The outbreak did not result in one hospitalization of students or staff. The reason this wasn't reported cannot be blamed on the information not being available at the time. It's right there, in paragraph five of the study on which the initial reporting was based. It's also worth highlighting that more than half of the infected students had no symptoms at all.

There was such a focus in the camp and school outbreak stories on cases, and the unsupported notion that children were driving transmission, that the effect of the virus itself—so benign to kids as to not even be noticed by a majority of those infected—was deemed irrelevant.

An assumption was baked into all of these stories that the social, academic, mental health, and physical costs to children, some of which would yield long-term or permanent damage, resulting from mitigations were automatically worth it.

Megan Ranney, the emergency medicine physician, who turned herself into a COVID pundit extraordinaire, appearing relentlessly in a list of major news outlets, including the *Times*—where her opinions on everything from masks to vaccines to epidemiology were featured in more than fifty separate articles during the pandemic—the *Post*, the *Atlantic*, CNN, NBC, CBS, and so on, expressed a common sentiment that summer when she tweeted that "it would be foolhardy to keep schools open" if infection rates rose. Foolhardy for whom? Certainly not so for the children, since attending school offered so many benefits, being blocked from attending school caused known harms, and all available evidence suggested that schools did not lead to a meaningful increase in the likelihood of infection. And certainly not for adults, since there was no evidence that schools were a meaningful driver of community or family transmission. In fact, schools often had lower rates of infection than the community. This was not mere conjecture, and it is not knowledge only available through a historical lens. By the summer of 2020 the Swedish reports and the EU meetings had already made this information available.

We also had data in the US that dovetailed with the European findings. As early as the middle of July 2020, while schools had remained closed, nearly a quarter of adult New York City residents already had had COVID. And Black and Hispanic adults were at greater than a 30 percent infection rate by that time. Therefore teachers in New York City, along with the rest of the public, were getting infected at rates as high as or higher than in Europe, where schools were open.

Donald Campbell warned that "the quantitative results may be mistaken as the qualitative." The media launched into a frenzy over the Georgia and Israeli school outbreaks—recall that the Israeli school was a "petri dish for COVID-19," and the virus "rippled out to the students' homes," Pam Belluck wrote in her *Times* piece. The well-being of the students— their ability to get a good education, to interact in person with friends and teachers, to have physical exercise, to not be forced into solitude on computers at home—was, with unconcerned irony, made a secondary consideration to the number of cases, even though cases, as a number, were merely the surrogate.

Campbell's Law returns us to Alfred Korzybski's adage about confusing the map with the territory. There was a conflation of cases with what they were supposed to represent. Inevitably, cases themselves became the priority, which (its relentless scaremongering about risks to children notwithstanding) was exactly how the media framed the school outbreak stories.

17

THE WORST OF BOTH WORLDS, PART I

Amidst the summer miasma of moral panic around children and schools, and tribalist hysteria, New York's Andrew Cuomo once again was positioned as the heroic antitoxin to the poison of Trump. Unlike the president's unscientific all caps declarations for schools to open without any strings attached, on July 13, Cuomo announced his formula, with specific benchmarks for schools to reopen.

A sense of security and order was palpable among the media and smart set. Finally, a leader who was a man of reason, and who respected *science*, would make his decisions methodically, based on the facts. "We're not going to use our children as guinea pigs," Cuomo said. "Is it safe? You can determine that by science."

The president, Cuomo said in a July press conference, told us to

"just reopen the economy! There's no reason for any of this stuff, data, masks." Yeah, we saw how well that worked. On schools he said, "just open them up, don't worry!" He was wrong on economic reopening, he's wrong on schools reopening. You reopen if it is safe. How do you know if it's safe? You look at the data. You don't hold your finger up and feel the wind. Look at the data. If you have the virus under control, reopen. If you don't, then you can't. We're not going to put our children in a place where their health is in danger. It's that simple. Common sense and intelligence can still determine what we do.

Schools could reopen that fall if a region's daily infection rate remained at 5 percent or lower over a fourteen-day average, Cuomo explained. That meant the virus was under control. "It's purely on the numbers," Cuomo said, "it's on the science."

There is nothing wrong with creating benchmarks. In fact, basing reopenings on quantifiable metrics creates a helpful road map for administrators to follow and for citizens to know what to expect. But, like the models, Cuomo's formula was presented as a scientific truism, while being nothing of the sort. Science does not equal policy. Saying opening schools is based *purely on the numbers* and *on the science* has no meaning. "Science" does not determine when schools can open. Epidemiologists and biostatisticians can try to predict what will happen when schools open in different circumstances, how doing so may or may not increase transmission by certain amounts, but the decisions about whether outcomes from opening are preferable to the outcomes of remaining closed are "purely," to borrow a word, subjective. Yet this glaring fallacy behind Cuomo's statements—that his reopening plan was based on science—went entirely unchallenged.

The 5 percent threshold Cuomo referenced likely came from the World Health Organization, though it's for a *positivity* rate, not an *infection* rate. These are two entirely different metrics. A "positivity rate" is the rate of tests that are positive. The "infection rate" can mean either the number of people each COVID-positive person will infect, or it can mean the percent of the population, for example per 100,000, that is infected. The positivity rate is informative and important, but also greatly affected by the number of tests conducted and who they are conducted on, and for that reason has a limited usefulness as a metric on its own.

Beyond that, and more damningly, the 5 percent rate cited by the WHO was a benchmark for opening up an entire region; it was not specific to schools. Why, after New York had already opened up many aspects of society based on some other criteria, would Cuomo use a threshold only for schools that was intended for broad application? No media stories discussed this.

The text on the state's slides shown in Cuomo's press conference read "below 5 percent," yet Cuomo said "5 percent or lower." This distinction might sound minute, but, if they were going by whole percentage points, that's a difference of 20 percent, which would have massive implications for whether children can be in school or not. It was an ironic imprecision for a politician who spoke regularly with such confidence, or some might argue smugness, that his decisions were "purely on the numbers."

On top of all this, Jerome Adams, the surgeon general at the time, said in order for schools to open the community positivity rate should be under 10 percent. That fall, Mayor Bill DeBlasio shut down New York

City schools when the city's positivity rate reached just 3 percent as a seven-day average. In Arizona the magic formula included a calculation of two weeks below 7 percent. In Memphis and its surrounding area the benchmark was 25 percent. All of this was made up.

Despite its evident arbitrariness, this 5 percent metric assumed a near-platonic ideal of enlightened certitude. The media repeated the formula over and over, and many close watchers of the pandemic would recite it knowingly in conversations or Twitter arguments.

People were frightened, and anxious about which actions to take. Was going to the store reasonable? Was sending a child to school "safe"? Cuomo's claim that his decisions were based on "science," and, more specifically, his recitation of 5 percent, reassured many people that there was technocratic control over the situation. Amid the chaos of uncertainty, the precision of a specific metric served as a lodestar. It also lent Cuomo an authoritative air. Surely these numbers came from somewhere, presumably "scientists" who figured out a formula for safely opening schools, whatever that meant.

Numerous studies have found that statistical evidence, if presented well, can be more persuasive than other forms of evidence. Part of the reason for this is addressed in a paper titled "Persuading Audiences with Statistical Evidence," by Michael Kearney, an assistant professor in the School of Journalism at the University of Missouri, where he explained that people tend to associate statistics with expertise. That the statistical benchmark Cuomo based school opening on was subjective was irrelevant regarding its power to rally much of the public behind it.

*   *   *

The 5-percent benchmark merely allowed schools to open. It did not determine whether they *would* open or under what conditions. Those decisions in New York, and many other states, were left up to individual districts.

Over the summer New York State instructed its roughly 750 school districts to compose and submit fall reopening plans for three scenarios: full-time in-person school, full-time remote learning, and a hybrid model in which students attend part time. Governor Cuomo said as long as a district was below the state's threshold it could open its schools. However, because New York State's guidelines required six feet of distancing between students, this meant that, with the exception of very few districts, schools would not be able to be open full time. To maintain this amount of space between students, nearly all schools could, at most, only operate at half capacity. Asking for three scenarios was a feint. The state knew that full-time in-person school was all but impossible for most districts.

As was often the case, particularly in blue states or regions, a recommendation from a health authority was interpreted as or converted into a requirement. The CDC's advice for schools was for students to keep six feet apart "when feasible." The federal agency's guidance implied that six feet was an ideal to be weighed against the severe cost of keeping kids out of school. Yet, like acolytes trying to prove their worth to the priest and other congregants, New York's health department tightened the CDC's permissive "when feasible" into more absolute language of "must maintain" in its guidance.

This pattern happened not just with states maximizing federal guidance, but was often repeated at the local level, with districts maximizing state guidance. Though New York didn't require barriers, for example, many individual districts nevertheless saw fit to mandate them. And after the mask mandate was removed in New York in spring of 2022, some districts continued to require them. Scattered schools throughout the country forced children to eat meals without speaking even though silent lunches weren't recommended at the state or federal level. And so on. When I asked a New York State health department spokesperson in the fall about the legality of my kids' district requiring barriers on every student's desk I was told that schools could "always do more."

Health authorities at the federal and state level did not seem to realize—or they did realize and were glad to relieve themselves of the responsibility—that without specific language prohibiting certain interventions states, and then districts, in an effort to appear "safe," were often predisposed to do more. This dynamic led individual districts and schools around the country to implement a wide and wild array of rules that were not recommended at the state or federal level, from forced outdoor lunches, even in the rain, to opaque desktop barriers, penning children's heads inside three-sided cardboard boxes all day. Most consequential, though, were New York and many other states turning the CDC's somewhat loose six feet "when feasible" suggestion into an inexorable requirement.

Administrators and facilities managers dutifully brought tape measures into classrooms, measuring the space between desks with a carpenter's precision. Cuomo said he was giving districts the power to do what worked best for their communities. Except the state's guidance did not allow for much autonomy. It was like an architect giving a contractor a project in which every major parameter was fixed—the height, the square footage, the materials, the design—but the contractor had to figure out how to execute it. There was autonomy, but only in how to actualize the blueprints.

But six feet between students was the best and most reasonable way to keep everyone safe, right? Any logical person would conclude that having schools open full time at normal density would lead to more transmission, right? Like Kim Prather would have said, this is basic physics! Obviously there was solid science upholding this policy, and there was no evidence to the contrary, right? And, as always, the mission of reducing transmission should take precedence over other concerns, right?

Alas, no. The ill-considered fetishization of an arbitrary metric that was seen with Cuomo's 5 percent rule similarly manifested with this other, far more consequential benchmark. Countless experts detailed, and copious research showed that absolutely nothing magical happens between five and seven feet. Some media reports, such as one in the *Washington Post*, suggested the origin of six feet might go all the way back to a German scientist named Carl Flügge, who, in 1897, found that bacteria-laden droplets could travel from a person up to two meters (roughly six feet). If so, this was an awfully tenuous form of evidence on which to hang such a consequential policy. (Indeed, I had a German scholar of environmental medicine review and translate for me a Flügge document that was cited in several academic papers, presumably the source for the media reports. It did not contain evidence related to bacteria droplets traveling two meters.)

In a radio interview, a Yale epidemiologist named Albert Ko suggested the six-feet guidance was derived from studies of transmission on airplanes. I corresponded with Ko and reviewed two airplane studies he referenced. One of the studies concluded that transmission was concentrated in the three rows in front of the index patient, which the authors had measured to be 7.5 feet. The other study was a modeling paper that mentioned that two rows on a plane was the WHO criteria for a "contact" of an infected person. Yet the WHO paper that was cited as the source of that claim did not provide evidence explaining how the two-row metric was arrived at. Regardless, two rows is roughly five feet, not six.

These and other likely apocryphal origin stories are perhaps why Scott Gottlieb, the former commissioner of the FDA, said "nobody knows" where the six-feet metric came from, and that the CDC initially wanted ten feet but compromised on six with a Trump official who had told them ten feet was "inoperable." In 2024 testimony before Congress, Anthony Fauci—who had repeatedly promoted the value of six feet of distancing during the pandemic—admitted that six feet was likely not based on any data and that "it just sort of appeared." In yet another post hoc admission, Francis Collins, Fauci's former boss and the head of the NIH during the pandemic, said in a 2024 interview that he could not recall any science or evidence that supported six-foot distancing. (In an exchange with a CDC representative, the agency refused to answer my request for clarification on the origin of the six-foot guidance for schools. More on this in endnotes.) Millions of signs, in stores, public buildings, even outside in parks, and yes, in schools, around our vast country all commanded us to keep six feet apart. And most of the public complied and didn't ask questions. The media outlets that tried to suss out the origins of six feet gave half-baked explanations like the citing of the German scientist or airplanes, and the CDC refused to provide answers to me, even after I filed a public records request. Like masks, and like school closures, there was no evidence behind this rule, yet we were obligated to follow it, and the media were largely uninterested in trying to get to the bottom of it.

Whatever the genesis of the six-foot guideline, more importantly, and most damningly, there was an overwhelming amount of real-world evidence from open schools throughout Europe where, in many instances, just three feet or no required distance at all bore no obvious ill effect.

Without any known evidence behind the benefit of six feet of distancing in schools, evidence to the contrary from Europe, and somewhat

THE WORST OF BOTH WORLDS, PART I

moderate language from the CDC regarding its implementation, why was New York's and many other states' militant distancing guidance accepted?

Despite the seeming arbitrariness behind the metric, and, worse, the refuting wealth of observational evidence from European schools—where there was no discernible difference in transmission rates between schools with two meters (roughly six feet) of distancing versus one meter or no specified distance—the six-foot metric was nevertheless exhorted with pounded fists on tables by American public health officials. It's not surprising then that most school administrators, pundits and many regular citizens didn't just tolerate but vociferously defended this as the necessary distance between students. That is what the experts told them to think.

Beyond the tribalism and media distortions I've already detailed, one of the reasons for the cheerleading behind this nonevidence-based intervention likely has to do with how statistics are used in communication. As noted, statistics lend an air of expertise to those who cite them. Asserting rules with confidence, particularly those with figures, can be enough to get people to buy in without too many questions. "Oftentimes, we are given numbers of high precision with no discernible basis," said Dr. James Zimring, a physician at the University of Virginia and the author of *Partial Truths*, a book about how statistics often deceive the public. For instance, he told me, you might see an "advertisement for a certain brand of shampoo, where they say it has been shown to make your hair, for example, 68 percent softer. 68 percent? Really? Not 67 percent or 69 percent? And how did you measure this? Do you have a soft-o-meter from the bureau of standards and measures for hair care that you put hair in?"

There is a fair amount of cognitive psychology research into how people can be manipulated with number presentation (size of number, round numbers vs. decimals, etc.), Zimring said, but most of it is in behavioral economics and focused on consumer manipulation. Yet we see the same principles play out with public health. Zimring, who has expertise in blood biology, shared a story about how when mad cow disease broke out in the UK people who had visited England for a period of time were barred from donating blood. The question was how long did the visit need to last for the potential donors to be excluded? A month? Two months? What if you were just passing through Heathrow? The authorities chose six months. The legend is that they calculated the amount of the blood supply they were willing to lose based upon excluding donors, and then back-calculated how long a stay in England would translate to that number. The number wasn't capriciously chosen, but it also wasn't based on safety data regarding contamination of the blood, as people likely presumed.

From a communications and operational perspective providing somewhat arbitrary benchmarks isn't wrong, per se. At times they may be necessary or at least helpful for administrators and the public to have some parameters to aim for. A nonspecific instruction like "keep your distance" could lead to chaos among school districts, and arguments between administrators and parents as they tried to figure out what, exactly, that meant. But, just as with the models, the harm was in the degree of certainty within which distancing guidelines were presented. The charade that they were based on something concrete led to myopically strict compliance, the consequence of which was keeping children out of school.

There was a condescension toward and derision of those who rather than a narrow focus, took a more panoramic view, wondering about costs and benefits of strictly enforcing six feet. This arrogance from health officials and politicians largely shut down debate, because to question the wisdom of six feet was to question "the science." And so, throughout large swaths of the country, from New York to California, at the state or district level, adherence to six feet of distance took on a religious fanaticism. And I use the word "religious" here figuratively but also purposefully, because the unyielding adherence to six feet in the US while millions of children in Europe and, later, in parts of our own country, were in school at much closer distances without evident harm required the denialist blind faith and compartmentalization typical of those devoted to scripture.

The distancing recommendation was also based on a premise that *seemed* logical, but was faulty. The real-world evidence from European schools showing otherwise should have trumped the theory that this distance was necessary—like so many of the schools policies, the insistence on six feet represented an epistemology that favored theory over empiricism.

Beyond the dismissal of evidence from Europe indicating that six feet, and in turn a hybrid schooling model, conferred no benefit, was the false assumption that kids were not interacting outside of school, and this was especially so after so many months had passed. At the end of July, William Hanage, an epidemiologist at Harvard's T. H. Chan School of Public Health, said in a public radio interview, "The hybrid model is probably among the worst that we could be putting forward if our goal is to stop the virus getting into schools." Jennifer Nuzzo, Dimitri Christakis, a pediatrician, epidemiologist, and the editor in chief of *JAMA Pediatrics*, and Martin Kulldorff, at the time a biostatistician at Harvard Medical School, all echoed that view in a *Wired* piece I published in the first week of August on the foolishness of the hybrid school model.

Because of the potential for so many interactions outside of school, Christakis said the hybrid model could actually advance the spread of the virus. In Christakis's view,

it would be preferable to have 30 kids in a classroom, even if there weren't sufficient space for 6-foot social distancing, than to switch off groups of half that size. In the latter scenario, each of those students would likely be exposed to more people overall. Their teachers, too, would be at higher risk—since instead of teaching one cohort every day, they'd be in charge of two.

It should be noted, for some people the takeaway from the article about the likely failure of hybrid schooling wasn't that schools should be open full time, as they had been in Europe, but, instead, that they should remain fully closed.

In many regards hybrid schooling would lead to the worst of both worlds—no discernible reduction in transmission or cases overall, and kids still unable to attend school on a normal schedule. In many instances a hybrid schedule meant children were in school far less than even half the time. This was either by design, such as in New York City schools, or because of holidays and frequent shutdowns—in New York City, for example, entire school buildings were forced to close for ten days any time two unlinked cases were found. In a number of hybrid districts the schools were only open a maximum of four days each week (with students attending at most two of those days) because one day every week—in my district it was "Flex Wednesdays"—was closed to any in-person learning so teachers could do "continuing education" to advance their remote teaching skills for all the students not in the room on any given day.

That the distancing requirement—from Cuomo, the CDC, and other authorities—had no evidentiary basis behind it appeared to make no difference to school administrators and those who argued for unyielding compliance. And this led to an extraordinary consequence: tens of millions of American children were kept out of full-time school. In many districts, such as New York City, schools were considered "open" under these hybrid schedules, yet many students attended just once a week or even less. In the aggregate, by spring of 2021, my kids, along with millions of others, whose schools were considered officially open by politicians and administrators, nevertheless missed half a year or more of actual school.

None of this mattered. Cuomo, Fauci and others benefited from what's known as a "halo effect"—elite society's already favorable impression of them, generally earned via a comparison to Trump, spilled over into everything they advocated for. In essence, the halo effect is the opposite of what happened to Trump, a storm cloud effect, if you will. Instead of making the effort to ask for and consider the evidence, much of the public health establishment and elite society relied on inference, in both directions—commendation for anything proposed by Fauci, and condemnation for anything proposed by the White House. As a consequence, school policies that were divorced from evidence were championed then implemented then defended, while suggestions of a more holistic approach, taking into account the costs of school closures and mitigations, and questioning their benefits, were demonized and dismissed.

As problematic as the six-foot requirement was, there was a much more peculiar manifestation of unquestioning adherence to an evidence-free benchmark. In the summer of 2020, I conducted an investigation for *Wired* on a little-known but widely employed distancing metric that I found in the reopening plans of numerous school districts. It was placed there by a security consulting firm.

Through a farcical series of errors and dubious assumptions one firm, which counted dozens of school districts as clients, had recommended that a 44-square-foot moat of space surround each student in their classrooms, a figure bizarrely disconnected from, and far higher than, what was necessary to maintain the benchmark of six feet of distancing. Even at a most basic and conservative calculation of six by six, each student would need only 36 square feet around them. (And that figure is markedly overgenerous, considering half of that square footage is not needed for students whose desks would be positioned against walls around the perimeter of a classroom.)

Trying to understand why my village's schools were only going to allow children in the buildings on a hybrid schedule of two days a week when it seemed there was plenty of space for students to attend more frequently and still comply with the required distancing, I took a deep breath and dove into my district's reopening plan, a 130-page colossus of flowcharts, graphs, color coded tables, and details on everything from safety drills to budgetary concerns. It was there, buried amid hyperspecific bullet points on social distancing, including the directive to measure and record room dimensions, that I first came across the 44 square feet rule, which I later learned the district's security consultant had recommended. Troublingly, but perhaps predictably, my district, along with many others, adopted this nonsensical 44 metric into its plan without questioning its logic. Either that or the administrators who ostensibly prepared this leviathan of a document never actually read what was in it. It's unclear which is worse.

Curious about how prevalent this faulty metric was, at a cursory look I found districts in North Carolina, New Jersey, and throughout New York with the 44 square feet rule in their reopening plans. The result of this error was that an untold number of children were kept out of school because it led to unnecessarily sparse attendance. For example, performing some basic geometry, along with the help of my editor and an illustrator at *Wired*, I diagrammed tilings and tessellations of desk configurations for my own district, based on its average classroom size, and found there likely was sufficient space for all students to have attended school full time while still maintaining six feet of distancing. This was especially so considering that a percentage of students had opted exclusively for remote learning, meaning fewer total kids in the buildings and extra personal space for those attending. (The *Wired* piece gets into the nitty-gritty of the calculations, and explains how the security firm that consulted for so many districts, including my own, arrived at this incorrect number, but I won't delve into that here.)

In the end, tens of millions of American children were kept out of full-time school because of an arbitrary distancing metric the CDC contrived. (And evidence from Europe that closer distances, or no specified distance at all, led to no overt ill effects was ignored.) This arbitrary metric of six feet was then recommended or, in the instance of New York and many other states, required in school buildings, resulting in hybrid programs in which, at best, only half the students were allowed to attend at a given time. Then, as if this metric weren't bad enough, other parties introduced additional errors, like the 44-square-foot minimum surrounding each student, which meant even fewer kids could attend school.

There was zero evidence that six feet instead of five-and-a-half feet, or four feet, or three feet between desks would make a lick of difference. Yet six feet was treated as though Zeus handed it down from the top of Mount Olympus to the mortals. Facilities managers, administrators, and teachers across the country carefully wielded yardsticks and tape measures around classrooms like fastidious set designers to make sure desks were properly distanced. To be clear, authorities providing benchmarks or rough parameters for school administrators to aim for would have been reasonable, even essential. The problem was, like so many of the public health establishment's pronouncements, these metrics were presented with unearned certainty, which led to them being followed with undue deference and robotic adherence. The earnest zeal with which the measurements were followed with such precision would have been comical had it not been so disheartening. Had the distances been presented by officials for what they were—mere guesses at what might reduce transmission by some unknown amount—and suggested as aspirational goals, rather than precise benchmarks, they might have been striven for but not at the expense of preventing children from attending school.

* * *

With my kids at camp, playing and interacting physically with peers, like kids always do, like kids *need* to do, as the summer wore on an increasing sense of dread overcame me. They'd come home from a day rich with activity, and as I looked at them, tired, sweaty, happy, "this is all going to end" kept running through my mind. The closure of schools lasting more than three months the previous spring was a failure. All of that time at home, zombified in front of screens, faded them, like a once vibrant tie-dye that had been submerged in bleach. I was worried about the fall.

With the state's six-foot rule I knew that my kids, along with millions of others, would at most only be in school part time, with no end point in sight. Indeed, during the summer my district announced that it planned to implement its hybrid model from among the three plans it had to submit to the state. This bode very poorly for the coming school year. Was there any way around it?

In July, the *Times* ran a fascinating piece on the popularity of outdoor classes around the country at the beginning of the twentieth century that were initiated, in part, as a precaution against tuberculosis transmission. The article featured old timey black-and-white photographs of kids bundled in thick overcoats and hats while sitting at desks or tables in class in a variety of novel locations—a ferry in the East River of New York City, on a rooftop, under a tent. In New England, during an especially punishing winter, children burrowed in wearable blankets called "Eskimo sitting bags," with heated soapstones at their feet. The project was deemed a huge success.

This seemed like a brilliant idea. It was already well known that evidence of outdoors SARS-CoV-2 transmission was close to nonexistent. Because of the European data I wasn't worried about indoor classes, but if "open air schools," as they were called, is what it would take to mollify those who were concerned about transmission so kids could attend school full time in person, then so be it. Not to mention being outdoors had other long-observed benefits, namely improving mental health and academic performance. It would be a win-win.

I sent an email to a handful of parents in town suggesting we propose outdoor classes to the district administration. Unlike the urban examples I had read about, we didn't need to use roofs or ferries. There was an expansive green in front of the elementary school and numerous athletic fields for the middle and high schools. News of private schools in the area buying large tents, the kind used for weddings, was circulating in texts and on social media. There were rumors of supplies running out. There was no reason we couldn't do this too, and the sooner we locked it down, the better.

Within a day close to 100 parents had signed on to a group letter that I then emailed to the superintendent and the BOE. It was a significant number, especially in that amount of time, for our tiny district of around

1,600 students. In the days after I had submitted the letter, more and more parents who had belatedly gotten wind of it emailed me, asking to be added to the list of supporters. People really wanted their kids in school, and they were eager to get creative to make it happen.

After the initial email there was much back and forth between the administration and me, and others. The superintendent said the idea was problematic because outdoor classes lacked sufficient internet access, and therefore children who stayed home would not be able to livestream classes. Yet, along with other tech-related gear for remote learning, the district had planned on purchasing hotspots, which enable internet access from anywhere. (It was also suggested that the elementary school could avoid streaming outdoor classes by having one or more teachers in each grade, whatever number was needed, teach from indoors exclusively to the remote students.) Knowing tents or related materials would be a non-trivial expense, we offered to do a fundraiser. This offer was declined. The administration raised issues about safety. They said a child theoretically could wander off from a nonwalled environment. Parents volunteered to act as chaperones and guards to prevent this improbable circumstance, but that offer was dismissed. At one point student allergies to grass and pollen were brought up. There even was mention that outdoor classes would run afoul of fire codes. Fire codes for outdoor classes! I couldn't wrap my head around how, exactly, children were at risk of harm from fire while being outdoors but, nevertheless, I assured the superintendent that the district could come to an understanding with the local fire chief, or, if necessary, other regulators. This suggestion was ignored.

There seemed to be no excuse, no matter how farcical or contrived, that the administration couldn't conjure to not pursue this option. And every single idea or solution that parents came up with was shot down or ignored. And the administration brought forth no ideas of its own to get kids into school.

What exactly was happening? Where was the American roll-up-your-sleeves, can-do spirit? A significant portion of the parent community was engaged, enthusiastic, and offering ideas, money, and even volunteer labor so our schools could open "safely." Yet the superintendent clearly had no interest in pursuing this course.

It's important to stress here that the school district, along with thousands of others, had the ability to open fully *and be in compliance with the guidelines*—yet chose not to do so. The absence of logic and honest dialogue surrounding the outdoor classes ordeal portended all that would follow.

My school district's intransigence was not an anomaly. Parents in other towns in my county, along with parents throughout the New York metro area, and in Virginia, Maryland, and California, among other states, all recounted similar experiences. Private Facebook groups and direct message groups on Twitter were formed. Doctors, including many pediatricians, around the country who wanted schools open in their communities networked with each other, sharing news articles, studies, and talking points, hoping to make change at the local level.

With the prospects of normal school looking dim, some families began pursuing the possibility of starting "pod schools," where a privately hired teacher would instruct a small group of children each day, usually in someone's home, a phenomenon I wrote about for the *Times*. The novelty and expense of pods (many of the programs cost $25,000 and up per student for the year) were a news sensation, and enraged many readers. Some blamed the parents. Others blamed the schools for not being open and said parents had every right, indeed obligation, to do what they could for their kids. However one came down on the topic, one thing was clear: pod schools were yet another option and advantage available only for certain children.

A small group of parents in my town put together a petition advocating for schools to open fully in the fall. The petition was based on the premise that we did not even need outdoor classes for school to run full time while still being compliant with distancing requirements. This is because the state guidelines contained a little-acknowledged clause: the New York Department of Health guidance document for schools released that summer stated that students had to maintain six feet of distance from each other *or* there needed to be physical barriers between individuals. In the petition we noted that there was no ambiguity about what the word "or" means. And we knew that the district had already purchased 1700 desktop barriers, one for each student.

Importantly, any families who wanted to keep their kids home were welcome to do so. We noted the evidence from Sweden, where lower schools had been open full time (not to mention, unlike our district, without masking or barriers), and found that teachers were at no higher risk of infection than the average professional. We said that staff who had particular vulnerabilities should be permitted to work from home. (Perhaps they could handle the bulk of off-site instruction for the students whose families wished for them to remain remote.) What rational objection could there be?

The petition also noted that the proposed hybrid schedule was not necessarily any safer, and potentially more harmful, than full-time school. We explained with an example:

As soon as the hybrid model was announced a flurry of texts was exchanged between hundreds of parents seeking to join their children together on the "flex" day, and, to whatever extent possible, on their primary "remote" days. Joining children from both the gold and green cohorts, and from different classes, of course undercuts any theoretical benefit of the hybrid model as a limiting factor for viral spread.

(The "flex" day was to be every Wednesday, when no instruction would take place in person or online, so teachers could receive additional time to improve their remote educator skills.)

Within a few days we had amassed close to 300 signatures, and ultimately garnered more than 500. Three days after submitting the petition we received a boilerplate response from the Board of Education thanking us for sharing our thoughts. The district wound up starting the school year entirely remote, for reasons not entirely clear, before shifting to a hybrid model that, as promised, included no instruction at all on Wednesdays. (Eventually, after an outcry, the flex day was nixed, and the two cohorts got to switch on and off two or three days a week of school, alternating Wednesdays.)

The children in the district would not attend school on a normal schedule until eight months later, and more than a full year from when they last attended full time.

It's worth pausing for a moment and reiterating that school districts throughout the state, and in many parts of the country, were given the authority to operate in whatever model their superintendent or whoever was in charge chose. Governor Cuomo specifically announced this, positioning it as an empowering enablement of autonomy to individual districts. Yet, unlike state health departments, superintendents and school boards of course had no epidemiological expertise. The ability to determine what was "safe" was wholly outside their purview. Yet when the state released guidelines most districts in New York—which had or could have ordered barriers, allowing a bypass of the six-foot rule—ignored the barrier clause and remained fully remote or in hybrid modes anyway. Just as public health officials and medical professionals had done so often in the past, school administrators implemented interventions without evidence of benefit, and even the potential for harm, based on intuitions and feelings and political considerations.

The experience in July and early August made me understand very quickly and clearly that I was approaching the situation from the wrong perspective. I viewed remote learning as a problem to solve. I wanted all kids to be in school whose families wanted them there. Solutions existed. But it was obvious that the largest obstruction to getting kids in school was not an outdoor fire code or cost of a tent or internet access. It was the administrators. They had decided it couldn't work and there was nothing, no logistical or financial answer, that would be accepted. Like the evidence from Europe, no amount of data seemed to matter.

It didn't matter that many parents wanted it. That the state allowed for it. That the district had the financial and logistical means of achieving it. And that children from families who were against in-person schooling had the option to remain home.

The reality is that evidence is irrelevant when political, professional, and social forces all point in the other direction.

18

BAD INCENTIVES

It is irrational to expect students will be able to learn in any reasonable manner, when their teachers and classrooms are constantly conveying the need for vigilance in mask-wearing and social distancing. The constant need for vigilance cannot help but be internalized as fear and anxiety. At best, schools will be more similar to a well-meaning prison than an actual rich learning environment where thoughts can be shared and joy can be expressed.

Computers are sterile imposters that rob the experience of the richness of our relationships with our students.

If you read the above passionate, colorfully articulated arguments and assumed they were written by anti-mask and open-schools advocates you would be forgiven, but mistaken. The text, along with warnings about the dangers of hybrid schedules, is from a joint letter posted in August 2020, signed by the heads of teachers unions in more than fifty districts in four neighboring New York counties. Despite the above sentiments, the letter was not an appeal for schools to open.

On the contrary, the letter also called for a list of preconditions for a "safe" opening of schools—HVAC units in schools to have a specified level of filtration; "prioritized supply lines" for PPE; mandatory fourteen-day shutdowns if a school closed for a COVID-related issue; and so on. Notwithstanding all the text pronouncing the harms of mitigations and remote learning, the letter suggested that if the provisions weren't met the only appropriate action was for schools to remain closed. The anticipated in-person experience with masking and distancing, described with such grim acerbity, was intended as an argument *against school*, not an argument against the mitigations. And the unproven benefit, let alone the potential for increased harm, from a hybrid schedule was also intended not as an argument for full-time in-person classes but, rather, for fully remote learning.

Regardless of its implication that schools should remain closed without specific measures in place, reading the August 2020 letter now, as I type these words years later, I'm struck by its candor about trade-offs and the explicit costs of school closures and NPIs in the classroom. Its vivid acknowledgment of the inferiority of remote learning and the detriments of mitigations in schools was not universally expressed. Rather, the narrative espoused by a number of prominent voices in the education and public health fields, which took deeper and deeper root over time, was that masks were no big deal and that remote learning was fine. The examples are endless, but to take just a few: Megan Ranney, the emergency medicine physician and COVID pundit, mentioned in media interviews and repeatedly tweeted to her tens of thousands of followers impassioned calls for student mask mandates, dismissing those who had concerns about them by saying that "masks aren't harmful," "masks hurt no one," and "masks cause literally ZERO HARM." But: What is harm? Does the answer change over time? And who gets to decide? When pressed on her assertions, Ranney argued on Twitter that masks were merely an inconvenience. But many parents rightfully felt that a piece of material strapped to a six-year-old's face for eight hours a day, every school day for more than a year was, indeed, a clear form of harm.

In August 2021, the *New York Times* ran a widely scorned opinion piece titled "Actually, Wearing a Mask Can Help Your Child Learn." (Among the essay's arguments was that blind children still learn how to speak.) In January 2022, the American Academy of Pediatrics argued in a "friend of the court" brief in a mask mandate lawsuit that masking children caused no harm because masks were no worse than sunglasses in their effect on diminishing children's ability to read facial cues. (More on this unusual brief and the AAP's involvement in the lawsuit in endnotes.)

That same month, in response to a question about the drawbacks of remote learning, the head of the Los Angeles teachers union said, "There is no such thing as learning loss." She continued, "It's OK that our babies may not have learned all their times tables" from being out of school. "They learned resilience." In the spring of 2021, a professor of education at New York University argued, bizarrely, that assessments "students take this spring can't possibly demonstrate 'learning loss,' since they can't be compared to anything else," even though numerous analyses of standardized test scores pre- and postpandemic made this exact comparison and showed significant drops. (More on this later in the book.) A poem by an online teaching resource company, circulated as a social media meme, was titled, "What If Instead of 'Falling Behind' Lockdown Kids Are Actually Ahead?" Among the "what ifs" in its several hundred words of text against the backdrop of a cartoon rainbow: "What if they learn how to live with stress? What if they learn to be resilient and content?" The poem was shared in its entirety, and written about admiringly by an education consultant for Head Start and the CDC.

In contrast to what came later from some prominent voices in the education field, not only was the joint letter from the New York unions, which included among its signers the head of the teachers union in my district, honest about the costs of mitigations and school closures. Its preconditions were a modest plea compared to the actions and demands of some unions and teachers elsewhere in the country that summer.

In July, United Teachers Los Angeles, the teachers union for the LA unified school district, the second largest in the country, with just under 600,000 students in spring 2020, released a seventeen-page document titled "The Same Storm, but Different Boats: The Safe and Equitable Conditions for Starting LAUSD in 2020–21." It is a remarkable artifact. It reads, even for those sympathetic to the political ideology behind some of its demands, as a fantastical manifesto. By way of introduction, it declares the United States a "profoundly racist society." Among its demands: a 100 percent testing rate of all symptomatic people in Los Angeles, a city with nearly 4 million residents; zero community spread; paid sick leave for parents; no standardized tests that infringe on instructional time; $250 million in additional funds to the district, which would not include the cost of investments in remote learning; Medicare for all; a special wealth tax on California's billionaires; a separate tax for California's millionaires; defunding the police; a city ordinance preventing evictions; housing the homeless; and a moratorium on charter schools. The document concludes that "the United States leads the world in the number of coronavirus cases and deaths—and not coincidentally, also leads the world in number of billionaires and per capita energy consumption," among other categories.

It's important to see the document through the lens of the cultural moment that summer, as America convulsed in the wake of George Floyd's murder. Demands for the recognition of systemic racism had taken over much of the national conversation. Teachers unions, by their own admission, were not just labor organizations but ideologically motivated groups, nearly uniform in their progressivism. Many of them felt this was the window of opportunity for all sorts of societal inequities to be redressed. And so, what should have been a sober assessment of the scientific evidence regarding risks and benefits of various school policies, instead turned into a cartoonish clarion call to rectify a catalog of grievances.

If nothing else, as an anchoring position in a negotiation it was supremely effective.

Public schools in Los Angeles did not open until April 2021, more than a year after they initially closed. (I know this has been mentioned many times in the book, but it's worth meditating on it again for one moment. Healthy children in Los Angeles were barred from school *for more than an entire year.*) When the doors were finally unlocked, the staggered hybrid opening saw some students at some schools attending just one day a week for the remaining six weeks of the school year. Some middle and high school students in Los Angeles did not set foot in a classroom until the beginning of the 2021–2022 school year, seventeen months after school buildings closed in March 2020.

At the same time as the LA union's Different Boats launched, a coalition of teachers unions, including those in Chicago, Boston, Milwaukee, and Oakland, under the moniker Demand Safe Schools, called for canceling rents and mortgages, and for moratoriums on evictions, foreclosures, voucher programs, charter schools, and standardized testing. Also on the requirements list was a "massive infusion of federal money to support the reopening funded by taxing billionaires and Wall Street."

Randi Weingarten of the AFT, among many other union leaders at state and local levels, argued at the time and continued to argue years later that the criticism that they didn't want schools to open was false. Rather, they argued, they did want them open, "safely." But the bar for "safely" was set somewhere in the exosphere.

Against the backdrop of panic created by health authorities and the media, educators across the nation launched campaigns of lavish histrionics. In Washington, DC, teachers piled body bags and placed fake tombstones, inscribed with "RIP Favorite Teacher," among other epitaphs, outside school system offices. In Milwaukee, the teachers union tweeted "paying tribute to those whom undoubtedly will die" accompanied by photos of gravestones featuring "Here lies a third grade student from Green Bay" and "RIP grandma caught Covid helping grandkids with homework" that art teachers had created for a car caravan. In Haverhill, Massachusetts, dozens of pairs of shoes were placed on the steps to City Hall, along with mock coffins, to symbolize the students and educators who would die if schools opened. (At the time, Haverhill had fewer than four reported COVID cases per 100,000 residents over two weeks.) An Arizona union created a template for its members to make fake obituaries for themselves to send to the governor in protest of schools opening there. At a rally in New York City, in addition to the obligatory coffins, was a teacher carrying a skeleton with a blood-dripping "Welcome Back to School" sign hanging from its neck. Many of the teachers used the hashtag #OnlyWhenItsSafe in their protests. This practice continued into the fall, after schools in much of the country had reopened, either in full or in hybrid models. The Prince William Education Association, a teachers union in northern Virginia, used child-sized coffins strapped to roofs of cars during an October protest caravan against opening schools there.

At the same time as the summer teacher protests media outlets around the country were reporting on teachers getting end-of-life affairs in order. "How horrible is it that one of the things on the list to do is to have a plan for students and teachers dying?" a teacher told CNN. In the same piece another teacher said that in addition to preparing a will she was looking into supplementary life insurance. Still another teacher said she had "extreme anxiety about death," while breaking into tears. Many teachers took to social media with similar sentiments. One tweeted: "I'm working on writing my will. I turned 27 last week, but I'm a teacher and I'm scared." Another: "I need a lawyer's help writing my will because we are being forced back into school in the midst of a pandemic." Randi Weingarten tweeted an article about a law firm offering free wills for teachers returning to school. A thirty-three-year-old Florida teacher posted a mock obituary for herself on Facebook, a stunt that was covered by *USA Today*, *People*, *Newsweek*, and the *Today Show*. The *Times* ran an opinion piece by a teacher who said going to school would be like her and her family taking a bullet.

The NEA and AFT, the two largest teachers unions in the country, both posted articles about teachers making wills. The AFT said it would support any local chapter that wanted to strike over reopening schools. After the Chicago Teachers Union threatened to hold a vote to authorize a strike the city's mayor, Lori Lightfoot, walked back her plan for schools to open with students attending two days a week to instead beginning the school year fully remote. The mayor said the change of plans was related to following "the science," even though the city's health commissioner said she was in favor of opening the schools and that the risk of spread was not significant.

The same media outlets that helped create the fear to begin with, now amplified the voices of those they had made afraid. A feedback loop of a frightened public, in particular teachers, that was both the news audience and its content—and its promise of increased "engagement" or "traffic"— proved too enticing an incentive for media producers to adhere to any decorum. No amount of hysterics was off-limits, and the stories featuring teachers expressing abject terror rarely contextualized their comments with data on the actual risks.

The information environment public health officials, politicians, and the media created, from both exaggerating the risks of schools opening and fabricating a certainty of benefits of school closures, in effect demanded action from union leaders such as AFT's Randi Weingarten. With so many union members throughout the US expressing that they were in a state of terror, Weingarten and local union leaders' role and responsibility was to battle for the rank and file.

The narrative of potential impending death for teachers, and that requiring in-school work was the height of immoral imprudence, was succinctly articulated in the "taking a bullet" Times piece, which referred to opening schools as a "massive unnecessary science experiment." Yet, remember that teachers had already been back at work in person in more than twenty countries throughout Europe, teaching millions of students. There was no evidence that teachers there were at an elevated risk relative to other professionals, and the Swedish report that explicitly looked at these data formally concluded the same. Keeping tens of millions of children out of school for months on end was the experiment, not the other way around. This is the point that the various philosophers and medical professionals I interviewed had made. The intervention (in this case, school closures) must show evidence of benefit outweighing harms. Otherwise you must default to the norm (schools being open).

In modern history conservatives have been the party often associated with believing in American exceptionalism. Yet, ironically, it was progressives and the liberal establishment that so deeply bought into this notion during the pandemic, viewing American schools, children, and teachers as unique, as somehow so radically different from their peers that it was a science experiment for them to do what had already happened elsewhere.

This dismissal or simply non-acknowledgment of real-world evidence from thousands of schools in Europe that showed opening did not lead to noticeably higher case rates allowed teachers unions to make their claims of looming catastrophe often without much official rebuttal from the districts that employed them. The failed information environment created by health authorities and the media gave school administrators a pass to not have to debate the merits of teachers' and their unions' claims.

Many teachers who were not at great risk nevertheless were sincerely frightened (due to being grossly misled by trusted sources in the media, government, and the public health establishment). And the union leaders, such as Weingarten at the national level, and countless others at the local level, were essentially required by their fiduciary responsibilities to push for the mitigations and restrictions that their members and the "experts" said were necessary. Union leaders often gave perfunctory remarks about protecting children, but the leaders' constituents were the teachers. The leaders' sole incentive was to fight for the perceived interests of union members, not the well-being of children. (The portion of teachers who truly were at grave medical risk were reasonable to request remote work for a period of time. Though it's worth noting that since schools did not present a unique risk, working remotely was unlikely to offer any advantage after a brief time except for individuals with a truly exceptional commitment to isolation.)

For all of the blame, rightfully, apportioned to public health leaders and the media for terrifying teachers, the acquiescence of many school administrators and government officials to union demands was, at its essence, political. Going back at least thirty years, more than 94 percent of political donations from teachers unions went to Democrats. Moreover, contributions skyrocketed from $4.3 million in 2004 to more than $32 million in 2016. In the 2022 election cycle the numbers climbed even higher: the NEA and AFT donated a combined $47 million—99.95 percent of which went to Democrats—together, placing teachers unions in the top ten largest political contributing organizations in the country. In 2020 they contributed $65 million in soft money to political action committees. In 2021 the unions also spent $4.5 million just in lobbying fees. And in 2022 the AFT's political action committee alone ranked number eleven in PAC contributions to federal candidates (100 percent went to Democrats).

The symbiosis of the teachers unions relying on Democratic politicians, and Democratic politicians relying on the unions, is well established. But the Biden administration made sure the relationship was explicitly, brazenly clear: First Lady Jill Biden's first official event, the day after her husband took office, was a meeting in the White House with Randi Weingarten, of the AFT, and Becky Pringle, of the NEA. "Joe is going to be a champion for you," Jill Biden, a longtime, proud member of the NEA, said. "You will always have a seat at the table." Photos of the trio, their cloth masks color-coordinated with their outfits, circulated widely.

A paper analyzing public schools' responses to COVID, coauthored by Michael Hartney, a political scientist at Boston College, who has a research focus on the influence of interest groups and unions on public policy, concluded:

Contrary to the conventional understanding of school districts as localized and non-partisan actors, we find evidence that politics, far more than science, shaped school district decision-making. Mass partisanship and teacher union strength best explain how school boards approached reopening.

Hartney's finding is succinctly evidenced in the data compiled by the analytics firm Burbio, which tracked schooling modes during the pandemic. The top ten states with the highest in-person school percentage were Republican, and the bottom ten states were all heavily Democratic.

The political association with in-person school percentages was so strong that it went deeper than the state level. Hartney's data set showed that even in red states, blue areas *within* those states stayed closed longer than the state average. Going a step further, because he had access to precinct and school district level voting records, Hartney found even at the county level blue districts within counties that had multiple school districts were below the county average for open schools.

In yet another data point showing a disconnect between school openings bearing any epidemiological underpinning, Hartney and his coauthor also found that districts were sensitive to the threat of students unenrolling and decamping for private school. "Districts located in counties with a larger number of Catholic schools were less likely to shut down and more likely to return to in-person learning," they found in their analysis.

Even without shared political affiliations, teachers unions don't control school districts. But the superintendents and other administrators who run the districts have to work with the unions. If you are a superintendent or schools chancellor or a board of education and the teachers union in your district is organizing rallies with child-sized coffins, it is, needless to say, an extraordinary challenge to compel them to come to work. (Some administrators did in fact do this in the fall, though, and I'll get to them and how they did it in the next section.) But because administrators were often in the same tribe as the unions, in many instances there wasn't much, if any, adversarial role for administrators to play since many of them shared the unions' aversion to opening the school doors.

When I spoke with Hartney, one of the topics we touched on was the bars-before-schools mentality in many states. "Look, bars and restaurants bring in tax revenue," he said. Schools, on the other hand, get money from taxes. How much this influenced policy is not clear, but it would be naive to exclude this financial incentive for governors and its potential impact on the hands-off approach many of them took toward allowing schools to remain closed if local authorities so chose.

*   *   *

One of the critical aspects that allowed for poor policy decisions on schools was a structural protection from accountability for nearly every decision maker. Superintendents claimed that they couldn't operate their schools without giving in to union demands; otherwise they risked teachers not showing up. The unions claimed that their demands were based on health experts' counsel. The experts presented their views as being in line with the consensus, which was often aligned with the CDC's positions. The CDC claimed that its school recommendations were just that, mere recommendations (which included plenty of "when feasible" semantic hedges), and that only state authorities could legislate actual policy. Governors and their state health departments in turn often explicitly based state policies on CDC guidance, sometimes upping the CDC's language from suggestions to requirements, in other instances leaving decisions up to individual districts as an ostensible gift of autonomy. And at the district level, even if not in an adversarial role with the unions, administrators often said that, despite the responsibility thrust upon them, none of the major decisions related to opening their schools or necessary mitigations were actually up to them. They were just following the state guidance— after all, who wouldn't follow a safety recommendation?

Governors not only left districts to decide what measures to implement in many circumstances, but districts had to figure out *how* to comply with whatever guidance they chose or were required to follow. It's here that we return to the security consultants. The firms, some of which had been hired years earlier by districts to design plans for dealing with school shootings and other catastrophes, swiftly moved into advising districts on infectious diseases mitigation. For school administrators this not only added yet another layer of insulation from culpability, it introduced yet another layer of potential blunders and bias. Which, as I detailed earlier, is how you end up with a nonsensical recommendation that every student be surrounded by 44 square feet of space.

None of this is to imply that security firms made incorrect calculations or harmful recommendations maliciously. Rather, it's that the benefits to the security consultants did not align with benefits to children. The security consultants were, of course, hired to help make the schools "safe," which in this context meant a lower likelihood (or, more accurately, a lower perceived likelihood) of COVID transmission in the buildings. If you're running or working for one of these firms your concern is not the harms incurred by a five-year-old, for whom English is her second language, who is unable to learn how to read via the three days each week she's home on an iPad, working with a glitchy software program neither she nor her parents understand, or the two days she's in school and she, her peers, and her teacher are all in masks with their voices muffled. You're also not paid to be concerned about the fourteen-year-old with ADHD, who is incapable of paying attention to the lesson on his Chromebook for more than two minutes and who spends his days playing video games instead. Nor will a twelve-year-old who developed an eating disorder from the isolation and misery of remote learning show up on a COVID case dashboard.

When thinking about incentives influencing policy decisions it's important to understand that there was virtually no upside to a security firm to push for *fewer* mitigations and for more kids to be in school. The security consultants' success was not going to be measured in child happiness or academic achievement or long-term well-being. It was going to be measured in COVID cases, or, even less directly, measured simply by the appearance of how much the district was "doing something." The costs to children from disrupted learning while in school buildings—from barriers, masks, and other interventions—and, worse, the academic, physical, and socioemotional harms from being blocked from attending school were largely downstream and too nebulous to ever be pinned on the firms. All motivations pointed in the other direction. The firm had no incentive to question the illogic of 44 square feet per student because reducing that number to one that more accurately matched the required six feet of distancing would have meant potentially increasing the number of students in school, which would have given the appearance of being less safe than recommending plans that compelled fewer students in the rooms.

Superintendents, principals, school boards, and other administrators had far more power and influence than security firms, but they were prey to the same incentive structure. None of them wanted to be the next Cherokee County, Georgia, chided by the experts and dramatized by the media with barely concealed schadenfreude and contempt as a nightmare example of red state folly. Though the education bureaucrats knew they were more culpable than a security consultant for what they would have viewed as externalities—the learning loss, the socioemotional harms and physical costs of time out of school, and a degraded experience while in school—during the pandemic, in the information environment created by the public health establishment and the news, nearly all of the rewards lay in enacting policies that projected the *appearance* of reducing risk of transmission. In blue localities in particular, administrators were incentivized to appease the fears of the community, or at least its loudest members, many of whom were frightened and misled by the media and health authorities regarding risks to children and teachers, and regarding the purported benefits of NPIs to reduce those risks. The incentive was for a maximalist and monomaniacal approach to school "safety." The more cases that were present among students or staff, the more the leadership would be questioned about whether they had done enough to keep people "safe." Therefore, the superintendents and administrators were incentivized to behave like a doctor overprescribing antibiotics, doling them out to every patient with a sniffle or sore throat who demanded them—maybe the amoxicillin would help, maybe it wouldn't, but the doctor would be credited if the patient got better, and would only be blamed if the patient got worse and no medication was given. If a patient had a reaction, well, these things happen. It was a fair price to pay for attempting to treat the illness. And antibiotic resistance was for someone else to worry about down the road. "Playing it safe" in the present is often at the expense of the future.

Beyond the superintendents, principals, security firms, school boards, unions, mayors, governors, and the entire political/bureaucratic apparatus related to schools, no one was more incentivized to promote a maximalist approach toward reducing transmission than the public health establishment, and most specifically, perhaps, Anthony Fauci, the figurehead of the pandemic response in the US. Fauci was not unique in his stance on schools, but rather embodied and amplified the consensus view, and validated it with his imprimatur. Therefore, an attempt to explicate his incentives for certain actions and outcomes that he supported is important.

Though Fauci lacked any legal authority to implement policy, because of his omnipresence in the media, his frequent designation as "America's top infectious disease doctor," and, most instrumentally, from a government perspective, his senior role in both the Trump and Biden White House pandemic responses, Fauci can be seen as the apex representative of the public health establishment (not unlike the *New York Times* being seen as representative of the legacy media). Fauci worked directly with

Deborah Birx in crafting and influencing the White House's positions during the Trump administration, including the hard push for the initial closures and the push for the longer extension immediately following the first fifteen days. And he was chief medical adviser to President Biden on COVID-19. With nearly forty years as the head of NIAID, the multibillion-dollar federal agency mandated to study infectious diseases and respond to emerging public health threats, Fauci's opinions on how to handle COVID were treated with great reverence by Washington insiders, those in the research and medical communities, and regular citizens. Publicly, his postures during the pandemic, expressed with extraordinary frequency in news interviews and press briefings, and otherwise referenced ubiquitously (his name appeared in 2,378 articles in the *New York Times* between January 1, 2020, and January 1, 2023—two-and-a-half times more than the combined mentions of the CDC directors during the same period), set the tone for how many Americans thought about all matters related to the pandemic.

The measure of Fauci's success would be based exclusively on the country's ability to "control" or appear to control the virus's spread. All of his credibility rode on whether, under his leadership, this viral menace could be tamed.

Fauci's report card would not include the vast and in many cases devastating harms from the policies that he advocated for to curtail the spread of the coronavirus—from people's inability to earn sufficient income as a result from various restrictions that wrecked millions of businesses (Black-owned small businesses were hit especially hard, with one study finding they had a 41 percent drop in spring 2020) to the epigenetic impacts from isolation and loneliness.

For the most part, Fauci's stance on school closures, like much of the official line from health authorities, was that schools should be open—if done "safely" or if the virus was "under control." Given his positions on masking, distancing, and interventions in general, this effectively meant schools would remain closed or, at best, operate at limited capacity for an extended period of time. It's important to note that Fauci explicitly advocated for school closures in the spring of 2020 when, in March, he cited their closure as a necessary mitigation. As I've discussed, initial closures may have been reasonable in some locations, but the absence of an explicit exit plan doomed them to continue beyond a reasonable time. In the middle of April, when New York City's mayor, Bill de Blasio, decided to keep the city's public school system shut down for the remainder of the school year, the *New York Times* reported that Fauci, informed of the decision ahead of time, gave de Blasio "his blessing." (At the time, cases were beginning to trend downward in the city, and there were still two months left of the academic year.) In May, in a heated exchange with Senator Rand Paul, Fauci warned that we "really better be very careful" when it came to children, and he mentioned the inflammatory syndrome, despite those who, unlike Fauci, had firsthand clinical knowledge of the syndrome having said there was no indication that it was a cause for broad concern. That summer Fauci advocated for a hybrid schedule in areas even with low levels of virus circulating, and said schools should be closed entirely if community levels were high, and that this could mean students would be in remote learning for months.

But Fauci—and the entire public health community—would not be graded on the immediate and long-term effects not only to children but also their families from school disruptions and closures that were advocated for. Just one example: At the onset of the pandemic, nearly half of all working mothers of school-aged children stopped actively working. Almost a year later, in January 2021, 35 percent of working mothers—more than 10 million of them—were still out of the workforce, an extraordinary figure the repercussions of which would require armies of economists and others to tease out. To put a fine point on the connection to school closures: the US Census Bureau reported that one in three moms were not working specifically due to "COVID related" childcare issues. In April of 2022, the US Chamber of Commerce released a report that estimated one million working women were still missing from the labor force.

The cascade of second- and third-order effects resulting from mitigation and containment measures, too voluminous and unknown to catalog completely, would largely be considered outside the public health domain. Although he was far from oblivious to or unconcerned with these effects, like the superintendents and mayors and governors, ancillary consequences were not Fauci's prime concern. But unlike the others, for whom COVID was but one of many considerations, stopping or slowing the spread (or at least giving the appearance of doing so) was Fauci's only visible responsibility. It was his mandate. All of his incentives aimed in one direction.

Fauci even admitted as such in one of his many acrimonious debates with Senator Paul, who, in May of 2020, questioned Fauci's singular domination of the narrative around what Paul viewed as aggressive and myopic COVID policy decisions. "I'm a scientist, a physician and a public health official. I give advice, according to the best scientific evidence," Fauci said. "I don't give advice about economic things." Yet, of course, "economic things" also affect health.

Fauci and the endless list of epidemiologists and others in public health who opined on the wisdom of various interventions were incentivized to value "doing something" over not doing something, as the survey of health professionals found. And they were incentivized to *believe* that doing something was beneficial because their professional worth, to no small extent, relied on this being true. After all, this is the very essence of their job—recommending interventions that improve public health.

In July 2022, more than a dozen researchers, from Harvard University's schools of public health, education, and medicine, and Boston Children's Hospital, among other institutions, published a fascinating paper. Low-income mothers, on average, have worse outcomes with pregnancies than wealthier mothers (this includes higher rates of stillbirths, preterm births, lower birth weights, and maternal health problems). Mothers in lower income households also tend to be less educated about pre- and postnatal health, and health in general. The relationship between a lack of education and poor health outcomes is clear. With this in mind, the researchers had conducted a large randomized trial of more than 5,600 low-income pregnant women, which sought to assess the benefit of regular home visits by a nurse who provided education related to prenatal health and child development. The visits began during pregnancy and continued for two postnatal years. Two-thirds of the women received the home visits, and one third were the control, meaning they simply had access to usual services and a list of resources.

The result, after nearly five years of total study, was that there was no benefit at all of the intervention. Outcomes for maternal and newborn health were the same whether the mothers received regular home nurse visits or not. (The moms who received the home visits actually had a marginally, though not statistically significant, worse outcome than those who didn't receive visits.)

Upon the study's publication, one of its authors announced that this was disappointing news. A doctor responded to her on Twitter, "I'm so sorry," and said that we still don't understand enough to intervene to prevent outcomes like preterm births. Michael Barnett, an associate professor of health policy at Harvard's T. H. Chan School of Public Health, mused, "Why didn't this common sense intervention work?" He guessed that "the results emphasize that the health system has only so much power to 'brute force' health outcomes."

A 2021 "megastudy" of more than 61,000 participants, conducted by 30 scientists from 15 different US universities, tested the effect of 54 different interventions to get people to exercise more often. The result: only 8 percent were effective after the study's rewards program stopped. More intriguingly, the study asked regular people, 156 professors from "the top 50 schools of public health," and professionals of behavioral science to predict the benefits of the various interventions. They overestimated the benefits by *nine times*. Even more telling, regular people's predictions were far more accurate than those by the professors and the scientists. The public health professors at the top schools were a distant third for accuracy.

There are two takeaways here. First is that, as I've detailed extensively by now, we simply don't know what interventions will or won't work. What may seem to be a patently obvious solution to a problem often does not bear out in real life. The world is more complex than what our intuitions tell us.

Second is that the surprise and disappointment by experts after the low-income mothers study publication, and the unrealistic overestimation of benefit of interventions in the exercise study, exemplify the natural bias among public health professionals toward believing interventions will be beneficial. Wanting to help improve health outcomes, especially for underprivileged people, is a noble goal and professional calling. But with this mission comes a belief, an ideology really, that orchestrated programs through government and institutions are an effective vehicle for eliciting good outcomes and solving public health problems.

For Fauci and the public health establishment to admit a lack of control over and lack of knowledge about outcomes would not have provided the sense of agency, for both officials and individuals, that much of the population understandably seemed to crave.

The nurse home visit study and the exercise megastudy illustrate why we *must* conduct trials or demand other high-quality evidence to find out if interventions that experts *think* will be beneficial actually are beneficial, and, if so, to what extent and at what cost.

Compounding Fauci and the public health community's bias toward action was that to advise healthy young people to "do nothing" would have gone against the tribe, in which the more aggressively one responded to COVID, the more one demonstrated their virtue—and leftist membership. To be seen as soft on mitigations one risked alignment with Trump and the "anti-science" Republicans and Libertarians.

The final incentive for Fauci and the public health community relates to how the costs and benefits of pandemic policies were seen and catalogued. Like the security firms, the metrics of Fauci's job performance in the public eye were relatively easy to measure. Even though cases on their own were not evidence of harm but merely a marker for potential harm (see: Alfred Korzybski, map/territory)—and for children a largely illusory one at that—cases became the scorecard. It was quite simple: If the case numbers were too high then things were going wrong. To Fauci's benefit, this was often marketed as a result of people not listening to him. "Fauci Blames Virus Surge on US Not Shutting Down Completely," from Reuters in the summer of 2020, was a typical headline. Belief in the effect of interventions, and blaming the public for viral spread—that all evidence suggested was largely out of the public's control—was not exclusive to Fauci and health professionals. Politicians and the media regularly parroted this sentiment. Cuomo, in his usual matter-of-fact delivery, said in a May 2020 press conference: "You tell me how well New Yorkers socially comply with distancing, and I'll tell you what that infection rate is doing. It's that simple."

COVID-related hospitalizations and deaths were also tallied and observed. Though more appropriate than cases as indicators of actual harm, these data, too, left out the non-COVID harms.

The NPI burdens were unevenly distributed, arguably inverse to the distribution of harms from COVID. Children were at the least risk yet, by and large, were burdened with the most disruptions. In aggregate, NPI-related harms were not necessarily any less damaging than COVID itself, and for many people they were much worse. Many of the NPI harms were much harder to quantify than COVID harms. But the scoreboard of cases, for months ever-present on cable TV news screens and the homepages of the nation's news outlets, which dictated the societal mood, media coverage, and a perpetuation of policies, did not make this differentiation.

Recall Campbell's Law—Fauci, naturally, was incentivized to focus on trying to affect the simple metrics that everyone could see easily and immediately. And in this the media and part of the public health establishment greatly aided him.

Throughout the pandemic the *New York Times* featured various COVID dashboards—pages of maps, graphs, and tables of cases, hospitalizations, and deaths by country, state, county, and so on—as a permanent fixture of its content. Johns Hopkins University's Center for Systems Science and Engineering featured an entire website of interactive global and domestic maps and numerous data visualizations on COVID. Visitors were met with scrolling lists of cases and deaths, by country, on the screen's left column, and a large world map in the center, pocked with red dots of varying sizes, depicting the extent of COVID cases, where one could zoom in and click a dot to get more granular data on the location.

The attention and deference paid to the *New York Times* and Johns Hopkins dashboards, along with the many other dashboards and tallies provided by state and local governments, the CDC, and media outlets were the primary lens through which much of the public was trained to see the pandemic. It was a reinforcing feedback loop: the more focus there was on these simple metrics, the more Fauci's asymmetric approach to the pandemic was validated; the more validated his approach became, the greater the justification for a focus on these metrics.

The country was operating in an information ecosystem based on a reductive quantification (and with the interactive maps something bordering on gamification) of success and failure, as people watched the numbers and graphs each day waiting to see what country or state was winning or losing. This isn't to say the availability of these data wasn't useful, and as a journalist covering the topic I found them extremely valuable. But, in aggregate, the ever-present displays of data became entertainment, offering an element of suspense, like a sporting event or horror movie. The graph bars growing and shrinking, the red dots on maps expanding and contracting, the cumulative numbers ticking ever upward—all of it was gripping material, in the way of rubbernecking an accident.

A regular person does not need to know the S&P 500 value each evening. Yet, nevertheless, many years ago TV news began providing these numbers as if this was something everyday people—the millions of pensioners and index fund investors who don't actively trade, not to mention the millions of people who don't hold any stock at all—needed to know daily to tell them how they should feel. People similarly did not need to know the daily COVID counts. Still, we were given, and many people craved, this information. Every time "the numbers" went up, they were tweeted, and texted, and posted on Facebook; mentioned behind masked faces in grocery store checkout lines; fretted over during calls to relatives; and emailed to superintendents and boards of education by certain anxious parents and others.

The *New York Times* decided that these numbers, every day, all the time, were important for people to think about and to impact how they should feel. The running counts and their various visual depictions, like a Vegas sports betting room with scoreboards in eyeshot no matter where you turned, conferred on COVID a place of prominence in the public mind. Now imagine if the *Times* instead, or at least in addition, had featured dashboards of "Days of School Closure" averages by state and county, and a "Child Misery Index" based on weekly pediatric mental health surveys conducted by the CDC. For that matter, imagine if the *Times*, the *Washington Post*, and every cable news network showed a tally of cardiovascular deaths, which is the number one cause of death in the US, permanently on homepages and chyrons on TV broadcasts. How might that influence how, and how much, we as individuals and as a society think about heart health?

Recall Bent Flyvbjerg's work on decision making in a society: powerful interests get to determine the parameters of what is considered important. While plenty of people, tragically, were directly touched by the death of a loved one or close acquaintance from COVID, many more people were not. Three full years after the onset of the pandemic the total number of people in the US who died with (though not necessarily from) COVID was a little more than one million, out of 330 million citizens—in other words roughly one out of every 330 people. The fact is it was statistically very unlikely, on a population level, for most individuals to directly know someone (rather than just knowing "of" someone, e.g., a friend of a friend or a distant acquaintance) who died of COVID. This isn't to say the deaths didn't bring great sorrow to many bereaved loved ones, or that COVID is not a genuinely horrible disease. The point is that one of the harms of the dashboards' prominence and eminence was that millions of people eventually witnessed a great disconnect between their personal lived experience and the ever-presence and, indeed, tyranny of these metrics to which they had no meaningful relationship. Ultimately, for a significant portion of the population, the empirical reality of their lives rendered all of these COVID data a statistical abstraction.

If a tornado rips through a town in Mississippi, every resident will see and feel its aftermath. They don't need the news or authorities to tell them that it was bad. They already know this from personal, direct experience. But with COVID many people knew it was terrible largely only because the media, the public health establishment, and "the numbers" told them it was terrible.

Even a TV executive admitted the disconnect between the media's constant focus on the scoreboards and people's reality. In a candid 2023 interview with the *Atlantic* Chris Licht, who took over as CNN's CEO in the spring of 2022, said of viewers' distrust of the network:

In the beginning it was a trusted source—this crazy thing, no one understands it, help us make sense of it. What's going on? And I think then it got to a place where, "Oh wow, we gotta keep getting those ratings. We gotta keep getting the sense of urgency."

COVID, COVID, COVID! Look at the case numbers! Look at this! Look at this! No context. And, you know, the kind of shaming. And then people walked outside and they go, "This is not my life. This is not my reality. You guys are just saying this because you need the ratings, you need the clicks. I don't trust you."

George Orwell wrote in *1984*, "The party told you to reject the evidence of your eyes and ears. It was their final, most essential command." Of course his novel warning about totalitarianism and surveillance differs in a great many ways from the circumstance I am describing. But this passage resonates because it speaks to the disunion regular citizens encountered from what they were being told was the reality.

The lived experience and the legacy of the COVID pandemic for many people was not a terrible outcome from the disease itself but rather the consequences of the mitigations imposed on them and their families. And these mitigations were in no small part dictated by arbitrary benchmarks that were based on metrics that were trumpeted to the public on dashboards through easily quantifiable counters and graphs and maps, infused with the symbolism of danger.

Parents watched their healthy children become sequestered in their homes for weeks, and then months. Athletics programs were canceled, playgrounds roped off with caution tape, swings chained together just in case anyone got any ideas. Skate parks were shut down, one of them in California bulldozed with thirty-seven tons of sand. Many families refused to allow their kids to have playdates with friends because that was the "right" thing to do. Once allowed back in school, masked students sat at desks with their heads burrowed behind plastic and cardboard barriers, unable to see or hear each other clearly. At lunch kids were spaced apart at sparsely attended tables, the cafeteria like a sad wedding reception waiting for more guests who would never arrive. Many children were barred from speaking during meals, still others made to eat outdoors, including elementary schoolchildren in the New York City winter, sitting on concrete in near-freezing temperatures. All for a virus that posed no greater harm to them than any number of other dangers for which their lives were never impeded. Little kids forced to eat silent lunches for a year (while adults could dine and chat indoors at a restaurant down the street) was not Fauci's concern. It was not reflected in the dashboards.

IV

PROGRESSIVE DOGMA AND NARRATIVE CONTROL

FALL 2020 AND BEYOND

19

PARENTS ADVOCATE FOR OPEN SCHOOLS

Through the eyes of some members of the Arlington Public Schools community things were worrisome well before the school year even began. In June 2020, in reaction to the district's plan to operate on a hybrid schedule that fall, a coalition of parents, educators, and other concerned residents in this wealthy Virginia county outside Washington, DC, formed Arlington Parents for Education (APE) to advocate for the schools to open fully instead.

The next month the planned hybrid opening was scrapped, but not for the schedule APE had hoped for.

The saga that would follow over the coming school year for parents and students in Arlington echoes that of countless towns and cities throughout the US. In some details—specifically, not opening in full until the fall of 2021—Arlington, along with many districts in California and those in a number of other states, was on the extreme end. But the approach to policy decisions, the often willfully abstruse communications from administrators with the parent community, and the lack of influence and power of parents—despite being organized, motivated, knowledgeable, and engaged—to affect change in Arlington was a story that played out around the country.

On July 16, Francisco Durán, Arlington's recently hired superintendent, announced a change in plans: there would be no in-person school at all at the beginning of the school year for the district's 27,000 students. His statement came less than a week after the local teachers union had sent him and the Board of Education a five-page, single-spaced letter, dense with fear and threats. In its first section, the letter stated that since case numbers were falling opening the schools would be like "cutting the

parachute the moment the descent has slowed." MIS-C (the inflammatory syndrome that was treatable and extraordinarily rare), the death of
a retired school custodian, that "every person is at risk of death or lifelong consequences," and that in-person learning "will most likely sicken
and possibly kill members of the APS community" were all mentioned.
The letter closed urging a virtual-learning-only model until it could be
demonstrated that schools would not contribute to community spread of
the virus.

When the first day of school arrived technology problems kept thousands of students from accessing remote learning. Plans were announced
for a phased opening of hybrid learning, beginning in October. But October came and went, and the schools remained closed.

During a board meeting that month Durán said that people should
not be critical of teachers who wanted to stay in a virtual-only model
because they were working hard. Around that same time APE launched a
postcard campaign from Arlington kids asking the district to please open
the schools.

In the first week of November, 230 (out of 27,000) students—only
those with disabilities who required direct support—returned to "in-
person learning." This was a misnomer, however. They did not receive
in-person instruction. Instead, they were given tablets and were super-
vised by staff while continuing with virtual instruction. An additional
150 students, including those of APS staff, were also allowed to return for
in-building remote learning. Images of the "in-person" learning, show
masked children spread far apart, their desks islands amid vastly empty
rooms, sitting silently, earbuds and headphones plugged into devices, as
a bored adult looks on.

This bizarre circumstance—of students physically in school buildings yet still only receiving virtual instruction—ultimately took place at
countless schools around the country, from New York to California. It
became known pejoratively as "Zoom in a room." (Though "remote learning hub," the sometimes official term for the practice, is more accurate
since much of the virtual instruction was not conducted live via Zoom or
another conferencing service.)

The inanity of allowing children—albeit in Arlington, very, very few
of them—in the school buildings yet still compelling them to do remote

learning was, of course, self-evident. If the building was safe enough for children to sit inside and do remote learning, why wasn't it safe enough for actual in-person instruction?

The program's absurdity and cruelty ran deep. One Arlington parent shared her daughter's story: her child, who has Down syndrome, was part of the small group of students permitted in the buildings. She had been in APS for preschool and was now in kindergarten. The child, along with a few others, sat in a room with an adult monitor, often a stranger who simply observed, while attempting in vain to engage with the teacher on a small laptop.

"We would get notes home with staff expressing frustration that our daughter wouldn't listen to the teachers via the laptop," the parent said. Remarkably, the girl's teacher was right down the hall, conducting remote learning from within the building but in a separate room, a practice a number of teachers carried out. "What a joke," Alison Babb, one of the APE parents, said, reflecting bitterly on the situation. "Imagine an autistic kid alone with an adult they don't know on an iPad for six hours."

According to several APE parents, there was one special ed teacher, who ran a class for disabled elementary students, who, along with an aide, went back into the building before teachers were allowed to do so because she refused to teach pre-K disabled kids on a laptop. The arrangement was kept hush hush, and all the parents who eventually found out about it quietly heralded the teacher as a hero.

In a November board meeting Durán said that he was committed to transitioning more students to in-person learning as soon as "health considerations" would allow. The general education students were scheduled to return in a multiphased plan, beginning in January, with exact dates "TBD."

APE parents were apoplectic. Over the previous four months they had distributed newsletters, submitted editorials to local media outlets, and held a rally. At one point APE even bought an ad in a local paper. Their Facebook group had one thousand members. All to no avail. Month after month, from June through the summer and then the fall, hundreds emailed everyone from the secretary of education on down to the school board. But the replies, when they got a reply, often just clouded the waters with lengthy nonanswers. A September 11 reply from a school

board member to an APE member's email was typical. It contained a laundry list of items that the district was "working on," including temperature
checks, ventilation, personal protective equipment, physical distancing,
cleaning and disinfecting, response procedures, contact tracing, access
to testing, and more. What exactly needed to be done with each of these
items was not explicated. Was there a delay in acquiring PPE or cleaning
supplies? Did the district not already have this gear? If not, why not? And
when would it arrive? The inclusion of ventilation in the list, in particular, was mystifying—and a worrisome tell—because a slide from a board
meeting presentation from September 10 read, in bold: "All classrooms,
including interior classrooms, have outside air ventilation according to
building code." One couldn't help but wonder about the rest of the items.

During Zoom board of education meetings parents were given just
two minutes to talk, and as policy board members wouldn't respond to
any speaker. To make matters worse the BOE would often turn off their
cameras.

The schools were closed. As the months wore on the parents became
increasingly worried and frustrated. Yet the best they could expect from
their inquiries about when the schools would open—when they got
responses at all—was a demoralizing stream of robotic responses or vague
language about safety: "Depending on the nature of your comments and/
or concerns, you may expect a reply. If a reply is required, it may take
between two days and two weeks to provide you with a thorough
response." And: "APS will continue to consult with the Arlington County
Public Health Division, Virginia Department of Health and CDC to monitor the COVID-19 situation. While many of the details are in development, the health and safety of our staff, students and community remains
our priority." And with BOE meetings conducted remotely and without
the opportunity for dialogue, there was no channel to meaningfully communicate with the powers that be. Month after month, their kids kept
out of school, despite their repeated pleas, parents could never get coher-
ent information on why the schools remained closed or when they'd
reopen. From every angle they were met with obfuscation.

At a base level, the circumstance seemed not just dystopian, but un-
American. As citizens they had the right to petition the government for
a redress of grievances. It seemed, at least in spirit, should that not also

include the right to a response? These were *public* schools after all, paid for with taxes.

Desperate for specifics, APE advocated for the district to provide metrics for when the schools could open, Babb told me, "because all we kept hearing was 'when it's safe,'" even though "safe" wasn't clearly defined. They were told that the district was monitoring metrics from the Virginia Department of Health. When they pressed for what the benchmarks were for opening, they were told that local decision makers "can" (with the word bolded) consider different indicators, but that they were broad guideposts.

At a certain point APE created a medical steering committee, which included an FDA infectious diseases expert, pediatricians, and the doctor who had treated the first swine flu patient in America. It didn't matter.

In November, APE initiated a slogan, "If they can do it, why can't APS," in reference to neighboring school systems—including Loudoun, Prince William, Chesterfield, Chesapeake City, Fauquier, Culpeper, Frederick County, Roanoke, Stafford County, and Spotsylvania—that had returned, even if just partially, to in-person learning. The Virginia Department of Education reported at that time that almost 100 of Virginia's 137 school districts had returned multiple grades of students to at least some in-person learning. Arlington—now months into the new school year, and more than half a year since the last normal school day—conversely, was steadfastly fully remote, notwithstanding the few hundred kids they allowed in the buildings, who weren't getting in-person instruction anyway.

Though Arlington stood out among some of its neighboring districts, it was hardly an anomaly. Among thousands of schools in districts around the country that did not even have a hybrid schedule, but rather had a full closure with zero in-person instruction, was APS's nearby peer DC suburb, Montgomery County, Maryland. The 160,500 students in Montgomery County Public Schools were also blocked from attending school. It wasn't until March 1, 2021, a whole calendar year after the initial closure, that just 730 students—less than one-half of one percent of the total enrollment—were permitted back in the MCPS school buildings.

In early September 2020, more than 60 percent of K-12 schools in America were closed entirely, with hybrid and full-time-in-person models

2020/2021 SCHOOL YEAR IN REVIEW
US K–12 Learning Mode Trends

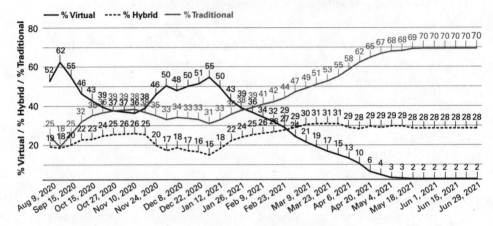

US K–12 Learning Mode Trends. Burbio School Opening Tracker.

at roughly 20 percent each. The percentage of fully remote schools fell through November to around 36 percent, before rising back to a peak of more than half of all schools in December and early January. (Looking at community case rates in the winter of 2020–2021, there is no correlation between areas that shifted from fully open to hybrid models or that closed schools entirely having any reduction in cases relative to similar districts that did not do so.)

*　*　*

Despite all the evidence that opening schools was fine, or perhaps because of it, advocates—from Arlington to Brooklyn to Evanston to LA—for kids to be allowed back in school had to contend with perhaps the most charged accusation in modern American culture.

In July, a *Washington Post* piece titled "The Racist Effects of School Reopening During the Pandemic—by a Teacher" set the tone, and, oddly, this general assertion did not temper as time wore on and the evidence mounted against it, but became instead more strident, more righteous, more indignant.

By December 2020, the Chicago Teachers Union tweeted the following: "The push to reopen schools is rooted in sexism, racism and misogyny." The sentiment from the union, which deleted the tweet at some later point, was not unusual, but rather a key narrative that emerged during the pandemic schools debate.

Devon Horton, superintendent of schools in Evanston, Illinois, told parents in his district who had voiced concerns about their kids being out of school for such a long time that they were exhibiting "white supremacist thinking." This was in January of 2021, when, ten months after the onset of the pandemic, the schools in his district had still not opened for in-person classes. Horton, who is Black, signed his emails to the parents he accused of white supremacist thinking "Unapologetically, Dr. Devon Horton."

In response to a 2021 school reopening plan in Cambridge, Massachusetts, a group called Educators of Color Coalition released a letter that stated the plans that the district "put forth for reopening, are rooted in white supremacy norms, values, and culture."

In January 2021, during a board of education meeting in Pasco, Washington, Scott Wilson, the president of the local teachers union, said, "There are decisions to be made. You stand on the lawn of the US Capitol as people break down barriers and head to the doors. Do you follow? We must not ignore the culture of white supremacy and white privilege. No one wants remote learning, but it is the right thing to do. We know the equity concerns." Wilson went on to say, "They complain their children are suicidal without school or sports. I find these statements an expression of white privilege."

The union had started a petition a month earlier, on December 16, demanding elementary schools return to fully remote learning, which was the only equitable option.

Megan Ranney, the emergency medicine physician-cum-COVID-pundit, tweeted an article on January 26, 2021, titled "The 'Reopen Schools Now!' Debate Is Rooted in Racism." Ranney, who after the pandemic became dean of the Yale School of Public Health, wrote in her tweet that racism was at work in many debates about reopening schools. Unaware or unbelieving of the copious evidence that schools did not drive transmission, the article's author rehashed fallacious arguments based on the premise that since Black families, on average, were at higher risk from COVID, their children attending school put their families in greater jeopardy, especially those in multigenerational homes. The article said that parents even seeking a "choice" for their kids to return was a "dogwhistle" for exclusion.

Beyond the extensive evidence that schools were not driving transmission, meaning that kids going to school were not "bringing the virus home" at an appreciable difference from when not in school, multiple studies suggest that exposure to children and the common cold coronaviruses they carry was actually *protective* for adults. One study, of more than 3 million individual health records, found that adults living with young children had lower rates of severe COVID than matched adults (those with similar age, health factors and demographics) who did not live with young children. Another study found patients who had tested positive for some of the common-cold coronaviruses had an 80 to 90 percent reduction in the likelihood of testing positive for SARS-CoV-2 infection. Essentially, in many cases, a kid with the sniffles from a common coronavirus may have acted as a COVID vaccine for those he infected with his cold. These findings also specifically cast doubt on the claims, promoted by Ranney and other prominent health professionals, that minorities living in multigenerational homes were at greater risk because of children cohabitating with elderly relatives.

Although these studies were published in 2022, Dr. Jake Scott, an infectious diseases specialist at Stanford University, said their findings were in line with basic immunology and existing literature. These findings—which upend the ubiquitous framing of schools and children as uniquely risky viral vectors, and both published in the prestigious *Proceedings of the National Academy of Sciences* journal—should be explosive and unsettling to a layperson. But among those with expertise in the field, they're unsurprising. "This hypothesis was aired since the beginning of the pandemic but was viewed as dangerous," Dr. Francois Balloux, an expert in the epidemiology of infectious diseases, said. "People avoided talking about this in polite circles." And so, with those who are well-versed in this corner of medicine generally staying silent about the science, public challenges to assertions that tied racism to open schools were largely absent.

Even as late as spring of 2021, after vaccines had come out—for which many teachers had been given priority—after tens of millions of children had already been in school full time in the US and Europe, after large swaths of society had returned to normal, when major league baseball teams were playing in stadiums in front of tens of thousands of fans, there were still charges that wanting to open schools was racist. In March 2021—a full calendar year after schools had closed—the head of the Los Angles teachers union said reopening schools at that time was "a recipe for propagating structural racism."

Similarly, a proposal to open schools in a San Diego County school district in April, based on teacher vaccination rates, was said to be part of a "very white supremacist ideology," by Charda Bell-Fontenot, the vice president of the school board. Bell-Fontenot, who is Black, said even putting the issue up for a vote was wrong. Forcing people to comply, she said, "That's what slavery is."

"You keep throwing out the racism, but I am Hispanic," Minerva Martinez Scott, one of the board members, responded, "and we have four adopted children, and we look like the UN. So, when you throw out racism, I don't understand that part." Martinez Scott said, "My child has also been affected by not being in school. My kid is in a facility because he had a hard time not being in school. I was able to find resources to get him the help needed. I want all the kids back in school."

That spring, parents in New York City held a rally for schools to open. Kaliris Salas-Ramirez, the president of her district's community education council (official groups that influence school policy in the city), organized a counter protest. She said that the rally was "white supremacy at its best." The counterprotesters hung a giant cloth banner with a crying white teddy bear and the words "White Supremacy with A Hug."

All these accusations of racism were against the backdrop and aftermath of mass protests around the country after the murder of George Floyd, an unarmed Black man, by the police. Quickly, many areas of life were enveloped by the wave of concerns about racism, and, perhaps most frequently, "systemic racism," a type of racism, it was charged, that wasn't overt but rather covert, woven into the systems of American society. Within this context it is easy to see how opening schools—which was falsely assumed to lead to more morbidity and mortality, with a disproportionate impact on Black people—was positioned as emblematic of *systemic* racism. A cornerstone of antiracist philosophy, as defined by antiracist figurehead Ibram X. Kendi, is that all racial disparities are evidence of racism. So if some white parents—and parents of Asian, Indian, Latino descent—wanted schools open, against the preferences of some Black parents, this was, by definition, racist. (The fact that President Trump, who was deemed a racist, also wanted schools open only served to calcify this argument.)

It was the nuclear option. The mere accusation of racism, particularly in the wake of the Black Lives Matter protests, was enough to brand people and destroy careers, social standing, and lives.

Making sure minority voices are heard is, of course, appropriate and a legitimate concern. But it is hard to see the sincerity—or at least the logic—behind claiming it was racist to want to allow Black children in school when white children (and other Black children) were already in school in thousands of districts. Even if the people making these charges genuinely believed Black families were at greater risk because of a child going to school—a mistaken belief made possible by the misinformation from so many public health officials and the media—parents didn't have to send their child to school. It was fantastical to claim that simply having the *choice* to send a child to school was racist, but removing that option was somehow just.

Moreover, given the substantial evidence that remote learning was inferior to in-person schooling, and that over time school did not increase anyone's risk of morbidity or mortality, an argument could be made that kids shouldn't just have had a choice to attend school in person, but, with rare exceptions, by the fall of 2020, and certainly by the winter—let alone spring 2021—it should have been compulsory. After all, for more than a century school had been compulsory in every state in the country.

The common thread among the accusations that advocating for opening schools was racist was a conflation of historical injustices against Black people with wanting to allow schools to open. What Ranney and many others seemed confused by was that it was not mutually exclusive to acknowledge past harms to the Black community, which were a legitimate cause of distrust and unease, and also acknowledge the bald truth: that, despite its many failings, school—for nearly all children—was a net benefit, and that staying home, especially for Black children, was a net harm.

I think it's fair to also entertain the possibility that at least some portion of the racism accusations should not be taken at face value. Consciously or not, the appearance of (ostensibly) defending the interests of a minority group, and simultaneously indicting white people in the process, carries enormous social capital in some communities, including much of the left-leaning fields of public health and education.

Further, the idea that schools still presented a unique and extreme danger, particularly as late as the spring of 2021, after the arrival of vaccines and much of society had been running, was so divorced from evidence and empirical reality that one would be remiss to not acknowledge that at least some union leaders were simply fishing for reasons to keep schools closed. I don't make this accusation flippantly. The wish lists that many teachers unions issued before they would return to school, some of which I covered earlier in the book—with their reverie of demands regarding tax policy, housing policy, and additional funds for teachers and schools in matters wholly unrelated to the pandemic—suggests that there was much more riding on schools remaining closed than mere claims of "safety." Consciously or not, fighting to prevent schools from opening gave leverage for more demands to be met.

Lastly, there were plenty of Black and brown families who did want their kids in school. For medical and public health professionals and union leaders and others to treat an entire race as having monolithic views was itself quite racist. And by doing so they denied the agency of the Black and brown families who wanted schools open.

Renee Bailey, a Black parent of three children, two of them school-aged, told me she and her children were devastated by the school closures in Los Angeles, where they lived. Her son had significant learning challenges and an IEP. "When school closed in the spring of 2020 they sent him home with a packet of blank paper, which was hilarious because he doesn't really write," she said. "They said he'd be back in two weeks. He didn't return for a year and a half."

His IEP entitled him to behavioral interventionists at all times, Bailey said, to encourage good behavior and help him stay on task. "Without it, he can't function," she said. Instead, Bailey became the behavioral interventionist herself, despite the fact that she had to work full time. She wound up hiring someone to look after her son at her own expense. Remote learning led her son to become reclusive. He developed social anxiety and self-injurious behaviors.

Bailey was outraged when the UTLA president, Cecily Myart-Cruz, said publicly that it was wealthy white parents who were pushing for schools to reopen. "Black and brown people don't want to be generalized. We don't want to be stereotyped," she said. "To say reopening schools is structural racism—that's wrong."

"People trying to say that people speaking out are only white. That's not true. I am a public-school-educated mother," she told me. "I always stood for public schools. This situation has changed my perspective greatly. I am pregnant now and this child will not set foot in a public school."

Maryam Qudrat, a Los Angeles parent, who is of Afghani descent, said that after speaking out to try to get schools open she was targeted by the union. On February 19, 2021, Qudrat received an ominous email from an employee of the UTLA. It began by referencing the several news articles in which Qudrat was quoted speaking in favor of opening schools, and then asked her to tell him her race for "a research project."

"Their conclusion was if you want schools to reopen right now, then that means you are racist against African Americans and Latinos," Qudrat said in a news interview at the time. "I think that they are very clearly case building, they are trying to collect data on folks like me who have been quoted in the *LA Times*, and they're trying to say that if you are in favor of the kids coming back to school, you're racist." Qudrat, an educator herself, said she stood with the teachers on strike in the rain a few years earlier when they wanted a pay raise. Now, she said, the union was turning school opening into a race issue, trying to pit Black and brown people against whites and other racial groups.

During remote learning Bailey worked with her daughter while someone else worked with her son. "She was in kindergarten! She had no idea how to stay on a computer, learn letters online, etc. It was a mess. It was so terrible." Bailey's daughter had live instruction from 9 to 11. "After that, she was supposed to do online assignments, apps like Schoology. The teachers would upload worksheets or activities, but the reality was she couldn't do it because she couldn't read it!" Bailey said the TV babysat her kids. School, she said, is a "stairway out of poverty, so every day that our kids aren't in school, that's just a day closer to poverty for them."

Bailey was deeply bothered by the narrative that schools should have remained closed because the Black community was so afraid of contracting the virus. While, surely, some people of color were exceptionally worried about the virus and were taking extreme measures to isolate themselves, just as many were not. "My husband was born and raised in Watts," she said. "I can tell you firsthand, those parents, those were the essential workers—at fast food restaurants, warehouses. When their kids were out of school, those kids were at home by themselves, and when not on Zoom they were running around playing with other kids in the hood," she said.

In Baldwin Hills (an affluent Black neighborhood in LA), she said, "they were still having block parties and art shows and community events. All this was happening but school was the problem? Come on."

Bailey's cousin Lamar Freeman coaches youth sports for underserved kids all over LA. Some of these kids were on track for college scholarships and even professional sports careers before they were completely derailed by closures. Freeman, in a 2021 TV interview while schools were closed, said the parents who he spoke to wanted schools open. "The parents are upset," he said. "They're kids, they need some kind of structure." He said 80 percent of his kids used to be honor roll students. With remote learning it dropped to 20 percent.

Bailey recognizes she was an outlier in her community when she spoke out about schools to the media. She said other parents agreed with her but were afraid to speak out, particularly white parents who didn't want to be seen as racist. "I could speak, but they couldn't," she said.

Bailey also said some of the perceptions about Black parental preferences were misleading. "The school where my son went, the parents there also wanted schools open. But they were focused on survival, paying the bills." A lot of these people weren't answering surveys, she laughed. "They wanted the schools open but fighting the system ain't never worked for us before so people felt there was no sense in trying to organize."

Despite the accusations against them, parents—and others—continued to advocate for schools to reopen. To them, not only was school clearly safe, and being prevented from attending school an obvious harm, but school was something their children, all American children, were entitled to.

20

RIGHTS AND RESPONSIBILITIES

Such wildly divergent outcomes between school districts around America over the course of the 2020–2021 school year raises some fundamental questions. Namely, what rights did families have to in-person schooling, and what professional responsibilities did schools and teachers have to provide it?

In the spring of 2020, when schools throughout Europe began reopening without notable impacts—while schools across America remained closed—it was an occurrence of exceptional significance, a feat of illogic impossible to overstate, and, one would have thought, impossible to overlook. Yet much of the American media and public health establishment dismissed the bald disparity with blithe postulations about Europe being different in one manner or another from the US, which, it was falsely claimed, negated any comparison. Whatever differences there were between the schools themselves, and the cities and towns between the continents, there was no evidence the differences were epidemiologically meaningful.

But as exceptional as the divergence between schools in the US and Europe was in the spring, in the fall of 2020 the course of events in America took a far more consequential turn: At the beginning of the academic year millions of American children began going back to school, while millions of other American children did not. This was an extraordinary development. Though it was never epidemiologically defensible, keeping schools closed in the US in the spring while their counterparts opened in Europe at least adhered to a domestic parity. As ill-conceived as the extended spring closures were, there was a perverse equity in all American children facing the closures. Now that equity was gone.

That fall, within a short time, many schools in states such as Georgia and Florida, among others, had children attending all day, every day, while millions of children in California, Virginia, Maryland, and other states did not set foot in a school building for more than a year.

There was wide variation of what was offered within states as well. A child could find herself in school full time, while her best friend down the block, in a different district, was confined to her bedroom, alone for hours each day, staring at a Chromebook. Millions of other children were enrolled in a vast experiment of "hybrid learning," in which schools were listed as "open," yet students attended only part time, some as infrequently as one-half day each week. Notably, millions of children who were enrolled in private schools attended in person while their peers in the same cities and towns did not. (This infamously was the case for California governor Gavin Newsom's four children, who attended a private school in person, while millions of children in his state, including most of those in Sacramento County, where the governor resided and his children attended school, were shut out of their buildings.)

All of this raises a crucial question: Is school an essential service?

Considering our government deems school to be so fundamentally important that it is illegal for a child to not attend, it would strain credulity to argue otherwise.

Therefore, we must accept that our officials at the federal, state, and local levels actively and overtly created, allowed, and perpetuated a brazenly inequitable circumstance: For more than a year, our country systematically denied an essential service to some children while providing it to others.

That the authority to deny this service for an extended time was handed over by many governors to local bureaucrats and administrators is perhaps the most consequential suspension of laws for American children in the last century, defying both legal precedent and our social contract.

The opportunity for a free public education is a long-cherished right, and an ideal deeply embedded in American history, even if its implementation has been, and still is, imperfect.

Laws requiring an opportunity for children to attend school are foundational to the nation. They even predate America's independence, going as far back as the mid-seventeenth century. In 1647 the Massachusetts

Bay Colony passed a law that compelled every town with fifty or more families to hire a teacher. Towns with 100 families or more had to support a local grammar school. Since this was a Puritan community, the prime purpose of the teachers and schools was to give children the ability to read scripture, though the law also stated the intent to prepare them for university. Other New England colonies adopted similar acts thereafter.

The act of 1647, according to historian David Carleton, established the core principles of public education we follow today: basic education is a public responsibly; the state can require communities to fund schools; and day-to-day operation of schools should be run at the local level.

The project of formal and free public education was so successful that more than a century later, John Adams said "a native of America who cannot read or write is as rare as a comet." A European clerk in the Caribbean in the 1790s marveled that he could give a pen to American sailors to sign documents, while French sailors didn't know how to write. As the journalist Anthony Brandt detailed in "Do We Care If Johnny Can Read?," his history of literacy in America, anecdotes abounded of foreigners from around the world over the next hundred years impressed by America's exceptionally literate population. During the Gold Rush in San Francisco in the 1840s, even though living conditions were generally quite primitive, a visiting Englishman named Frank Marryat observed in amazement that there still was a public school.

By the time of the American Revolution a number of cities and towns across the northeast had free local schools paid for by town residents. The Founding Fathers believed a thriving democracy depended on the citizenry being educated. And though women were denied the right to vote, many leaders, nevertheless, specifically supported educating girls.

There are no hard data on literacy during the early years, so Adams's remark about the comet, naturally, should be taken loosely. And, alas, state education did not extend to all groups equally, notably enslaved people in the south were largely denied a formal education, and a child's ethnicity, gender, and geographic location also were potential disqualifiers. But the early American attempt at public education (however flawed its lack of universality at the time) was fairly remarkable.

After the Revolution, Adams, Thomas Jefferson, and other leaders proposed the creation of a more formal and unified system of publicly funded schools, according to a report by the Center on Education Policy at George Washing University. By the 1830s Horace Mann, the Massachusetts legislator famous for championing education reforms, began advocating for free public school available to all children. He also lobbied for schools to move away from overtly parochial Christian doctrines, and instead adopt the teaching of broad moral themes (though still underpinned by religion). Educating the poor and middle classes was also a priority so they could get good jobs and help the American economy. But education was also seen by some as a means for people to achieve happiness and fulfillment. And for Mann, education for the lower classes was a means toward the social and political virtues necessary for national unity and a functional democracy.

By the end of the 1800s nearly 80 percent of young children were enrolled in public schools. And by 1918 every state had passed legislation making school compulsory. Constructing schools, and funding them through taxes, built a sense of community. The centrality of schools in communities cemented over time, and they not only served to educate children but to hold gatherings and meetings. The buildings themselves became critical locations for public functions, especially in rural communities.

This isn't to dismiss the discrimination of access to education based on race, gender, religion, and against immigrants. This is one of the reasons Catholics created a system of private schools. Nevertheless, public schools taught waves of immigrant children in the nineteenth and early twentieth centuries English and enabled them to assimilate into the broader culture (though often not without prejudice).

In the last half-century or so, the Elementary and Secondary Education Act of 1965, the Individuals with Disabilities Act, and various court rulings helped ensure all children, regardless of background or disabilities, had access to free public education.

Of course, even in the best of times American schools have been, and still are, vastly unequal. But when the option of school was taken away from only some children during the pandemic it did not remedy whatever inequities that already existed. It exacerbated them.

As innumerable data show, some of which I will detail later, for many economically disadvantaged children, in addition to those with academic and various personal challenges, school closures only served to widen the scholastic divide between them and their peers. The schools and children that were underperforming before the pandemic, by and large, only did worse after the closures. This is to say nothing of the noneducational hardships that only certain children had to endure while being locked out of school.

But even for children with financial means, and other advantages, remote learning was still plainly inferior to school. This was obvious very quickly to families, and many of them who had the resources sought any means they could to supplement "distance learning," or to get out of the system entirely.

The 2020–2021 school year saw a 3 percent drop in enrollment in K–12 public schools, more than 1.2 million children, the largest drop since World War II. The youngest grades saw the sharpest downturns, with the greatest concentration among kindergarteners. Not surprisingly, the largest declines in enrollment were in schools that were fully remote. For anyone arguing that, in aggregate, remote learning was successful or a sufficient substitute for real school, the enrollment declines suggest many parents felt otherwise. Data on where all the children went are unclear, but it's certain that a portion of high-income families pulled their kids out of the public system and enrolled them in private schools. The National Association of Independent Schools, a nonprofit that represents 1,600 independent and private schools in the US, reported that more than half of its schools saw an increase in interest in enrollment the summer of 2020, before the school year began. There were also extensive anecdotal reports in the media of many private schools and boarding schools maxing out their classes. CNBC reported in November of 2020 that as the pandemic wore on through the fall, more families were "seeking out schools that are fully in-person rather than remote—and, for many, that means switching to an independent institution, despite the cost." Emily Glickman, the president of Abacus Guide Educational Consulting in New York, told CNBC that her phone was "ringing off the hook with New York City public school families applying to private middle and high school." As of mid-October, 60 percent of private schools were operating in person, and just 5 percent were fully remote. Some polls found a substantial number of families began homeschooling their children. In Fairfax

County, Virginia, a survey found half of unenrolled students shifted to homeschool. An analysis of 22 jurisdictions found an increase of 30 percent of homeschoolers.

A report by the Urban Institute, a social policy think tank, found that only two-thirds of the enrollment drop could be explained by private school, homeschool, and demographic changes. In California alone there was no explanation for more than 150,000 students who unenrolled. The report author theorized that some of these kids had likely skipped kindergarten, were unregistered homeschoolers, or, troublingly, became truants.

Similarly, there were reports from around the country of children who simply disappeared—for any number of reasons they never participated in remote learning, yet weren't homeschooled or in private school either. Principals and other administrators drove around neighborhoods, knocking on doors trying to find out what happened to these kids—where they were, what they were doing. Some were nowhere to be found, others were home taking care of younger siblings, still others were working. The notion that it was safe for a fifteen-year-old to work at Target but not be in school was, of course, nonsensical and indefensible.

* * *

Much of this book is focused on epidemiology, science, and evidence—or lack thereof—related to NPIs. But setting that aside, and viewing school closures and their inequities purely through an ethical and legal framework raises some specific questions: Since schools are essential why should this service be denied, especially to only some children and not others? And what were the societal implications when unelected superintendents, rather than citizens, were empowered to enact this denial of service?

Though teachers unions have long argued that their work is essential, the message that closed schools—especially while bars and restaurants and malls and liquor stores and casinos were open for adults to patronize and enjoy themselves at their whim—sent to children and the community at large was, of course, that schools and teachers were not essential.

Some have argued that these other parts of society could be open because people weren't forced to go there, whereas school was not a choice. But, remember, nearly all districts that offered hybrid or full-time in-person school still gave families the option to keep their children home. The only people who would have been obligated to attend in person were teachers and staff.

What obligations do essential workers have to society? Healthcare workers were still expected to show up at hospitals and medical centers, and were honored for doing so. Cashiers were still expected to be at their retail stores. The specialists who repair and maintain the electrical grid, gas lines, and other vital infrastructure were still expected to do so. No other group of essential professionals en masse fought—and succeeded—to not have to show up to work. This isn't to say a great many teachers and education administrators didn't work incredibly hard conducting remote learning. But remote school, by nearly everyone's admission, including that of union leaders like Randi Weingarten, was, predictably, a woefully insufficient substitute for actual school.

Ethics ought to inform policy, just as science does, but neither is reducible to the other. It is a moral question about how much risk we ought to take, Dr. Daniel Sulmasy, a physician who also holds a PhD in philosophy, and is the director of the Kennedy Institute of Ethics at Georgetown University, told me.

"There is a moral duty to take reasonable risks," Sulmasy said.

"This sense of 'I didn't sign up for this,' that we heard some teachers say as a defense for demanding schools remain closed, represents a breakdown. It's a misunderstanding of the idea of what it means to be a professional," Sulmasy said. He lamented a lost sense of working toward the common good, especially in a profession afforded privileges—as was seen with its vaccine priority—and charged with overseeing children. We are called to take precautions, but we are also called to service, he said.

While schools of course were not a zero-risk environment, there was no evidence that schools were an exceptionally risky environment either. There was no evidence that all of the teachers who taught in person in thousands of private schools had any higher rates of infection or severe disease than the teachers in their neighboring public schools that remained closed. And, as was seen in the Swedish study, and observational evidence throughout Europe, there was no evidence that teachers working in person were at any higher risk than average among all professionals.

Despite the unexceptional risk they faced, and not having to show up in person, in some instances teachers received extra commendation and consideration. In Fremont, California, the *schools didn't open at all* in the 2020-2021 school year, yet an editorial in April 2021, nevertheless, called for Fremont teachers to receive hazard pay. The state of Michigan set aside $53 million for additional pay to teachers for the 2019-2020 school year, remarkably with "hazardous conditions" as one of the eligibility criteria, even though no teachers in Michigan worked in school buildings at all that spring after the onset of the pandemic.

*　*　*

The pandemic school closures demonstrated a profound shift in how a teacher's responsibilities, specifically those for caregiving, were seen. The word "care" here is not just colloquial; it carries specific connotations within ethics and feminist theory. It is here, in a reflection on morality and responsibility, that Joan Tronto, the feminist scholar referenced earlier in regard to safetyism and the paternalism of "protective care," is especially instructive.

Tronto, who is a professor of political science at the University of Minnesota, and coauthor of a highly influential 1990 essay, "Toward a Feminist Theory of Caring," has been at the forefront of care ethics for three decades. She defines an ethic of care as "an approach to personal, social, moral, and political life that starts from the reality that all human beings need and receive care and give care to others." This is what marks us as humans, she says. The core message is that we are interdependent beings.

Tronto's primary concern is that as women are decreasingly held back by certain barriers to join men in the workplace, the work of "care" would be passed on to poorer or lower-class women and to men of color. "My nightmare was that the women's movement would succeed and the positions that women traditionally held would become classed, rather than gendered," she told me.

During the pandemic the meme "teachers are not babysitters" circulated widely, in blog posts, editorials, and on social media. There were even T-shirts for sale with the slogan. Parents who advocated for kids to be back in school were maligned, with people calling them lazy, and saying "You just want a babysitter!" The title of a July 2020 post by a teacher on a website for education professionals was typical: "Teachers are not babysitters and I'm not returning back to school."

But this viewpoint does not reflect reality. The fact is, academics is not the sole function of school—as an institution or as a physical place. Part of the function of school in America is to provide a safe place for children to go. Parents—particularly those in families who do not have a parent or guardian at home during the day, a luxury unavailable to many families—rely on school for childcare. Though teachers, foremost, of course, are educators, they specifically *do* provide care, even if many of them declared this was not the case.

Tronto believes that teachers don't necessarily understand their role as caregivers. "Teachers have worked hard to dissociate themselves from babysitters, daycare workers, etc.," she said. Those are seen as lowly roles in our society. They're paid worse than a ditchdigger. In one sense the desire for this dissociation is understandable since there is such a disregard for care in our society. (One exception is nurses, who have professionalized their status, whereas they used to just take orders from doctors.) Still, demanding that the public pretend that this crucial and very real part of a teacher's job didn't exist was a denialist ruse.

But it worked.

During the pandemic, even through the spring of 2021, we wound up with Zoom in a room in schools around the country—from New York City to Los Angles and points in between—where, typically, low-wage workers were hired to oversee the children, while the teachers were off-site. Teachers passing on part of their responsibility to others in order to protect themselves was a perfect example of the exact problem Tronto had been studying, writing about, and fretting over for thirty years. It was a privileged irresponsibility, she said.

John Dewey, the great American philosopher and education reformer of the late nineteenth century and first half of the twentieth century, argued that school should be a place for fostering democracy and social reform. For Dewey, education, and school in particular, were about something more than just preparing people to be workers, cogs in the capitalist system. It was about teaching people to care for one another. But, according to Tronto, there has never been a proper discussion about schools as a place of care. The acceptance of Dewey's vision was never fully realized. Alas, this failure, perhaps, has not been better exemplified than by teachers unions' advocacy for long-term closures of schools in the US during the pandemic.

It is an inescapable irony—and one could argue for the stronger *hypocrisy*—that during the pandemic, teachers, who almost universally reside on the political left, through their unions—themselves bastions of collectivist leftism—acted out an individualist ideology. A significant portion of them urged schools to remain closed. Yet everyone knew that remote learning for a great number of kids would be a disaster, academically, socially, psychologically, even physically. There was never any doubt that some portion of kids *needed* the haven of school, and that when it was denied to them they either would be left on their own (with all of the expected harms of isolation), or the duty of caring for them would be foisted onto others—parents or guardians who might have had other vocational duties they had to tend to; or low-wage workers in daycare centers, YMCAs, and those Zoom in a room sessions (often in the very schools that apparently were too dangerous for teachers to work in but were fine for these other workers).

While there was much ire from groups of parents and others directed at the unions, a good deal of it justified, it's worth raising a flag here for a brief moment: none of the proceedings with the unions could have happened without the cover provided by the public health establishment, and by extension the media, (mostly Democratic) politicians, and, ultimately, much of the public. The health authorities, from Anthony Fauci on down, through their myopic focus on mitigating the spread of a virus (or at least a performative impression of mitigation), and their misleading claims that "no one is safe"—when, in reality, the risk to a healthy adult, and even more so a child, was not exceptional—allowed unions to craft outlandish lists of demands that needed to be met for schools to open in full. The distancing, the barriers, the HVAC upgrades—there was no evidence behind any of these measures having a meaningful effect. Nevertheless, they were touted repeatedly by health officials, and in turn cited by unions as requisite for schools to open and to operate "safely." Knowing the called-for safety benchmarks were all but unreachable, teachers ensured their responsibility for providing care would be passed on to others.

21

THE WORST OF BOTH WORLDS, PART II

To what extent union demands for mitigation measures, without which many schools were prevented from operating fully, were cynically employed, versus sincerely believed as necessary, is impossible to know. Regardless, the result was that millions of children were barred from attending school full time or even part time.

Compared to the twenty million children in Arlington, Montgomery County, Los Angeles, San Francisco, Baltimore, and countless other districts where schools were fully closed for all or most of an entire year, my district, with its hybrid model, made out relatively well. Still, it was an unnecessarily miserable experience for my kids and millions of others. And plenty of parents were frustrated, concerned, and resentful as time wore on and no advancements toward normalcy were made.

Like Arlington, my district was set to open in hybrid on day one, but, for vague reasons, instead began the year fully remote. That the superintendent, board of education members, and other parents had the attitude of "What's a few more weeks? It's not a big deal," demonstrated the chasm between how different families had experienced remote learning the previous spring and, more broadly, how they felt about schools opening in general.

Posts on our private local parents Facebook group descended into acrimony. What baffled me the most was why there were certain parents who argued so vociferously for the schools to be fully remote (and once we were in hybrid to either revert back to fully remote or to remain hybrid and not progress to full time). They could keep their kids home! What did they care if other people wanted to send their kids to school? The notion that other children attending school would somehow endanger their children, who ostensibly were ensconced at home, did not make sense. And any abstract argument that schools being open would drive up cases overall, thereby indirectly endangering others in the community, was belied by the evidence from Europe and elsewhere. I don't recall by that autumn there being vehement opposition to restaurants or stores being open. People who felt patronizing them was unsafe simply didn't go to those places. But schools—a place, too, where their children had the option to not go—were an emotional focal point.

As a coauthor of the petition to open the schools in my district I became somewhat of a local figurehead for that movement. And with that position came admiration from some and, in the Facebook battleground, scathing condemnation from others. I was asked in one post, "Why are you all so eager to murder children?" I found out one of the people who was particularly nasty toward me and others who were advocating for schools to open didn't even live in our town, but was a teachers union representative a few towns over. In one of her threads a like-minded commenter fumed about people "petitioning for our public school teachers and staff to go into the slaughter house."

These types of comments were common around the country. The Arlington parents were called the "Open Caskets Now" crowd by their opponents, and an Arlington teacher wrote on a Facebook post to them "Stop trying to make me die." Less overtly acerbic was the insinuation that parents who were advocating for schools to open were simply lazy and didn't feel like supervising their children, a dovetail to the "teachers are not babysitters" meme. Andy Slavitt, who later served as a pandemic adviser to president Biden, tweeted in July 2020, "Some people want their kids back at school to get an education, but I think others don't want to be around their kids all day long. They have more passion for the issue." A reply to an open schools advocate's tweet was typical: "Maybe prioritize your kids over yoga class."

Some parents who argued for schools to close or to not offer full-time classes claimed that they weren't only, or at all, fighting for their kids, but rather they were fighting for teachers' safety. But that concern was hardly credible—or at the least it was ethically inconsistent—given that these same parents continued to eat meat prepared at slaughterhouses, staffed by shoulder-to-shoulder workers, that never closed, and without interruption received an infinite array of products delivered from Amazon that were packaged by teams of workers in warehouses.

Thankfully, unlike Arlington, some two to four weeks into the school year, depending on the grade, hybrid schooling finally began in my district. This delay may seem trivial, but for the children (and their families) who struggled mightily during remote learning that lasted for months the previous spring, every additional week that ticked by before the kids could be back in person was agonizing.

Some single-parent families or those with both parents who worked found their homes in a constant state of tension and rancor. Many of the parents, absorbed in their own work or obligated to Zoom much of the day, were unavailable or unable to help their kids with the inevitable tech glitches and communication issues that constantly arose with remote learning. Thousands, perhaps hundreds of thousands of social media posts from around the country, some with videos, painted a dreary scene of elementary-school-aged children in states of extreme frustration from being mandated to spend hours alone in front of a screen for "school." Many tweens and teens simply turned their screens off and didn't bother engaging at all. Forcing kids out of school for all or part of every week brought a list of sufferings for many children—from learning loss to depression to the more gruesome, like physical abuse. But for many millions of children the harm was more ineffable, something less incendiary and more quietly devastating. Seven-, eight-, nine-year-olds, normally sparks of light and energy, instead were anesthetized under a blanket of ennui.

In many areas, like New York City, once schools did eventually open, the absurd scheduling was hardly better than fully remote. Politicians, like Mayor De Blasio of New York City, and, later, Joe Biden after he took office, liked to boast about schools being "open." But the reality for many students was a few hours in the building one or at most two days a week, often spent on a screen with virtual instruction.

A section of a *New York Times* article on open schools advocates memorably captured the circumstance:

Among parents who have been fighting for open schools all year, Rachel Fremmer, an out-of-work librarian and the child of two New York City public school-teachers, has been one of the most vocal. Her daughter, a student at LaGuardia, which specializes in the arts, is in the building only on Thursdays and just for two hours and 45 minutes. On Mondays her remote school day is over at 1:10 p.m. On Tuesdays there is only an hour of online Italian. This term her daughter is receiving no math or English instruction at all.

Recently a friend with children in private school noticed Ms. Fremmer's daughter in Riverside Park in the early afternoon and was confused. "Anyone who doesn't have a child in public school thinks schools are open," Ms. Fremmer said. "If a store had hours like this, with random, nonconsecutive times for online shopping, you wouldn't call it open." I asked her what her daughter and her friends were doing with all of this free time that they didn't necessarily want. "They're teenagers, so they are sleeping and watching Netflix," she told me.

It was no wonder that so many families chose to continue with fully remote learning—going in to school for a few hours of Zoom in a room was hardly worth the trouble. Yet some teachers, union leaders and others strategically pointed to the percentage of fully remote students as evidence that those families preferred remote learning to being in school full time, when the truth was they preferred remote learning to the mangled schedule that hybrid schooling offered.

Compounding the frustrations of hybrid schedules were extremely aggressive quarantine rules that repeatedly locked students out of school if they were deemed a "close contact" of an infected individual. The students in quarantine could have no symptoms at all, or even not be infected, but they still had to stay home. The "close contact" rules varied from place to place, and were borderline inscrutable, requiring the focus of a Talmudic scholar to interpret them in each potential case. If parents felt their children were wrongfully quarantined there was little recourse for grievance. To attempt to find answers and appeal the decision was to take a Kafkaesque odyssey to nowhere.

The CDC's rule, which my district, among thousands of others, followed, was that if a student was six feet or more from an infected individual then they were not considered a close contact. One time we were alerted that my daughter got nabbed in the quarantine trawler net. I asked the administrators, "Considering the classes are all half empty, and it's the rule that kids are six feet apart from everyone at all times, how is it even possible that she is a close contact of an infected person?" The school said it was possible that a teacher walked around a classroom, briefly breaching the six-foot space as they passed by students. Except, I countered, in order to be a close contact required not just being closer than six feet, but it had to last for fifteen minutes or more. The school then said that although the close encounters were brief, *in aggregate* they may have totaled fifteen minutes. Due to privacy laws, they wouldn't say who the infected person was so there was no way to ascertain the truth. So without proof, and through a process that was secret, the school forced my daughter into quarantine.

New York City had a "two case" rule, in which two unrelated cases would trigger the closure of the entire school, which, inevitably, became a common occurrence. Children who technically were attending "in-person" school, in actuality found themselves with wildly erratic attendance that was out of their control. Even though schools were "open," it was not unusual for a student to have been in the building just two or three days over the course of the entire fall.

* * *

After a number of weeks of fully remote learning, my kids' hybrid schedules finally began, with my daughter in two days a week, and my son, his fourth-grade class divided into morning and afternoon cohorts, in each day for two-and-a-half precious hours.

My wife and I were both working full time. Nevertheless, I stepped away from my desk repeatedly to help with remote learning. But the larger problem was what to do with all the down time. After his "school day" ended in the late morning, my son was at a loss as to what to do the rest of each day. Yes, he drew pictures. Yes, he read. Yes, he and my daughter went outside. That all took care of an hour or two. Then what? Nearly all the families in town were adhering to strict distancing rules, so playing with other kids was out. I took time off when I could for bike rides, board games, and whatever else we could think of. But, like most Americans, my wife and I have to work or we can't pay our bills. We couldn't just not do our jobs. She would get fired, and I, as a freelancer, would stop making money.

My kids' foreign language classes were taught by teachers in masks, making learning new words and pronunciations near-impossible in the building. But on the remote days of hybrid, trying to learn another language from a teacher whose mouth you couldn't see, with a muffled voice, carried over a glitchy Google Meet connection was an exercise in farce and frustration.

What was the district's plan? What was the holdup? My son was nine years old. Two and a half hours of school is the schedule of a three-year-old in nursery school. That was not going to cut it. Nor were two days per week.

When they were actually in the buildings this was the setup:

Every student had a three-sided tabletop barrier on their desk. Its front panel was see-through but not entirely clear, like cellophane. And the sides were opaque cardboard, like horse blinders. The children were to sit with their heads inside of these barriers for the entire school day. Naturally, no one could hear each other easily, so the students would lean backwards, their heads outside of the boxes, to talk to each other, defeating the purpose of the barriers. Speaking through masks, they often had to raise their voices to be heard clearly, which, in theory, increased the likelihood of transmission.

Taking a belt and suspenders approach, in addition to mandatory masking, and the desktop barriers, the district took it upon itself to install floor barriers between rows of desks. They were composed of wooden

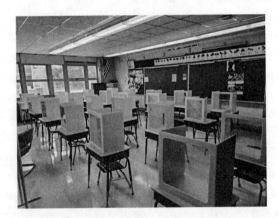

Classroom in Hastings-on-Hudson school district, prepared before the first day of school fall 2020. Once schools did open, the classrooms accommodated fewer than half of the desks visible in this photograph. *Source*: Hastings-on-Hudson school district.

frames and more durable plastic. The facilities staff of the district apparently worked extremely hard building the floor barriers themselves over the summer.

I, along with other parents—many of whom were among the more than 300 who had signed the open-schools-full-time petition—sent numerous queries to the administration asking why a plan for full-time in-person learning was not being implemented. One of the responses was that because of the floor barriers it would be too dangerous for classrooms to operate at capacity.

I emailed the superintendent and BOE again. I noted that the state guidelines did not require these giant floor barriers in addition to desktop barriers. "By implementing both types of barriers the district is, by its own admission, creating a roadblock to children being in school full time," I wrote. To be clear: the district installed additional barriers that were not required. And then it claimed the schools couldn't open full time because of the dangers posed by these additional barriers.

I also expressed how hard it would be for anyone, let alone kids, to sit with their heads inside the desktop barriers for seven hours a day, especially when they couldn't see out the sides. Though the state guidelines explicitly said barriers negated the need for six feet of distancing, my kids were still limited to two days per week as a result of a six feet of distancing requirement. The barriers not only provided no benefit for viral mitigation, their one potential benefit—allowing for a relaxation of the six-foot rule, which would enable full classes and full-time school—was not taken advantage of.

Though there shouldn't have been barriers at all since the kids were maintaining six feet of distancing and, as a consequence, stuck in hybrid, I recognized the district was not getting rid of the barriers anytime soon. Resigned to that reality, I sent the administration links to websites selling barriers that were clear all the way around. At least let the kids be able to see things other than what was straight ahead through a blurry plastic square. They were $60 to $90 each. Could the district please at least switch to those? I said I would organize a fundraiser, if needed. This was rejected. I also suggested to the superintendent and principals—who got to sit freely at their desks all day, unencumbered by any barriers—that if they were going to force the kids to sit with their heads inside horse blinders for seven hours a day, that the administrators, too, should do so, in solidarity. This suggestion was also rejected. I did not intend the suggestion sarcastically. I meant it sincerely. If the superintendent had to keep her head inside one of those barriers all day long, for as long as the kids were required to do so, I was, and still am, of the firm belief that the barriers would have come down. Just like the unmasked politicians at sporting events and clubs, and Governor Newsom dining at an elite restaurant while the citizens of California were barred from such gatherings, it seemed the burdens imposed by those in charge didn't apply to them. It was a case of rules for thee but not for me.

Like Arlington, my district's administration gave vague pronouncements about its plans. "Over the next month the Board and Administration will dynamically evaluate conditions in our schools, region, state, and country to continue to redefine the best path forward," a Board of Education letter in September stated. I asked what benchmarks the BOE was using in its "dynamic evaluation" to determine when schools could open. With the use of barriers and masks we already were able to open full time and be in compliance with state requirements. I was baffled why and how a local school board, with zero epidemiological expertise, could have the authority and impetus to prevent kids from attending school every day when the state of New York—which did employ a large team of public health professionals—already said we could open full time.

Moreover, I said that the positivity rate in our region had been below 1 percent for months. You couldn't get any lower than that. What, exactly, were we waiting for?

Lastly, I reminded them that there was evidence that hybrid models could *increase* exposure to students and teachers. I linked to my article in *Wired* from the summer on the risks of hybrid learning, and a tweet by an infectious diseases epidemiologist at Harvard Medical School suggesting as such. Was it guaranteed that hybrid would lead to more cases? No. But nor was it guaranteed that the hybrid schedule would lead to fewer cases. Without evidence either way, the default should have been for the kids to be in school. Since any family had the option to keep their child home for fully remote learning if they wanted, why not let the kids in school full time for the families that wanted that option?

The superintendent responded that there was passionate discourse and disagreement on all sides of the opening schools issue. She said the district had to consider "the fears expressed by faculty and staff regardless of the safety measures that have been implemented." If the schools opened full time, she said, some unknown portion of staff might not show up.

A week or two before the email exchange a parent whom I had gotten to know through the open schools petition reached out to me. He had connections with an influential teacher in the district, he told me, and he wanted to arrange a clandestine meeting between me and his contact. The three of us met one afternoon at the parent's home, sitting at a patio table. The teacher, who taught in the elementary school, said an informal poll among colleagues showed that all or nearly all of them were prepared to work with kids in the building full time. Most of the teachers hated hybrid, and, not surprisingly, found that teaching kids in the room and simultaneously to kids who were remote was a nightmare. They weren't able to service either cohort effectively.

I wrote back to the superintendent and told her what I learned about the elementary teachers. I also mentioned the names of several nearby towns that had at least elementary grades open full time. If they could do it, why couldn't we? I was told that the elementary school principal would respond to me. When she did, the elementary principal told me there were many perspectives among the staff and that the district wanted to proceed with caution. This was belied by the information I had gotten from the teacher, but there was no official poll to corroborate or challenge what the principal said.

The administration used the word "equity" repeatedly in its communications. An administrator's earlier email stated that "equity" was the obstacle to the elementary school opening full time because the middle school and high school were going to remain hybrid. The concept of equity meant that every student needed to have the same experience. So it would be inequitable for only the younger students to attend full time. (Never mind that since students were from a range of backgrounds, living in a range of circumstances, remote learning was already inequitable.)

My experience and concerns were not unique. The intransigence of school administrators; the not just dismissal of, but willful disinterest in

any data or evidence presented to them that pointed toward more schooling or fewer mitigations; their circular arguments and vague explanations
for how they would make determinations for opening the schools were
happening all over the country. I've highlighted Arlington and my own
district, but there were similar experiences in hundreds of school districts,
from major cities to small towns, from coast to coast. Whether it was for
hybrid or fully remote, the playbook was basically the same.

For all of the animosity I and others around the country experienced,
there also was a budding community of parents, doctors, public health
specialists, educators, and others who wanted schools open. Open
schools Facebook groups were sprouting up, composed of parents band-
ing together locally and nationally. New Twitter accounts kept appearing,
with names like @angrynycmom, of people sharing links to studies (from
outside the US, of course) showing that schools were not driving transmission, and that children were at exceedingly low risk. Private DM groups
formed on Twitter, made up of parents and others committed to the cause,
from California, New York, New Jersey, Texas, Illinois, Washington, DC,
Maryland, and Massachusetts. Parents from Georgia and other states who
had kids in school full time but felt so passionately about the issue that
they were fully engaged in the movement to help other kids. There were
even a few standouts on Twitter who didn't have kids and didn't work
in public health (and were not Republicans, so there was no political
motivation), who nevertheless fervently took on the cause of getting kids
back in school. A Manhattan art dealer named Eli Klein and a mystery
novelist and financier named Zac Bissonnette were particularly active,
relentlessly debating and prodding experts and media types, amassing
tens of thousands of followers between them. Bissonnette, a former non-
fiction author with many media connections, waged a behind-the-scenes
campaign, regularly private messaging dozens of high-profile journalists
at the *Times*, the *Washington Post*, and other major outlets, challenging
them whenever he felt their—or their publication's—coverage of schools
was misleading or wrong.

A dozen or so dads who became friendly through the open schools
petition and advocacy started periodic evening get-togethers in a parking
lot in town. We'd arrive one by one, by foot or car, carrying lawn chairs
and beers, arranging ourselves in a big circle. The nights would begin with

talk about the latest developments in the schools—new controversies and inanities related to remote learning, the complex hybrid schedules, quarantines, indecipherable word salad memos sent by the superintendent, Facebook fights, and so on. But the conversations would shift after not too long to all matters of interest. Home repair, movies, Foucault, The Simpsons. A continual topic was what was going to happen with kids' sports. As the weeks and months wore on, the meetings became smaller, and after the clocks rolled back, and nightfall overtook our village between four and five o'clock, we'd arrive in the dark, latecomers only finding the group by the sound of distant voices. By then, the core group of us mostly just shot the shit, skipping schools talk entirely. With social distancing and masking and all the rest, society in the New York metro area was still in a state of discomfiting abnormality and duress. No one in the group thought COVID was fake. We didn't bother with masks, but we still met outside, even in the cold, as a nod toward the norms of the time. There was a doctor at Columbia University, a tech guy, a corporate lawyer, an actor, a financial consultant, a think tank president, a few others, and me. Most or all were liberals of the classic variety, or Democrats, I think. We just felt that the schools should be open. That view didn't seem at all to be in conflict with most of our politics; there was nothing inherently illiberal about it, even though it was against the party line. Since the most vocal and active people in town were decidedly progressive and wanted the schools shut, it was hard to tell whether we were in a true minority, or perhaps the more vocal tip of a silent majority.

The camaraderie and relationships, both in-person in my town and virtually with others around the region and the country, were a salve. It was common to talk about the feeling of alienation, the newness of being in the "out-group" in decidedly blue areas, and of losing friends but also gaining new ones. Advocating for schools to open, and for reducing the various burdens on children, created communities of people who often had never been politically active before.

Though the friendships that resulted from the movement had been a joyous and curative force, its impetus was dark—a commonality of bewilderment and exasperation, resentment and alienation at how the personal liberties of children had been stripped away, and without any persuasive justification. If you could look past the hysteria of media coverage, and

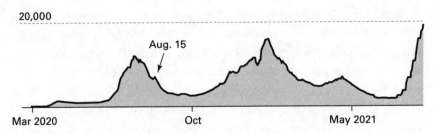

Florida COVID cases, March 2020 through spring 2021. *Source: New York Times.* "Aug. 15" and arrow added by author.

the authorities' messaging, by mid-fall it was clear that nothing special was happening in the places around the country where kids were in school full time. There was no discernible correlation between any of these attempted mitigation measures and outcomes.

To take but one example: Here is a graph of Florida COVID cases. Nearly every one of Florida's districts opened schools between August 10 and August 31. Yet cases in the state continued to fall and then remain flat for more than an entire month, until mid-October. Moreover, similar case-rate epi curves during the same period were seen in California and other states where significant portions of schools were closed.

Does this mean schools didn't contribute to the spread of COVID? No, of course not. What it shows is that opening schools did not lead to a catastrophic rise in cases. (Indeed, cases *fell* after schools opened for more than a month.) There was no correlation at all with school closures or openings and case rates. This was plain to see in real time. To the parents and others advocating for open schools, preventing kids from attending school full time by that point simply made no sense. It was absurd. Many of the children were hurting, some far worse than others.

DEEP DIVE: HARMS OF SCHOOL CLOSURES

The focus of this book is on the decision-making process behind school closures and interrupted learning, and, secondarily, mitigations within schools, many of which further interfered with children's well-being. As you surely have observed, relatively little time has been spent giving detailed narrative accounts of children and young people suffering from disrupted schooling. The harms of school closures are so manifest that continually cataloging them or weaving drawn-out anecdotes throughout the book struck me as unseemly and superfluous. A spotlight on the mechanics of how these poor decisions were made, of how the gears of society and culture turned, is, in my view, far more important as a historical record, and also as a sociological study. Nevertheless, it is worth taking a limited, intense tour of the evidence to remind readers of what was at stake from the actions of decision makers that this book so meticulously dissects.

The harms I will detail predominantly were known and observed in real time, or even known in advance, just as nearly all of the evidence I present in this book was known in real time or in advance. The single most important myth that this book seeks to debunk is the notion that various interventions—most specifically related to schools and kids—were reasonable or even necessary to be employed because "we didn't know" at the time about their lack of benefit, or the relatively benign course for children from the virus. On the other side of the coin, it was similarly false to say "we didn't know" about the harms that would accrue from these largely ineffective interventions. With that said, I will introduce a few data points and studies about learning loss that necessarily are retrospective. However, given the pre-2020 historical record of learning loss associated with an absence of schooling, it should have been anticipated.

*　*　*

Perhaps the most heartbreaking consequence of school closures is the association with increased child abuse. First, children in unsafe homes, who normally would have had the respite of school, found themselves instead essentially locked inside with abusive adults for extended periods. Many of these adults were out of work because of the mitigation policies, and those who worked from home or normally were at home anyway found themselves no longer alone during the day, but with a child, perhaps unwelcome, infringing on their solitude. It was a toxic mix.

But the larger and exacerbating problem is that educators represent the number one source of all official reports of child abuse or neglect. When kids were prevented from attending school teachers were no longer available to act as a safety net for children being abused. Once schools closed, around the country, from New York to Illinois to California, there were massive drops in reports of abuse. "They don't have a way of telling people that something might be happening, and that really, really scares me," said Dr. Norell Rosado, at Lurie Children's Hospital in Chicago, at the time.

At a Virginia safety center, calls plummeted by around 70 percent. And when the center did get calls more of them were for injuries so grisly that it was because an adult had to seek medical help for the child. A pediatrician who works with a children's aid nonprofit that serves underprivileged children who often are in foster care, unstable or unsafe homes in New York City, told me of one child she treated who, alone all day with an abusive step parent, was beaten with an electrical cord.

All of this was predictable. The critical role of teachers and schools as a leading reporting mechanism for abuse was known before the pandemic. And, as expected, evidence that the nightmare had come to pass arrived very shortly after all the schools closed in the spring of 2020. "We are seeing an over 25 percent decrease in calls to our hotline since schools closed. That means many children are suffering in silence," said Darren DaRonco, a spokesperson for the Arizona Department of Child Safety, on April 13, 2020. The sirens continued to blare as the months wore on. A highly comprehensive paper titled "Suffering in Silence: How COVID-19 School Closures Inhibit the Reporting of Child Maltreatment," in the *Journal of Public Economics*, explored in great detail the association between school closures and child abuse during the spring lockdowns. It was published in August of 2020. The authors of the paper estimated 212,500 allegations nationwide went unreported during the months of March and April 2020 alone. So not only was this grievous outcome foreseeable before the March shutdown, the extensive data in the spring and summer guaranteed that public health officials were well aware—or were remiss in not being well aware—that this inevitable horror would continue in places where school was fully or partially closed through the fall and beyond.

Another group of children and adolescents who disproportionately suffered because of school closures were those who required special education services. More than 7 million students between three and twenty-one years of age were covered under the Individuals with Disabilities Education Act (IDEA). These children receive an individualized education program (known as an IEP). Once schools closed, these services, many of which require an adult to physically work with a child, were greatly diminished or were terminated entirely.

Remote learning was challenging enough for general education children. But for many kids with autism, ADHD, cerebral palsy, and a long list of other cognitive or physical disabilities it was a nonstarter. Expecting a child with autism or ADHD to sit alone and learn math or how to read on a screen was, in many instances, to cruelly doom them to failure. Many remote learning programs did not even have what was termed "synchronous" learning, meaning live instruction. Instead, "asynchronous" lessons were assigned, in which a child was intended to engage alone with a software program or to watch videos or work on various assignments with no interaction or input from a teacher.

A mother of an eight-year-old son with ADHD told me, "This was never going to work." She and her husband both were working, so her son, frustrated at his inability to focus on the remote instruction, zoned out on YouTube and video games for hours on end each day. Eventually the mom quit her job and effectively became a full-time aide, helping her son with his virtual learning. "It was a nightmare. The loss of income, the fits of rage by my son," she said. "I have enormous respect for teachers and paraprofessionals. I can't do what they do." Like the circumstance in many families I spoke with, her son regressed without the proper supports. He began hitting his mother and breaking things, behavior that, through a lot of work, had ceased the year before the pandemic.

There are more than one hundred thousand children in the US who are deaf or hard of hearing. These students qualify for an IEP. Cheri Dowling, the executive director of the American Society for Deaf Children, talked with me about the impact of school closures and remote learning on this community. Some of these kids, especially those who use American Sign Language (ASL), and where the school provided ASL online, did okay with virtual learning, Dowling said. For others, it was "a total disaster." Some kids who were hard of hearing had an interpreter in the classroom but didn't have one online. Schools told these families that the kids didn't need one or that the school couldn't find one, so the child simply couldn't participate at all in online learning. Some families were able to help their kids. Other families, often with two working parents, were not able to help. The problems of NPIs extended even into the school buildings for these children. With everyone in masks it was deeply problematic for many kids who were hard of hearing. Masks muffle people's voices, which make it very hard to hear or understand them. Further, facial expressions are hugely important, Dowling said. "Just seeing eyes alone is not sufficient."

Dr. Sylvia Fogel is a psychiatrist affiliated with Harvard Medical School who specializes in treating the psychiatric needs of parents with autistic children. While the children themselves suffered, one of the lesser-told stories was the strain and terrible hardship school closures inflicted on families as a whole. This was especially acute within the autism community. When Fogel and I first spoke, in the fall of 2020, she told me many families with autistic children were "stretched to the breaking point." In normal times, raising some of these children, depending on their level of disability, is often extremely stressful. Some of these children cannot perform basic activities by themselves, like going to the toilet and getting dressed. They put dangerous things in their mouths, and so on. "There are enormous caregiving demands," Fogel said. "The degree of distress on these families, I'm not even sure how to convey this."

Fogel told me the story of one woman with an autistic teenage son who was considered middle to high functioning. When schools closed he became increasingly anxious and violent, hitting and scratching his parents, hard enough to cause bruising. He smashed the TV. They had to send their older teenage daughter to live with relatives for her safety. And the dad had to stop working and go on leave to take care of the son full time, while the mother, who is in the medical field, continued working. The family took a huge financial hit, which, naturally, increased stress. In families like this, Fogel said, they really needed at least one parent home full time, unless they had exceptional financial resources to outsource the caregiving. Many of the parents were so terrified of COVID that even some with the money for extra help didn't take advantage of it because they were too afraid of having a nonfamily member in the house. "The public messaging about COVID risks distorted their perspective on what was reasonable to pursue," Fogel said. But most families did not even have that option.

A number of Fogel's clients had new-onset psychiatric symptoms from the enhanced and unrelenting stress of the circumstances. She had to hospitalize one parent. While there are commonalities among many of these stories, Fogel told me there is a saying within the autism community: "You've seen one child with autism, you've seen one child with autism." Every family had its own unique challenges. Many of her families were able to send their children back to school in the fall, in particular because a large portion of them attended special schools. Except even though they were in the building, many of the children were still not getting the in-school services they needed, and the days were shorter for some of them.

"No one is thinking about the harms of these school closures," she told me at the time, "and the lack of normalization in schools, with the standard services not being offered that many children rely on." People were not having conversations about the downsides, she said, which were amplified for her population beyond the normal hardships that so many kids and parents were going through.

Eileen Chollet had a daughter in the Fairfax County, Virginia, school district. Her daughter, who has special needs, was unable to participate in remote learning. The district provided laptops but because of motor issues her daughter could only use a touchscreen, which the district refused to provide. The district began offering a perverse program in the fall. A small number of kids could come into school buildings but they had to continue with remote learning (in other words, Zoom in a room)—except parents had to pay for the privilege, up to $1,472 a month. The program wasn't even run by the school district, which had rejected pleas to require teachers to come in person. Instead, it was overseen by the county government, with county employees serving as staff. Chollett refused to pay, arguing the district should pay since her daughter was entitled, by law, to Free and Appropriate Public Education, known as the FAPE. Chollett ended up suing the district.

In November and December of 2020, a survey of 244 families in 30 states, in 125 school districts, with children who required in-person supports before the pandemic found that 88 percent of them were not receiving any in-person supports during virtual instruction. If this sample is any indication of the broader population of the millions of families with kids under IDEA, even if it's off by a large magnitude, the numbers are staggering.

Chollett was not alone in taking legal action. According to Patrick Donohue, an attorney who specializes in education law for children with IEPs, thousands of cases were filed by families against their districts for not following IDEA. Donohue was the lead attorney in a federal class action suit involving more than 500 families from over 25 states for a violation of their children's civil rights under IDEA. Part of the suit's claim was that school districts continued to take billions of dollars in Medicaid and other federal funds for IDEA, which were intended for providing specific services, even though the districts halted providing those services entirely, or in effect stopped providing them (you can't give physical therapy over the internet). "It was fraud," Donohue said, "on a massive scale."

Of course school closures, or partial closures through hybrid learning, affected the broader population of students as well. Accounts of physical and mental health harms, along with learning loss, are endless. Three out of five child suicides in Milwaukee County, Wisconsin, were triggered by the stress and isolation of remote learning, the county medical examiner's office reported. Reports from Colorado to Arizona to Washington State of children and adolescents killing themselves with either an indirect, or an explicit link—through comments made or a note—to school closures and the cancellation of activities made the news. The proportion of children seeking emergency mental-health services who required immediate hospitalization spiked from 2019 to 2020, and hospitals around the country reported not having enough beds for kids with mental health emergencies. It's important to note that for the decade leading up to the pandemic there were upward trends in a variety of mental health categories, such as sadness and hopelessness. Nevertheless, according to a CDC report, the rates appeared to jump from 2019 to 2021, particularly in female students, as did the rate of kids seriously considering suicide. In 2020, 581 ten- to fourteen-year-olds died from suicide; 32 died of COVID.

Multiple studies found an explosion in eating disorders in children and young people during the pandemic as well. "I've been in the field for over 35 years, and in 2020, I saw some of the sickest patients I've ever seen," said Dr. Neville Golden, MD, chief of adolescent medicine and professor of pediatrics, who treats patients in Stanford Children's Health's Comprehensive Eating Disorders Program, in a Stanford news release. The rise was not just from patients who already had eating disorders and found them exacerbated, but many young people developed eating disorders, he said. While weight gain does not necessarily indicate an eating disorder, a study published by the CDC found that the rate of body mass index increase in persons aged two to nineteen *doubled* during the pandemic. Echoing this finding, an analysis in *JAMA* found "significant weight gain" during the pandemic in youths, especially the youngest children.

Some public health professionals and others have argued that increased rates of mental health problems in children and adolescents during the pandemic should be attributed to the environment of the pandemic itself, rather than school interruptions specifically. Without a doubt, the overall circumstances contributed to stress and depression in many young people, as it did in many adults. Yet, if we look at the data, school interruptions were a direct and driving factor. In early 2021, the CDC published the results of a survey given in the fall of 2020 to more than a thousand parents of children aged five to twelve. The findings in nearly every category of inquiry were worse, oftentimes startlingly worse, for those who had children in remote learning or hybrid learning versus those who had children in school full time. With few exceptions, the less children were in school, the worse off they were.

Fully remote children had double the rate of decreased physical activity, and double the rate of decreased time outdoors than did children who were in school full time. Fully remote and hybrid kids spent less time with friends in person than kids in school full time. Perhaps surprisingly, hybrid and especially fully remote children, on average, also spent less time with friends virtually than children who were in school full time. This means the more time a child was physically removed from peers was not compensated for with additional time online with friends; on the contrary, less time in school meant less time a child spent with other children both in person and online. The effects of this isolation, predictably, were very bad for some kids. The survey found higher rates of depression and anxiety in fully remote kids versus those in school. The effects of remote learning also impacted parents, with higher rates of loss of work, concerns about job stability, childcare challenges, conflicts between working and childcare, emotional distress, and insomnia. (It's a fair conjecture that the higher rates of hardships and stress on parents caused by interrupted schooling created a feedback loop, further stressing the children in those homes.)

A survey of pediatric mental health professionals conducted by researchers from Harvard University, Johns Hopkins University, and the University of North Carolina, which I also coauthored, found that nearly 80 percent of respondents saw an increased demand for services during the pandemic. Increases in psychotropic medication prescriptions or higher doses of existing prescriptions were reported by half of prescribing respondents. But here is the salient datum: A majority of providers saw an increase in frequency or need of treatment sessions directly associated with education disruptions. The majority of practitioners indicated that half or more of their pediatric patients specifically blamed remote or hybrid learning for initiating or exacerbating negative mood. Nearly all respondents reported at least some improvement in patients' mood symptoms with increased in-person instructional time. The loss of arts and athletics (which associated with school closures) were also noted as drivers of depression and negative mental health. Patients with learning challenges, such as ADHD, autism, and hearing loss, saw these challenges worsen during remote learning. In a write-in section, one respondent said "a 7 year old child who is generally happily engaged at school and loves to talk and help peers became almost mute/talked like a baby." Another noted that any patient with ADHD "struggled mightily" in remote learning.

Arthur Samuels and Pagee Cheung, the cofounders and co-executive directors of MESA, a charter school in the Bushwick neighborhood in Brooklyn, told me about the toll remote learning took on their students. Due to cohorting rules the city imposed, which Samuels and Cheung felt the school wouldn't be able to follow, MESA stayed fully remote the entire 2020-2021 school year. One of their seniors, who was a high performing student, developed a severe video game addiction. He would log in to class, Samuels said, but then immediately start playing games. He stopped speaking to his mom and sister. He eventually became nonverbal entirely. "This was a kid who had been one of our top students sophomore and junior year," Samuels said. The student graduated but, Samuels said, he almost didn't make it. Another student, a former soccer player, put on what Samuels estimated was at least forty pounds (when Samuels saw him at an event in the spring). The student, who was "very bright," slowly stopped showing up to his AP class online and eventually transferred out. Anecdotes like these were representative of many stories I heard from parents, administrators, and teachers around the country.

An extremely important point to note is that school closures and interrupted learning were about much more than the schools themselves closing. They also impacted all of the extracurricular activities—from athletics to arts programs—that are so critical to children's development and happiness, and for some, a ticket out of an underprivileged circumstance.

George Lanese is a co-founder of a nonprofit in New York City called About U Outreach that works with student athletes to help them realize their potential in sports, academics, and life skills. Lanese said he knew in July 2020 that "inequities were going to explode" with the shutdowns. A lot of his kids rely on athletics, specifically football, to gain access to college. New York City not only closed its schools but ended all sports programs. "You took these alpha male types and didn't give them structure or exercise," he told me. "You have a teacher for one year. But you have a coach for three or four years." This important relationship for these kids was extirpated.

Lanese runs a football showcase of high school athletes for college scouts. Some of his kids have been recruited to Division 1 schools. A few might end up in the NFL, he said. But with the closures the showcase was canceled. Despite his pleading, the city wouldn't allow his players to even use an athletic field. Through a lot of fighting and networking, Lanese was able to get a private Catholic school to allow them to use its facilities so he could run the showcase in the fall. With the season canceled this would be the only opportunity for these kids to get seen by scouts. But one showcase can only do so much. By canceling football it wasn't just the elite athletes who lost the opportunity for scholarships, it was also regular kids who lost the outlet to have fun, be on a team, stay out of trouble, and hopefully learn some valuable life lessons.

The kids were at a far greater risk from a list of harms and downstream effects from being prevented from taking part in sports than they were from COVID, Lanese said. The notion that ending the season was for safety made no sense. You had kids in the projects, with tens of thousands of people, hanging out with other teens all the time, Lanese said. The city did not have an appreciation for what a closure meant for kids in housing developments, with no place to go, and twenty thousand people around them, versus a closure in the suburbs. It was devastating, and stupid.

Lastly, academic performance, predictably, suffered dramatically during school interruptions. For years educators had evidence of the "summer slide"—the tendency for students, especially those from low-income families, to lose some of the achievement gains they made during the previous school year. Closing schools for three months in the spring, on top of the standard summer break, was guaranteed to lead to serious declines in achievement for many students. Reports in fall of 2020 saw massive drops in assessment scores. In Fairfax, Virginia, for example, failing grades increased 83 percent during remote learning in the first quarter of the 2020–2021 school year versus a year before. To the extent that it was being monitored, the drop in academic performance was seen by teachers immediately during the spring shutdowns. The downstream effects of poor academic performance are vast. There is a wealth of evidence that shows a correlation between educational attainment and earning potential.

Much of the media covered drops in scores on National Assessment of Education Progress tests (NAEP). Misleadingly, it was often reported that there wasn't a clear association between the scores and degree of in-person learning. Yet this conclusion was based on crude state comparisons. Learning models differed extensively *within* states. And multiple robust and in-depth analyses of scores between districts, which is the appropriate comparison level, indeed found straightforward correlations—the less children were in school, the worse they performed. The results are unequivocal.

An analysis by Vladimir Kogan and Stéphane Lavertu at Ohio State University found that "districts with fully remote instruction experienced test scores declines up to three times greater than districts that had in-person instruction for the majority of the school year." Moreover, their research showed that "disadvantaged students had disproportionate learning declines during the academic year."

An analysis of student assessments by Andrew Ho, a psychometrician and education professor at Harvard University, found college and career readiness "declined substantially among California students in grades 3–8 from a 2019 pre-pandemic baseline to 2022." He found that "the magnitude of learning loss was greater in California school districts that serve more low-income students." And he found that the state chose a "biased calculation" of the data, which favorably misrepresented the degree of disparate impacts of learning loss.

A paper by economist Emily Oster and coauthors at Brown University, published in the journal *American Economic Review: Insights*, found that pass rates on standardized tests during the pandemic declined compared to prior years, and that these declines were larger in districts with less in-person instruction. They found that moving a district from fully virtual to 100 percent access to in-person learning would have reduced pass rate losses in Spring 2021 by 13 to 14 percentage points in math, and 8 percentage points in English language arts (ELA). Having 14 percent more students fail math because of remote learning, who otherwise would have passed, is a devastating finding. They found more in-person learning in districts with higher baseline pass rates and fewer Black and Hispanic students. Put differently: districts with more historically underserved students were less likely to have access to in-person schooling. The result was that pass rate declines were larger in districts serving a higher population of Black students. The authors are very clear: pandemic schooling disruptions amplified a "disparate impact" on Black students.

A figure in the paper is a dramatic illustration of the findings. The pattern couldn't be more stark: On average, all students experienced test score drops because of the pandemic. But the percent of in-person schooling was directly correlated to how bad those drops were. And districts with the highest share of Black students had the largest drops. The correlations are apparent in ELA, but in math they are astonishing.

A thirty-six-page report by Dan Goldhaber and coauthors at Harvard University's Center for Education Policy Research, based on data from more than two million students in 10,000 schools, found that remote instruction was more prevalent among Black and Hispanic students, and that it was a primary driver of widening achievement gaps. They also found that high poverty schools spent more weeks in remote instruction during 2020–2021 than low- and middle-poverty schools.

A number of public health professionals and parents claimed not only a preference for remote learning (presumably out of fears of in-person school), but said it offered distinct advantages. Theresa Chapple, a Black epidemiologist who was very active on social media and with a large following, wrote in praise of remote learning that "overwhelmingly, Black parents said our kids can learn at their own pace, less stressed, kids aren't getting into trouble." There also were anecdotal reports by individual students of a preference for remote learning. One, published on the blogging platform Medium, by a fourteen-year-old girl, noted that by being home she was "spared some of the common social pressures" associated with high school. Her district was extremely competitive, she noted, so not being around other students reduced her anxiety of comparisons with her peers, and she was able to concentrate more on her work.

There is no doubt that by removing the social dynamics of school, children would experience fewer of the downsides that come with in-person interactions with peers. The relief that some students felt was real, and is an important data point for future study about ways to improve schools. But there is a strong argument to be made, as the psychologist Jonathan Haidt and activist attorney Greg Lukianoff did in their book *The Coddling of the American Mind*, that experiencing and confronting many of those downsides, ultimately, leads to building stronger, healthier adults. Socializing and academic competition *are* stressful. But, to some extent, they serve a beneficial purpose, even if they are not always enjoyable in the

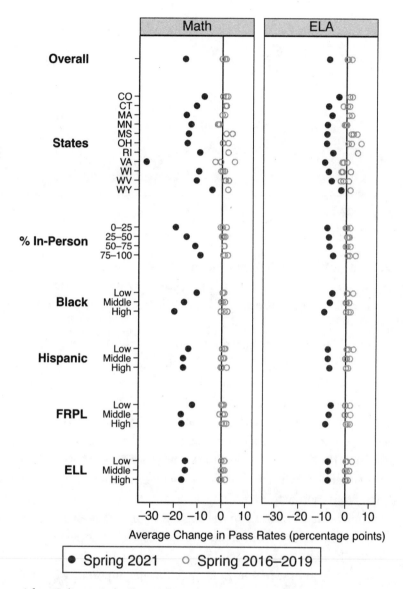

Figure 1 from Rebecca Jack, Clare Halloran, James Okun, and Emily Oster, "Pandemic Schooling Mode and Student Test Scores: Evidence from US School Districts," *American Economic Review: Insights* 5, no. 2 (June 2023): 173–190 © American Economic Association; reproduced with permission of the *American Economic Review: Insights*.

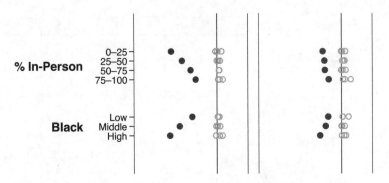

Excerpt of figure 1 from Jack et al., "Pandemic Schooling Mode and Student Test Scores." ©American Economic Association; reproduced with permission of the *American Economic Review: Insights*.

moment. Even though some students subjectively preferred the experience of remote learning, that doesn't necessarily mean it would yield the best results for them as people. Needless to say, kids' preferences are not always aligned with their best interests.

Some highly motivated students, particularly once they've reached high school and a degree of maturity, might perform better academically by working alone, at home, and might favor the experience. If that is the lifestyle these students and their parents want for them, home school or state-run programs that enable remote learning (outside of a direct relationship with the in-person scholastics in one's home district) might be an option they should pursue. But the evidence for K–12 students overall is very clear about the advantages—academic and otherwise—for being in school, in person with peers and teachers.

If you've made it this far in the book, you know I am skeptical of modeling projections, so I will spare you the dozens of papers that predict specifically how lower academic performance and achievement correlates with a host of worse life outcomes. But the importance of education for a better life—from finances to physical health—is a well-established and well-evidenced truism across cultures around the world. The consequences for kids—disproportionately those with fewer resources—who, because of lower scores and missed education, were unable to attend the tier of college they otherwise would have, who wound up not going to college at all, or who dropped out of high school, will be life altering.

* * *

Like many parents, I witnessed what the isolation in the spring had done to my kids. Yes, part-time in-person learning the following school year was better than no time, but being home five out of seven days, remanded to their rooms to sit alone, staring at a Chromebook was simply not compatible with anything even remotely resembling a healthy experience. I knew from my own kids, but more so from other parents in town and, increasingly, from parents reaching out to me from all over the US, that their kids were really struggling. They were being set up to fail. For parents in these families even hybrid was a disaster; every single day mattered.

It is impossible to quantify how life trajectories are altered by an infinite number of downstream effects: the inner-city football player who lost his shot at college, the thousands of children who simply disappeared during remote learning and never returned, the teenager who developed an eating disorder that might stay with her the rest of her life. But although the harms cannot easily be quantified or even identified they are still real.

On that point, despite all of the data, it is important to emphasize that harm should not only be calculated or considered through the lens of long-term effects. During and even after the pandemic a common sentiment was expressed, often as a rejoinder to someone pointing out the harms to kids being kept out of school, that "kids are resilient." The specific word "resilient" was frequently used, as it connotes grit, an admirable and advantageous trait. This word was everywhere from teachers quoted in the *New York Times* and the *Washington Post*, among endless other news outlets, to innumerable social media posts and comments. Don't worry, they said, it may seem bad now but kids will bounce back. When Randi Weingarten, the head of the AFT, was asked in a February 2021 interview if there were a point that kids could be out of school so long that the losses were irrecoverable, she answered, "No. Kids are resilient."

Often dovetailing with the "kids are resilient" argument were comparisons made to earlier challenging eras. Look how well everyone turned out from that, was the line of reasoning. Dr. Jerome Adams, the former surgeon general, tweeted: "Why is it the young people who lived through the Great Depression (12 years) and WW2 (5+ years) came to be known

as our 'greatest generation,' but we look at the young people who lived
through pandemic shut downs (1–2 years) as irreparably harmed?" He
went on to say in a series of tweets that those greater, and long-lasting
challenges from earlier times were character building, and he questioned
how missing just a year of school and sports was something that couldn't
be overcome. Recall the tweet by the prominent epidemiologist Eleanor
Murray, in which she downplayed school closures because "mandatory
schooling is barely a century old."

These resiliency arguments are wrong for a few reasons.

Most importantly, children suffered in the present, and that alone
matters. This is a crucial point to understand, and one that has largely
been lost in discussions about the consequences of school closures. One
need not make an argument about or produce evidence of their long-
term harms. The entire topic of learning loss, for example, could be
eliminated, and the school closures and interruptions would *still* be devastating. If you get food poisoning and are on the floor of your bathroom throwing up all night, even if you ultimately recover and are fine,
no one would argue that this wasn't nevertheless a terrible experience.
If someone punches you in the face and the only physical injury is a
black eye that heals after a week, you still experienced a punch in the
face. Childhood is vanishingly brief, and more than a year of kids' lives
were damaged unnecessarily. Harms were endured even without literal or
metaphorical scars. Though the focus on learning loss and other metrics
is important, it obscures this basic truth.

Second, unlike during the pandemic, in the earlier eras that Adams
harkened back to children still attended school and, beyond that, physically interacted with friends, relatives, peers, and others. The attitudes of
some of these influential public health figures are telling as to why they
felt it was acceptable to close schools, and, more broadly, compel—either
by law or by norm—social isolation for most of the citizenry, including
children. The people with medical degrees seemed to lose sight of what
every regular person knows: human interaction, in person, is a bedrock
of society and personal flourishing, especially for children. This isn't to
downplay the hardships of growing up during the Depression or World
War II in the US, but during those times children were not physically isolated in the manner they were during the pandemic. With the exception

of Pearl Harbor, during a war that took place exclusively on foreign soil, American children spent time with friends, played sports, went to school, hugged grandparents—in other words, kids were still able to be kids. Comparisons to previous eras are often facile, given the complexities of each time period. Looking at the overall calamity of a war or Depression versus a pandemic is the wrong frame. Instead, as you push the lens in, the one critical difference was the imposed physical isolation.

Outside of studies and data are many far more nebulous effects. Many educators observed worrisome behavioral changes in their students after they returned to school, such as more acting out and more bullying. Other students became more withdrawn, their personalities different from what they had been before. Cheung, at the MESA school, in Brooklyn, said, "We grossly underestimated how big of a transition it was for back to school." The lack of socialization during remote learning, and the flagrantly abnormal environment in the buildings—with mandatory masking, distancing, desktop barriers, and so on—deprived many young children and adolescents of interactions they needed to grow.

22

AN ABSENCE OF LEADERSHIP

After having conducted research and interviewed experts for the article I published that summer on hybrid schooling, and not finding any data showing that it would yield a mitigation benefit (and reason to believe it may lead to more transmission), seeing my kids home three days a week, miserable and struggling, the life draining out of them with hours alone in front of a screen, I felt compelled to continue to try to do something about it. The sense that all of this suffering for them and millions of other kids was for naught consumed me. I could not silence the voice in my head that this was gravely stupid. The circumstance was an exquisitely painful irritation, like fiberglass splinters covering my entire body.

I contacted an editor at *New York* magazine whom I had worked with in the past. All of the coverage of schools was about things going wrong, I told him. What if I did a large feature on a couple districts that were open full time and everything was fine? He gave me a green light. The magazine even hired a photographer to join me. Off I went to Chappaqua and Bronxville, two well-to-do towns in Westchester County, just north of New York City. Both had kindergarten through eighth grade full time in person.

Much of the piece is a magazine-style anthropological study—the journalist parachutes in to a foreign land and reports back for the masses. I intended the piece as a historical document, a time capsule for future generations to see what some American schools looked like in the fall of 2020.

The Chappaqua buses had dash-mounted thermometers, ready to deny entry to any child with an elevated temperature. Bronxville had video kiosks installed at the front door that scanned and recorded each entrant's temperature, then displayed the number across the bottom of the person's image on the screen like a news chyron. "They can track forty kids a minute," Roy Montesano, the district's superintendent, said, observing me marvel at the device. Schools in both districts utilized every inch of space in their buildings. To comply with distancing rules, in addition to regular rooms, classes were held in gymnasiums and libraries so students could be spread out. In Chappaqua, many classes had students dispersed over two rooms, with the teacher bouncing between them, and video monitors giving a live feed to the students in both rooms and to students at home whose families chose to stay with fully remote learning. The school had commandeered art, music, makerspace, and other specialized rooms to enable the double-room plan for spacing.

A teacher in Chappaqua scurried around the expansive cafeteria, which had been turned into her classroom, with a wireless microphone taped to the end of a yardstick, which she held at a distance in front of individual students' faces any time they wanted to speak to her or the class. The room was so large and the kids were so spread out that without using the microphone and PA system they would not hear each other, especially with masks on. Classrooms with modular desks in strange shapes that fit together in pre-pandemic times for collaborative learning, now were broken apart like an exploded puzzle. The schools had directional arrows on the floors so foot traffic theoretically flowed without students physically interacting with each other. Teachers in Chappaqua wore buttons with photos of themselves unmasked so the children could identify whom they were talking with. An antimicrobial film had been applied to high-touch surfaces like door handles in Bronxville.

With the students sufficiently distanced, Chappaqua was able to do away with barriers. The Bronxville classrooms had them, but they were hard and crystal clear Plexiglass all the way around. A number of kids personalized them with stickers or graffitied drawings, including a very good rendition of the Simpsons. (Needless to say, I couldn't help but think about my district's cardboard desktop partitions, with opaque sides and a flimsy plastic window in the center—a small, distorted lens to the world.)

All of this seemed insane. Millions of kids in Europe were in school full time, without masks, without barriers, without six feet of distancing, or any of the bells and whistles. And schools were open right here in the US, in states like Georgia, without any of these measures either. I didn't blame the districts for doing this. Much of it had to be carried out to be in compliance with New York's state guidelines. (And they were the lucky ones—more than a third of the nation's public schools weren't open at all.)

Though drama programs were shut down, this was the ultimate theatrical performance. Histrionic media reports about Georgia and Florida notwithstanding, no one produced any evidence that any of this stuff made a meaningful difference. Did Bronxville have fewer cases because it had barriers while Chappaqua did not? Did anyone actually believe that a three-sided piece of plastic that topped out a few inches above a child's head, and was wide open in the back and above, actually prevented the spread of an aerosolized virus? Surely they were aware of the properties of air. Most importantly, what did all this distancing actually do? Did six feet of separation between desks—leading to the majority of schools in the New York metro area operating on hybrid schedules—actually reduce cases?

As part of the article, I ran a detailed analysis of forty districts in Westchester, roughly the entire public school system in the county. By October 19, 2020, when the article published, according to New York's "COVID-19 Report Card"—a dashboard of school district statistics—there were 8,801 students and faculty attending or working for full-time programs in Westchester public schools. Of those 8,801 students and faculty, there had been four COVID-19 cases since the beginning of the school year, or 0.04 percent. Among the approximately 155,162 students and faculty not participating in full-time in-person school, there had been 97 cases, or 0.06 percent.

My findings were not an anomaly. Emily Oster, the Brown University economist who had collected data and created dashboards for daycare centers and summer camps, was back at it with her most important project—collecting data on schools. Oster's data, of nearly 200,000 schoolchildren, in 47 states, showed a confirmed COVID-19 infection rate of 0.19 percent among students and 0.65 percent among staff who had been in school full time at full capacity. While higher than the hundredths-of-a-percent rates in Westchester, her data showed that full-time in-person schools had negligible case rates. (The rates in schools would rise later, mirroring the rises in their communities—or in many instances significantly lower than community rates—which further proved the point that was empirically obvious from the fall data: schools were not driving transmission.)

None of this should have been surprising, as it matched what was seen observationally in Europe in the spring, and matched findings of studies of past epidemics. While school closures, in conjunction with very strict societal lockdowns, might have a transient benefit if implemented extremely early in a pandemic, there is no evidence of meaningful benefit after that time. To take but one example: a 2016 study published in *Open Forum Infectious Diseases*, on the influenza season of 2013, concluded that "closing schools after widespread influenza-like illness activity did not reduce transmission."

I shared my article, and highlighted all of the statistical evidence, with my district's administration. 0.04 percent in Westchester and 0.19 percent nationally for schools that were open full time in person! It was close to impossible to get any lower than that! It had been a long, frustrating journey, but now it would finally come to an end. My kids, and hopefully millions of others, at least in the New York metro area, and perhaps around the country, would get back to school full time. The evidence from Europe had been dismissed for a list of fallacious reasons. But this was evidence right here in America, and even right here in my own county—when comparing my district to districts fifteen minutes away that had similar demographics to our own but were running full time in person, *the outcomes were no different*. It shouldn't have had to come to this, but it felt good to finally have the excessive proof that these people seemed to require.

Alas, my district administration was unmoved. The evidence meant nothing to them. This wasn't about evidence, I was told. It was about feelings. And some people didn't "feel" safe. (Pointing out the marginally higher rate of cases in schools that were *not* open full time did not persuade the administration against the hybrid model. They'd rather *increase* the risk of transmission and continue with hybrid if it meant supporting the performance of safety.) Similarly, Arlington, Los Angeles, Baltimore, Berkeley, and thousands of schools around the country—serving 30 to 40 million children—were still fully or partially closed, and would remain that way for a long, long time.

What was it about Bronxville and Chappaqua that was different from my town? Some people suggested that districts in my area that opened full time only did so because they were wealthier and had more resources. Surely, money helped (that antimicrobial film on door handles in Bronxville cost $40,000). And different schools had different floor plans and density issues. But plenty of wealthy districts in Westchester—Scarsdale, Rye, and Mamaroneck, to name a few—were not open full time. Conversely, Hendrick Hudson and Somers, where median home prices are less than half that of the aforementioned towns, were operating kindergarten through fifth and sixth grade, respectively, full time. Remember, the New York State guidance also allowed for less than six feet of distancing if barriers were in use. My district had barriers but still adhered to six feet. Even though my district ignored the exemption from distancing that barriers offered, the administration still chose not to utilize the gymnasiums, libraries, cafeterias, or specials rooms as was done in Chappaqua and Bronxville. It was clear the reason schools were not open full time was because the administrators didn't want them open full time. But why?

The superintendents of Chappaqua and Bronxville both exhibited a passionate drive to get the kids into school. To meet the distancing requirement, Roy Montesano, Bronxville's superintendent, knocked down walls in smaller rooms, and ripped out and carted away bookcases, file cabinets, and other furniture to make more space. "We took out about basically everything that wasn't a desk," he said. Then they swapped in older desks that were smaller, sometimes just college-style chairs with tablet arms, to grab a few more inches, further allowing for more desks while still complying with the six-feet rule.

That summer, when I had written the darkly comic piece for *Wired*, in which I attempted to track down the origin of a requirement of 44 square feet of space per student that was in the district's reopening plan, I drew countless tessellations and configurations of desks, trying to figure out how to pack as many desks as possible into a classroom while still complying with the spacing rules. I had a line in a draft of the piece about how I wanted to go into the school with a crowbar and rip out bookcases and shelving and anything else to make more room for more desks, but my editor told me I sounded like a crazy person, and we cut it.

After hearing of Montesano's actions I felt vindicated. Either you viewed this as a problem to solve, or you didn't.

In August, after the full-time in-person plan was announced in Chappaqua, teachers there held a motorcade rally advocating for a remote-learning-only start to the school year. But Christina Ackerman, the superintendent, pushed ahead with her plan anyway. And the teachers showed up. What got the schools open full time was leadership. Most politicians and education officials said they wanted kids in school. But they either didn't mean it, or didn't have the courage or skill to make it happen. Ackerman and Bronxville's Montesano got it done.

"From the beginning we were very worried about the harms inflicted on our kids by keeping them out of school," Montesano said. At the end of the last school year, the district psychologist told him that "anxiety among the kids was sky high." Moreover, "In the summer we saw that the science is telling us young kids are less likely to be infected," he said, "so we started figuring out how to get K–2 in full time. Then I thought, 'What about K–5?' Then K–8. We saw this as a problem to solve." Montesano was so committed to getting kids into school that even half-time hybrid for high school students wasn't acceptable to him. At the time of my article, he implemented a complex new hybrid schedule for the high schoolers, rotating them in the building two-thirds of the time. "Anything I can do to safely get kids, all kids, into school as much as possible, I will do," he said. It was a far cry from flex Wednesday.

Ackerman's team in Chappaqua started buying PPE and contracted for air filtration work back in April. "We had all that in place at the end of last school year, even though official guidance wasn't released until July," she said. "We brought in faculty over the summer to work with us," Adam Pease, Chappaqua's assistant superintendent for curriculum, told me. "Our attitude was, 'We need as many kids in school as safely possible,'" he said. "So we prepared models. Christine would not take no for an answer."

Ultimately, without leadership at the state level, it was left to superintendents in individual districts to open the schools. And the reality was most of them, while perhaps good people and competent professionals in normal times, simply lacked the skill set and mindset to do what needed to be done. When I pressed my district's administrators for explanations for certain practices or plans that were keeping the kids out of school, I oftentimes was told that the other nearby districts were doing the same thing, as if that somehow made it legitimate. Most bureaucrats simply don't want to stand out. They got to their positions by conforming to expectations and norms. And the norm was a maximalist performance of COVID safety.

It became clear to me that only the rare type of superintendent, like Ackerman and Montesano, had the leadership skills and mentality to go it alone, relative to their neighboring districts, and against pushback from teachers or others in their community. This approach was simply too much to ask of most superintendents. There needed to be leadership at the top level of the state, requiring individual districts to act, otherwise most would simply follow each other, sticking to nonsensical plans devised by a security firm with no expertise in viral mitigation, and that resulted in an overtly imbalanced cost-benefit for the kids.

As I wrote in the *New York* magazine piece:

An enormous weight has been dropped on school administrators. Andrew Cuomo, New York's governor, said that if the positivity rate was below five percent using a 14-day average, schools were merely *allowed* to open. Cloaked in language of community autonomy, Cuomo punted, leaving every superintendent on their own to make decisions about opening and, when cases inevitably arise, decisions about closing. In the absence of a requirement to open full time, it was obvious from the get-go that the vast majority of superintendents were going to choose what they perceived to be the most cautious path.

"If there was a mandate from the state that would have made things so much easier," Montesano said. "Superintendents are not health officials, yet we've been tasked with making health-related decisions."

The superintendent of another district in Westchester, which was not open full time, told me that even though they had barriers, which meant they technically could open full time, he had to meet what he perceived to be the interests of the teachers and community. "There's no way the board of education or I were going to choose the less conservative option."

The dynamic between the governor and local districts of course was not limited to Westchester. It took place around the country, particularly, though not exclusively, in blue states. Recall Arlington. Without a requirement from the Virginia governor demanding that schools open there was no amount of evidence, pleading, or cajoling that would move the Arlington schools administration.

For governors, particularly blue state governors, this was an easy move. Why take the political hit of forcing schools open when instead you could lay the responsibility at the local level? Of course with a significant portion of the population whipped into a frenzy of fear, in particular and especially irrationally over children, it was only the rarest of superintendents or schools chancellors who bucked the narrative.

Sonja Santelises, the CEO of Baltimore City Public Schools, told me that she planned to open her district of 75,000 students in hybrid in the fall but that her "families weren't ready for that," so the district operated fully remote instead. In late September, like so many other districts, Baltimore opened so-called student learning centers, aka Zoom in room, for around a thousand students from families that met certain criteria, in city recreation centers and—unabashedly—in schools themselves.

Eventually, in mid-November, Santelises pushed to open 27 (of the district's 156) schools for the most at-risk students—about 1,200 kindergarteners, children with special needs, and English language learners. The local union, part of the American Federation of Teachers, was furious, wanting all the buildings closed until everything was "safe" or the vaccine was widely available. When the plans were announced in October, the union publicly pleaded with parents to not send their kids in the next month. And, according to a *Times* piece, the union had also pressured teachers not to volunteer to go back in. The head of the union said they were fighting for the lives of students and staff.

As was the case in New York, where I detailed the differences between districts in Westchester County, and throughout much of the country, so, too, was it in Maryland. Without a state directive to open individual districts were left to fend for themselves, with all of the responsibility tossed from governors into the hands of superintendents and chancellors.

Santelises only opened the schools—even just for a tiny percentage of students—because she "led through the fear," she said. The majority of teachers and parents were not ready for schools to open, and confidence had to be built up and earned from the community, she said. She noted that the district was over 70 percent African American, a group that has a historical experience of malfeasance and neglect. Relative to many other inner-city superintendents, Santelises had the grit and social capital necessary to push back against the union and local sentiment. Still, it was a puny victory. It wasn't until March 2021 that kids only up to second grade were able to get back into the buildings. And it wasn't until April, more than a full year after schools closed, that all kids in Baltimore city schools were allowed back.

There is no doubt that the fears of many community members in inner cities and in left-leaning areas in general were sincere. And it has been argued that many communities—in particular communities of color in inner cities—that supported school closures were also the hardest hit by deaths and severe disease from COVID. Therefore, the logic went, it was perfectly reasonable for them to want the schools closed. "We'd rather have our kids be out of school than dead," was a typical sentiment (in this instance expressed in the *New York Times* by the head of an advocacy group).

This line of thinking, which dominated discussions over schools, was wrong on multiple levels.

First, there was no correlation between open schools and an increase in deaths or severe disease of children or adults who lived with them or in their community. It was incumbent upon public health leaders to disabuse people of this notion. But they did not. Instead, plenty of epidemiologists and other health professionals supported the sentiment from residents in inner cities who wanted schools closed. "If you're advocating for opening schools for the sake of mental health for students, where is your equity lens? Where will you be when students and families living in already marginalized spaces get Covid" was a representative tweet. Boston University epidemiologist Eleanor Murray tweeted her approval of comments suggesting that when minorities had lower attendance for in-person school it was wrong to refer to this as a problem of "school hesitancy" that needed to be solved.

So, against a preponderance of evidence that kids were at exceedingly low risk from the virus, that schools were not driving transmission—that kids were getting infected at the same rates over time whether they were in school or not, that adult household members were getting infected whether children in the household were in school or not—and that harms were accruing from remote learning, in particular for children of color, Murray and others, nevertheless, actively promoted the idea that children of color in cities should stay home (while white kids, increasingly, were in school).

Second, an analysis of local district reopening plans by researchers at Michigan State University found that decisions were more tied to local political partisanship and union strength than to COVID-19 severity. Because governors left the decision to districts it "opened the way for the influence of local political partisanship," the authors wrote. An analysis by political scientists Michael Hartney and Leslie Finger, in the journal *Perspectives on Politics*, similarly concluded that "partisanship and vested interests best explain the degree to which schools reopened." Democratic districts and those with stronger unions were far less likely to reopen, their data showed. Further, the authors wrote, "We find little connection between reopening decisions and indicators measuring the severity of the virus." So the idea that school closures in Baltimore or other inner cities were because the disease burden on the community was greater there than elsewhere, not because of ideology, was not borne out by the evidence.

As the map presented here shows, even on a crude statewide level this is apparent. The left-leaning West Coast, Mid-Atlantic, and Northeast had lower in-person percentages, and Florida, much of the right-leaning South and Great Plains had higher in-person percentages, even though COVID hit areas in each of these regions with a wide range of severity.

Third and most importantly, an analysis by political scientist Vladimir Kogan at Ohio State University reveals something fascinating and little-known or talked about in regard to parental feelings about school openings. The University of Southern California, as part of its "Understanding America Survey," began asking parents in November 2020 about their preferences of modes of learning. At the time, a majority of parents of color preferred remote learning, compared to only about 35 percent of white parents. This seems unsurprising, considering the political divide on the issue and that most people of color are democrats, and given the extensive media coverage about Black people incurring a disproportionate share of harm from the virus. However, Kogan discovered something that completely upends the narrative around parental preferences among Black and inner-city parents regarding school closures.

In-Person Index
(0=Virtual; 100=Traditional)

0   100

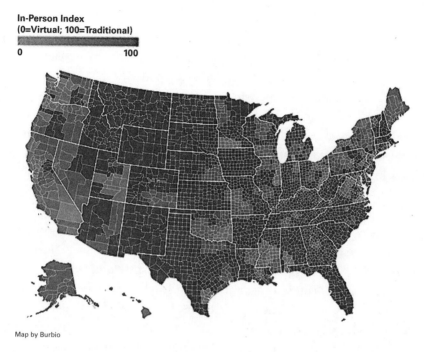

Map by Burbio

County-level in-person index, 6-21. *Source*: Burbio School Opening Tracker.

When he looked at the polling data over time—which were gathered and cataloged each month for more than a year—he found that parents became significantly more willing to resume in-person learning when their schools opened their doors. In fact, Kogan wrote, "One of the strongest predictors of attitudes toward in-person learning was whether one's own school was open or not." To paraphrase a famous quote—if you open it, they will come. A major reason why parents of color were opposed to schools opening was simply because their schools weren't open. Once their districts' schools reopened, parental opinions shifted in favor of them staying open. Political affiliation and whether one's schools were open, according to Kogan's analysis, accounted for nearly all of the difference in attitudes on school openings.

Kogan's finding was one of those rare instances when a researcher discovers something truly revelatory, a result that topples a commonly held belief. (It reminded me of when the medical establishment told everyone in the 1980s and 1990s to eat a low-fat diet, until, all of a sudden, in the

2000s, research became accepted that a high-carb low-fat diet actually made people fatter.)

"To what extent did the disparate health impacts of the pandemic contribute to racial differences in parent support for school reopening?" Kogan repeated back to me when I reached out to him. "The answer is none at all," he said. "Statistically controlling for all of the usual suspects—high-risk health conditions, living in multifamily households, knowing someone who had died from the virus, or people's subjective beliefs about how likely they would be to die or get hospitalized if they fell ill—did not explain any of the racial differences in public opinion on schools." There were only two factors that mattered: "Were you a Democrat or a Republican, and were your own schools open."

Where Santelises and so many other decision makers were mistaken was a belief that keeping schools closed (or mostly closed) was the right or perhaps only course of action because it reflected the desires of the community. This was true, but only insofar as the community's views merely reflected their present circumstances. When decision makers kept schools closed for this reason they unknowingly perpetuated a circular logic. The only way to break the catch-22 in these areas was for there to be a leader who was willing and able to *lead* the community.

One of the most oft-repeated responses I got from the administration in my district when I questioned the logic behind certain practices—desktop barriers, flex Wednesdays, the fully remote start, the hybrid schedule—was that this was what other districts near ours were doing. Frequently, the administrators didn't rebut evidence I provided that challenged these practices. They simply pointed out that this was the norm for the area. I said this was a chance for our district to be a leader in our region, to be *different* from the others near us. But this was not a compelling proposition to them. It didn't matter that a district fifteen minutes away from my own, with similar demographics, was open full time and its population experienced no different outcome with cases than my district did while operating in its two-day-a-week model. Even the most blatant observational evidence was irrelevant to the decision-making process.

Different districts faced different challenges to opening. Santelises no doubt faced far more community opposition to opening than Montesano and Ackerman, making the hurdles for her far higher. But it's worth remembering that Chappaqua's union held a rally to not open schools full time, and Ackerman did it anyway—and the teachers showed up to work.

School closures, hybrid schedules, and the myriad ineffective measures imposed within the buildings were the result of a complete abdication of leadership at multiple levels. By not mandating schools open full time, Cuomo, along with most other governors, ensured that some portion of them would not. The lack of leadership at the state level created the scenario in which schools not opening fully was unrelated to local disease prevalence or risk. It was inevitable that superintendents—who were ill-equipped and disinclined to make evidence-based decisions—were going to base opening model decisions on "feelings." No doubt a great number of superintendents and other district leaders are good people, smart, hard-working, and caring. But they are also bureaucrats, which means most of them, definitionally, are predisposed to not deviate from norms of their peers. It took a very rare type of education administrator to do so.

Although Sweden famously never closed its lower schools, it's not widely known that early on there was significant domestic pushback against this plan. Anna Ekström, Sweden's minister of education during the pandemic, who made the decision, told me that there was pressure from political parties and the public to close the schools. In March 2020 editorials appeared in the major Swedish papers pushing for school closures. Ekström went ahead and kept them open anyway, but, unlike in the US, she had the support of Sweden's main pediatric organization and of Anders Tegnell, the state epidemiologist for Sweden's public health agency.

The CDC technically does not have the authority to close schools. The agency is limited to giving guidance. Only governors, and if they chose to pass the authority to local or district officials—which was the case in the majority of states—could close schools and compel other interventions. With this arrangement, no one claimed ownership of or was held responsible for decisions. The CDC issued guidance, and then governors decided what to require based on the guidance. But while many governors, indeed, issued a list of requirements through their state health departments, such as mandated distancing and masks, the most important decision—whether schools needed to be open or not—was generally punted down to the districts. District administrators, in turn, said they were merely following the guidance of the state health department or the CDC or were doing what neighboring districts were doing. As a result, anyone trying to hold any of the parties to account was often met with a finger pointing to someone else. To seek answers from officials about why a school was closed, or why any number of school mitigation measures were in place, was to be thrust inside an M. C. Escher painting, forever ascending staircases, expecting that you would reach the final authority on the next floor, only to somehow always wind up back where you began.

During the pandemic, a meme surfaced that captured the dynamic perfectly:

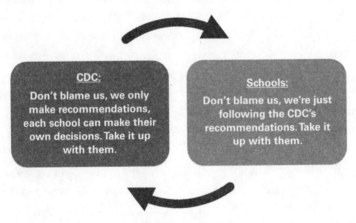

Meme of CDC's and school administrators' lack of accountability. Credit: Matthew Bring.

23

INSTITUTIONAL FAILURE

As I've detailed extensively, a key reason that schools remained closed and dubious interventions were imposed on kids was due to an incurious media that kept the public ignorant of information that would have called these policies into question. But in many instances, the health authorities were incurious as well. Though they control a vast research apparatus at the federal and at state levels, they didn't seek evidence to support their policy positions. And of the evidence that was formally acquired, the system was such that only evidence that aligned with preexisting official positions was published and promoted by the authorities, and evidence that conflicted was rejected or ignored.

The National Institutes of Health is the largest funder of biomedical research in the world. In 2020 it had a budget of $45.3 billion, of which the agency allocated $2.2 billion toward COVID-19 research. More than 90 percent of that money came from a special supplemental appropriation from Congress. Out of a total of 56,169 grants awarded by NIH in 2020, *six* were for research to study the efficacy of social distancing. There were zero grants dedicated to studying the efficacy of face masks on children.

"The lack of rapid clinical research funding to understand COVID-19 transmission may have contributed to the politicization of the virus," Dr. Marty Makary and coauthors of an analysis of NIH funding, published in *BMJ Open*, wrote. "Some of the most basic questions that were being asked of medical professionals in early 2020, such as how it spreads, when infected individuals are most contagious, and whether masks protect individuals from spreading or getting the virus, went unanswered." The authors went on to single out the pediatric population: "Significant restrictions have been placed on the nation's 52 million school-aged children, including school closures, 6-foot distancing requirements and outdoor masking while distancing; however, only a few grants were dedicated to studying these questions in this unique population."

In late spring of 2020 I reached out to Dr. David Coil, a microbiologist at University of California, Davis, to try to understand why playgrounds were closed and my kids' schools were sending emails about "deep cleanings." Coil had written a short post I came across where he said that detection of RNA is not the same thing as detection of infectious viral particles, which does not equal transmission risk, even though the media conflated the three things. At the time (and I suppose still now, years later), there was much uncertainty about how the coronavirus could spread. What I wanted to learn from Coil was why weren't there two dozen studies happening right then, or already conducted in April or May, looking into the possibility of transmission on surfaces, especially outdoor surfaces. I was baffled why if thousands of playgrounds were roped off around the country this wasn't being studied. Wasn't there an urgency within NIH to at least let the kids get some exercise and fresh air at playgrounds? Coil was surprised and frustrated himself at these same questions. "There's so much we don't know," he said. "And schools are being asked to make complex decisions on surprisingly incomplete information."

You might recall from early in the book I explained how I had talked with a highly placed person within the Cuomo administration. It was a huge opportunity for me to speak to a source from the inside so I could learn about the behind-the-scenes decision making about schools. How were they determining different benchmarks for when schools could open or close? Did the state's public health department review CDC guidance on distancing and come to any different conclusions? And so on. Yet his response was that they didn't discuss schools much at all.

What about the federal level? $45.3 billion, and NIH couldn't be bothered to spend a couple million on testing the duration of infectious SARS-CoV-2 on playground surfaces? Officials at the agency weren't curious about whether six feet actually reduced cases in schools versus three feet? Did barriers do anything at all? And what about masks? These interventions kept millions of children out of school, and when they were in school dramatically degraded the experience. Yet there was zero urgency to get high-quality evidence on the interventions' effectiveness. Instead, guidance and rules were kept in place and the authorities either pretended there was evidence behind interventions, or just shrugged and said "there's so much we don't know," while doing next to nothing to gain knowledge.

With so many questions unanswered about NPIs, in particular school closures and the distancing requirements that led to hybrid schedules, it slowly became clear to me that the people in charge—the politicians, and the public health officials—didn't actually want to know the answers. This is my own conjecture, but I believe that, in part, the more time went on the less incentive they had to find out. If a study found that six feet of distancing saved a certain number of lives, or that school closures led to a significant reduction in cases, neither would be all that validating, considering the public was already told that these measures were critical to save lives. Masks on kids, HEPA filters, the barriers on students' desks— none of this stuff had a strong evidence base, and it was clear by the allocation of funds that the powers that be didn't want to find out if it didn't actually work.

Not pursuing research to gain quality evidence was only part of the problem. Some of our health institutions, in particular the CDC, actively thwarted evidence that went against its guidance. The *Morbidity and Mortality Weekly Report*, known as *MMWR*, is the CDC's house journal. When it publishes studies they often receive a wave of press, with journalists uncritically reporting the findings. What most of the public does not know is that *MMWR* is not peer reviewed, which means there are no outside experts to look at the content of studies before they are published. The entire acceptance and editorial process happens behind closed doors at the CDC. There's something else even more surprising about *MMWR*: by policy, the journal will only publish research that supports current CDC guidelines. You read that correctly: if an outside researcher conducts a study that finds results that conflict with what the CDC has been telling the public, *MMWR*—by design—will not accept or publish that study's recommendations. It is not hyperbole to acknowledge that *MMWR* is essentially a propaganda journal. Yet, to most of the public, when they hear "a study published by the CDC" there is an imprimatur of quality and objectivity.

It's beyond the scope of this book to detail how poorly done many of the MMWR papers were during the pandemic, but suffice to say, in the absence of any outside review, and with a mandate to only publish material that supports the agency's existing guidance, many of its studies were of abysmal quality. I will provide just one brief story on this, though there are many:

In 2021, I wrote a widely read feature for the *Atlantic* about an *MMWR* paper that purported schools without mask mandates were three-and-a-half times more likely to have COVID outbreaks than schools with mask mandates. What the paper didn't reveal was that districts without mandates had a *longer* observation period in the study than districts with mandates. If you look at school A (no mandate) for five weeks, and school B (mandate) for three weeks, and then compare how many outbreaks the schools in each district had, obviously the districts without mandates that had data compiled over more time also had more opportunities for outbreaks. A thumb was on the scale. It was absurd. The study also had an impossible number of schools listed in the paper. I got the official number of schools from the state of Arizona, where the study was conducted, and those numbers conflicted with the numbers in the paper. I alerted the journal editors and the paper's corresponding author to these errors—which the author acknowledged—but they declined to correct the paper. I then asked for the data set they used, and the authors and the journal refused to provide it. Despite the fact that an author of the paper herself *admitted that its data were wrong*, and despite the fact that I had official numbers from the state that were different from the numbers in the paper, a communications officer for the CDC replied to me that there were no errors in the paper. It was pure gaslighting, like something I'd imagine out of a corrupt regime behind the Iron Curtain.

I interviewed a half-dozen infectious diseases specialists, pediatricians, and epidemiologists, including a former CDC staffer, and they all were aghast at the errors in the paper—there were many, many others in addition to those mentioned above. Several said the paper was so bad it never should have been published. To be clear: There were factual errors in this paper, the CDC knew it, and it didn't care. Rochelle Walensky, who became the head of the CDC when Biden took office, repeated the "three and a half times more likely to have outbreaks" line over and over.

She said it in TV interviews, in White House press briefings, and in print. Even after my exposé came out, Walensky continued to cite this erroneous figure. Did the CDC really need to persuade the public so badly that mask mandates in schools worked that it was willing to lie repeatedly? The answer is yes. To this day, the study remains in *MMWR* and is cited by journalists and others as evidence of the effect of school mask mandates.

During the summer of 2020, the chief of the Division of Infectious Diseases at Massachusetts General Hospital, who was also a professor of medicine at Harvard Medical School, emailed the mayor of her town in Massachusetts that if people in schools were masked, then three feet of distancing was both "safe" and "much more practical" than six feet. This was important because the CDC had been recommending six feet of distancing, and perhaps the advice of a highly credentialed professional might sway her district.

The author of that email was Rochelle Walensky. Yet when she became the director of the CDC, the guidance remained at six feet of distancing.

Under Walensky's leadership, the CDC released guidance for summer camps in 2021, which included the recommendation for masking *at all times*, including outdoors. There was a wealth of evidence by then that outdoor transmission was exceedingly unlikely, not to mention the fact that kids were at a risk lower than the flu, for which masking was never required, let alone outdoors. I wrote an article for *New York* magazine, in which I quoted several experts, including the editor in chief of *JAMA Pediatrics*, one of the top pediatric medical journals in the world, who called the rules "draconian." A source I quoted from within the NIH referred to the guidance as "cruel." A pediatric immunologist at Columbia University called them "irrational." Within forty-eight hours Walensky and Fauci were being asked about the guidelines after my article had gone viral. Why should a child who is playing tennis, Walensky was asked, and thirty feet away from anyone else, be forced to wear a mask in the summer heat? She had no answer.

In one of the triumphs of my journalistic career, within a couple weeks of my article the CDC changed its guidance and no longer recommended outdoor masking for kids in camp.

I have other examples. But I'll stop here. The point is that the CDC and NIH have the external appearance to some—they certainly did for me before the pandemic—of dispassionate scientists. Instead, what was manifestly clear is that the agencies were not sufficiently devoted to scientific inquiry or thoughtful application of evidence-based public health.

But this is not about just saying the CDC did a bad job. Its failures, along with those at NIH, were institutional features, not bugs. The fact that *MMWR* doesn't publish studies with findings that support recommendations that run counter to the CDC's guidance is scandalous, and that this fact is largely absent from media coverage of the CDC's studies is similarly scandalous.

Even when inconvenient evidence was published in other accredited journals it often was ignored by the media, and not incorporated into the authorities' statements to the public.

In May 2021, two studies, published in the journal *Pediatrics*, found that pediatric COVID hospitalization numbers were inflated by at least 40 percent. Because hospitals, as policy, had been testing every single admission for COVID many of the "COVID hospitalizations" were simply incidental—a child with a broken foot, for example, who just happened to test positive. Yet the COVID hospitalization numbers were constantly cited in the media, shown on dashboards in places like the *New York Times*, and referred to by politicians when discussing the danger of COVID to children. The number of children who were actually in the hospital "from" COVID rather than merely "with" COVID was roughly *half* of what we were regularly being told.

Also in the spring of 2021, the CDC published a study about COVID deaths, with a particular statistic that got very little notice. Unlike the PR campaigns devoted to its dubious masking papers, this *MMWR* paper was referenced in far fewer outlets. The top-line finding reported was that 375,000 deaths in 2020 were attributed to COVID. But buried in the paper, and not mentioned in the media coverage, was an astonishing finding: 35.2 percent of what were categorized as "COVID deaths" in children had *no plausible connection to COVID*. For example, some kids died of suicide, others were murdered, others died in car accidents, and so on, and they just happened, incidentally, to test positive for COVID around their time of death. Of course a child who died from a tragic fall but just happened to test positive for COVID before the accident should not be counted as a COVID death. Nevertheless, that's exactly what happened, and the CDC's own study said so. Like the hospital numbers, more than a third of the tally of pediatric COVID deaths were not actual COVID deaths. We're not talking about the pediatric mortality statistics being off by 5 percent. COVID deaths in children were overcounted by *more than 35 percent*. This type of assertion got people suspended from Twitter and kicked off Facebook. We were told that people who said such things were cranks, right-wing lunatics, QAnon conspiracists. But it was published by the CDC. Interestingly, this finding did not get repeated by Walensky over and over at White House briefings or in interviews. It did not receive the fanfare of the Arizona masking study.

We need to ask ourselves, and ask our officials, why that is.

The government's own data show that more children may have died of the flu in several of the last ten flu seasons before 2020 than from COVID in each of the pandemic's three years. Each year, more children die from drowning, from car accidents, and from suicide, *individually*, than they did from COVID over the first two years of the pandemic *combined*. The numbers aren't even close. None of these statistics were trumpeted by the authorities to provide context when imposing COVID interventions on children.

This isn't to say COVID posed no risk, but that its risk was no greater than background risks of life that children always face. Yet, as late as spring 2023, there were still perfectly healthy children whose parents required them to wear masks all day, every day. That same spring, *three years after the pandemic's onset*, a Montessori school in Ithaca, New York, in addition to all-day masking, still forced its students to eat silent lunches.

For many citizens not following the issue closely, it seemed that opening schools in their area was a foolish and irresponsible idea. After all, this was the implicit, and sometimes explicit, message they were sent from the health establishment, which then was amplified by the media and mostly Democratic politicians. The deliberate lack of evidence, and the disallowance of contrarian views, ensured that a particular narrative, both within and beyond the scientific establishment, would remain dominant.

In the monomania of the pandemic response in America, there were two key questions that were never appropriately reckoned with:

First, will the mitigation measures actually achieve the reduction in deaths and serious illness that the public health authorities say they will achieve? Second, even if the measures are guaranteed to achieve what they are said to achieve, are they worth all of the collateral damage?

More succinctly: Are these measures effective, and even if so are they equitable or wise?

Throughout this book variations of the word *moral* have appeared more than two dozen times. To understand why the above questions were not adequately considered requires recognizing that the marketing of morality was the connective tissue between the public health establishment's positions, the media's representation of those positions, and much of the public's internalization of just action. The phrase "out of an abundance of caution" and the word "safe"—both deployed ubiquitously throughout the pandemic to justify interventions—are imbued with emotional resonance. They alluded to an impending or amorphous danger, one that could be avoided through action. To not act, to not follow the experts' guidance and rules on how to make yourself and those around you "safe," would be immoral.

It is this moralizing of disagreement that was so damaging. In large measure it prevented an open debate between the Left and the public health community in America about NPIs, in particular those in relation to schools and children.

Recall Andrew Cuomo casting healthcare professionals as "soldiers fighting a battle for us," and saying that the pandemic was a war. Recall the "your mask protects me, my mask protects you" campaign perpetuated by Cuomo and many others.

The overall "fight" against COVID was set in moral terms. Who wouldn't support the soldiers fighting to protect society? Who wouldn't in any way possible join the "war effort"? Who wouldn't wear a simple mask that prevents harm to other people? Only selfish assholes, of course. (Never mind that there was no evidence that community masking reduced transmission.)

By framing NPIs as morally righteous, any opposition to them, in turn, was rendered immoral. Telling people that they were racists and murderers if they wanted their kid to be able to go to school epitomized this dynamic.

Yet this was not a war in which a country or people are under attack and the only reasonable or honorable option is to fight. SARS-CoV-2 is a highly contagious respiratory virus. Pathogenic viruses are a fact of nature (albeit in this instance, possibly made in a lab) that humanity has accepted through all of history. Acceptance doesn't mean doing nothing. It means having the humility to recognize the limitations of what we can do, the wisdom to balance potential benefits of interventions against their negative effects, and the foresight to understand the harms that can result from thinking our efforts are more effective than they actually are.

In October 2020, three scientists, Martin Kulldorff, the Harvard Medical School biostatistician whom I had interviewed that summer for my article about the downsides of hybrid schooling; Jay Bhattacharya, a physician and public health economist at Stanford University: and Sunetra Gupta, an infectious diseases epidemiologist at Oxford University, authored the Great Barrington Declaration (GBD), a clarion call for this exact type of prudence. It was a joint statement that argued for restraint from the military offensive that health officials and politicians had been waging, and, instead, advocated focusing protection on the most vulnerable in society and letting the rest get on with their lives.

The GBD was rooted in an understanding that, as the saying goes, a cure can be worse than the disease. In medicine iatrogenesis is the causing of harm through examination or treatment. Kulldorff and his coauthors argued that the NPIs—including, specifically and especially, school closures—aside from likely being largely ineffective, were an iatrogenic harm on a societal level. They wrote that keeping children, who were at close to no risk themselves, out of school was "a grave injustice."

Though its feasibility and details could be debated, the GBD's general premise was not out of step with mainstream epidemiological thought prior to 2020. Nevertheless, it was seen as a direct challenge to what had become establishment dogma, and the retaliation against the Declaration and its authors was swift and brutal. The *New York Times*, the *Washington Post*, the *Guardian*, *Scientific American*, *Nature*, *BuzzFeed*, *Vox*, the *Economist*, and CNBC all published scathing hit pieces. "I think it's wrong, I think it's unsafe, I think it invites people to act in ways that have the potential to do an enormous amount of harm," Rochelle Walensky, who would go on to head the CDC under Biden, was quoted in the *Times*. *Business Insider* included a statement from the Infectious Diseases Society of America that called the GBD "inappropriate, irresponsible, and ill-informed." *Vox*'s headline called it "an ethical nightmare."

An October 14 *Washington Post* article said the GBD strategy was "called 'fringe' and 'dangerous' by National Institutes of Health Director Francis Collins." In the *Times* and CNBC pieces Fauci referred to the GBD as "nonsense" and "dangerous." A blog post on the website for the Union of Concerned Scientists referred to the GBD as a "dangerous fringe theory."

Less than a week before the *Post* article, on October 8, Collins had sent an email to Fauci and a top deputy with a link to the GBD website and said: "This proposal from the three fringe epidemiologists who met with the Secretary seems to be getting a lot of attention." Collins then said, "There needs to be a quick and devastating published take down of its premises." He ended by writing that he hadn't seen any takedowns yet and asked if one was underway. (The email only came to the public's attention through a Freedom of Information Act request.)

Never mind that much their ideas were rooted in the basics of epidemiology, including those detailed in a famous 2006 paper co-authored by D. A. Henderson, possibly the most celebrated and accomplished epidemiologist in recent history. And never mind that the three scientists, who had extensive subject matter expertise, were at three of the most prestigious universities in the world. For their dissent from the orthodoxy, they were successfully demonized as "fringe," and their non-aggressive approach as dangerous, i.e. immoral.

Although more is most certainly not always better, the moral imperative to "fight" is nevertheless our foundational metaphor for dealing with illness and disease. (One has to "battle" cancer. And if the person dies, it's because they "lost the fight.") And it's not just on an individual level. Susan Sontag, in her treatises on illness, wrote about how disease becomes a judgment on the community. Indeed, during the COVID pandemic countries and communities were judged based on how aggressively they responded to the virus. Florida and Georgia were immoral death-cult states, whereas New York and California were "good." It wasn't even necessary to have lower COVID case counts to be viewed as morally superior. The results—how effective the NPIs actually were, and how much collateral damage they caused—were irrelevant. Rather, it was the amount of active intervention—of "doing something"—that made for a righteous culture. Many public health figures even cited the draconian, authoritative measures taken in China as morally correct.

The positioning of *action* as the only moral approach to the virus, and as a consequence dissenting voices defamed and dismissed, is one of the reasons why a sober assessment of the core questions—Will these interventions work? If so, to what extent? And what harms may be incurred because of them?—did not happen.

"Sometimes, a scientific consensus is established because vested interests have diligently and purposefully transformed a situation of profound uncertainty into one in which there appears to be overwhelming evidence for what becomes the consensus view," wrote Eric Winsberg in an article on the necessity of scientific dissidents. A key lesson here is that consensus is often manufactured, knowingly by some, unwittingly by others. We must always look for evidence, rather than expert opinion or the appearance of consensus. "This doesn't mean we should believe every heterodox thinker that comes along. But it means we should strongly resist the urge to punish them, to censor them, to call them racist." Instead, Winsberg wrote, we should simply "evaluate their claims."

Fall wore into winter and the portion of public schools in America open full time hadn't budged above around one-third. By the beginning of January 2021, roughly ten months after the initial shutdowns, more than half of schools were fully remote, and around 15 percent were hybrid. No amount of observational evidence from Europe, and from around the US, was enough to change the false narrative in large pockets of the country that schools were dangerous. The health authorities had not produced any quality evidence to show the benefits of distancing in schools and the resultant hybrid schedules, nor the benefits of closed schools. And since, against the norms of medicine, the burden of proof had reversed, and the default was now the intervention, the authorities had no imperative to pursue the matter.

But finally, inevitably, things had to change.

24

UNLIKELY HEROES AND THE EVENTUAL ACCEPTANCE OF EMPIRICAL DATA

The story of how kids around America eventually got back into school relies on some unlikely heroes. Where the government and the rest of the health establishment failed society, these professionals stepped into the void. They shared two simple traits: a desire for evidence, and the determination to produce it.

In the summer of 2020, a small-town pediatrician named Amy Falk, who lives and practices in the rural, dead-center of Wisconsin, wanted to find out whether opening schools actually led to an increase in cases, as so many people had been saying. She knew how important school was, wanted the kids to be able to attend, but knew she needed data. Falk had never conducted research before in her life. Her focus had always been seeing patients. But with the health agencies not studying the matter she felt she had no choice but to collect the data herself.

The NIH has a $45 billion budget, and our country had to rely on a random, small-town pediatrician with no experience doing research to initiate a study to get data on the safety of schools being open. "I wanted to find a way," Falk said. "My husband and I talk and say, 'Why us?' Other physicians were wringing their hands, and I'm like 'Let's get in there and do something.'"

Falk teamed up with Dr. Tracy Høeg, a physician and epidemiologist, who had grown up in Wisconsin, and who had experience conducting and publishing research, to run a study. "Why isn't the CDC paying researchers to do this?" Høeg wondered. "This is the most important question and the only people studying it are independent and, at least in our case, doing it for free."

During the study period, from August 31 to November 29, cases were sky-high in the Wisconsin community the researchers studied, with some positivity rates north of 30 percent. Though it was a rural area the schools were large, with more than 5,530 students and staff who opted for in-person school. Yet Falk, Høeg, and their coauthors found the case rates in the schools were significantly lower than those in the community, a dramatic 37 percent difference. Moreover, of the cases found in schools, only one in twenty was linked to in-school transmission.

Elementary students were divided into cohorts, within which there was no distancing. There was only distancing between cohorts. And in the high school there wasn't even distancing between cohorts. The kids ate lunch indoors together. Fifty percent of the schools had not installed new ventilation systems.

The finding was incredibly important. It demonstrated a clear separation between the community rate and the school rate of infection, even when the buildings were crowded with students who weren't distancing. Schools were not driving transmission.

"The results weren't a surprise to me," Høeg said, because they were similar to what was already seen abroad. But since these data were from within the US she was confident they would be more influential to get American schools open. "I thought, 'This is so great, now they'll see what's been happening in Europe,'" Høeg told me.

Shortly before Høeg and Falk's paper came out, also in January 2021, researchers at Duke University posted results from their own study of schools, in North Carolina. Over nine weeks, out of nearly 100,000 students and staff who were in person, there were just 32 cases of within-school transmission.

Remember, the preceding fall I had conducted and written about my own analysis of Westchester County, New York, where I found schools that were open full time did not have higher case rates among students than schools that were closed or hybrid. Emily Oster's national data were similar. But the Duke study and Høeg and Falk's study were set to have far more impact because they were published in academic journals, *Pediatrics* for Duke, and, most importantly, *MMWR* for the Wisconsin study. Høeg believes the only reason her study got published in *MMWR* was because, to her chagrin, the journal spun the paper's conclusion about low rates in schools to emphasize that students and staff were required to wear masks, a prime CDC guideline. Høeg felt this was an illegitimate assertion to make, given there was no control group without masks, not to mention European schools, many populated with maskless children, did no worse. (Indeed, a study out of Norway, published several weeks before the *MMWR* paper, where COVID was a significant presence in the community, also found low school rates even though masks were not required or even recommended in their schools.) The Duke authors, similarly, attributed their results to mask wearing, even though they had no control group without masks to compare to. Still, whether the CDC pinned the encouraging outcome on masks or not, the findings of low school rates relative to their community rate were clear.

Amazingly, despite the Wisconsin *MMWR* paper, that February, with Biden in the White House and Rochelle Walensky now heading the CDC, the agency came out with new school guidelines that in some ways were even more restrictive than before. There was now a complex scheme of a four-tier color-coded system, tying different community rates to whether it was safe to open schools in a given area. In February, according to the system, more than 90 percent of the country was in the most restrictive tier, meaning that elementary schools in those locations should not be open for full-time in-person learning, and middle and high schools should not open at all, even in hybrid, without screening tests.

Høeg was aghast. Her paper, published by the CDC itself, not only didn't immediately lead to all the schools opening in her current home state of California, but even coincided with more prohibitive guidance. But the interesting thing is the new guidance—perhaps, in part, due to some press about the Wisconsin and North Carolina papers—signaled the official loss of influence of the health authorities. Beginning with the new year, the percentage of schools with either hybrid or full-time in-person schooling began a steady rise, and fully remote a steady decline. These trajectories, which continued through to the summer break, were in defiance of the new guidance. Though millions of students were still blocked from attending school for the remainder of the academic year, many millions more were slowly coming back, even if just in hybrid. School districts, by the thousands, stopped listening to the CDC.

My kids in New York, along with millions of others around the country, were still stuck in hybrid, though. The six feet that children needed to maintain from each other, this distance based on magical thinking, had proved unbreachable. Untold numbers of children in Europe had been in full capacity classes since the previous May, eight months earlier, with no noticeable effect. But distancing and hybrid in New York continued. First, Emily Oster's data came out, with still no change. Now, in the winter of the 2020–2021 school year, we had a proper study conducted in the US, published in the CDC's own journal, with crowded classrooms and a lower rate than the surrounding community, yet the fixation on six feet remained. Given the flipped burden of proof, to get the kids back in school full time there needed to be some higher level of evidence, a direct comparative study in America between six feet and some lesser distance.

In July of 2020, Westyn Branch-Elliman, the Harvard infectious diseases specialist, got a call from Elissa Schechter-Perkins, an emergency medicine physician at Boston University. They lived in the same town in Massachusetts and knew each other from the district's health committee. "The town was initially proposing some crazy hybrid scheme of 2.5 hours in the mornings for two days a week because they were afraid of lunch," Branch-Elliman told me. "Elissa and I said to each other, 'No one knows what benefit, if any, there is for these various plans being floated.' It was really disconcerting."

That fall, the *Boston Globe* began tracking the school plans in every district in Massachusetts. "Elissa said, 'You've got to put all this together in a proper database and analyze it,'" Branch-Elliman recounted. "My plate was full. And I thought, 'Surely someone else is working on this. This is the biggest problem facing the country.' But over time Elissa and I realized no one was doing a proper comparison between schooling interventions. And without good data we—rightfully, it turns out—were afraid the kids wouldn't get back into school." So the two doctors got to work.

What made Massachusetts perfect for a comparative study of distancing was that, unlike most blue states, Massachusetts, at the time run by a Republican governor, Charlie Baker, allowed districts to go below six feet. Its department of education recommended a minimum of just three feet (mirroring the WHO's guidance of one meter), though most districts in the state stuck with the CDC's more aggressive six feet.

But cataloging the school plans was only half the job. They had exposure data—meaning how close the kids were to each other and how often in school—but they also needed outcomes data—the rate of infections. Branch-Elliman posted about their need on Twitter, and Emily Oster responded that she had what they were looking for.

The match was perfect for a proper study. "The gatherers of the exposure data were blinded to the outcome data," Branch-Elliman explained. In other words, she and Schecter-Perkins had no idea of the case counts (Oster's territory) while they organized the school interventions data. This helped eliminate the possibility of bias affecting the study outcome.

All in, the three of them, plus four additional coauthors, looked at more than 500,000 students and nearly 100,000 staff from September 24, 2020, to January 27, 2021. Like Wisconsin, the incidence of cases among students and staff was lower than the community rate, but shadowed it, yet again suggesting that schools were not drivers of transmission. At most, schools merely reflected what was happening in the community. In this massive data set, over this long duration of time, they found that six feet of distancing conferred no clear benefit over schools that adhered to a minimum of three feet. The graphs in the paper are striking—the lines representing case rates in schools with three feet of distancing almost perfectly overlap the lines representing case rates in schools with six feet of distancing.

This was about as close to irrefutable evidence as anyone was going to get that six feet of distancing—the rule that prevented tens of millions of American children from attending school full time for an entire year—was for nothing.

*   *   *

One of the main problems with conducting research on schools and children during the pandemic to try to gain quality evidence is that most states followed CDC guidance. If masks were mandated and kids were six feet apart there was no way to actually test whether either of these interventions worked because there was no control group of schools not doing these interventions to compare them to. It was a catch-22. The CDC is the authority on what is true, therefore you should follow the CDC. But the only way to test if what the CDC says is actually true was to not follow what the agency recommended. It's only in the states and locations that defied the CDC where researchers were able to conduct studies to actually test whether the CDC guidance was effective—and find out that it wasn't. Of course it's supposed to be the opposite. An intervention is supposed to have proof that it works *before* it's required and implemented. You're not supposed to implement an intervention on millions of children—let alone do so for a year—and have to prove that it *doesn't* work in order to rescind it. But that's what happened in America.

Moreover, the states and people that didn't follow the CDC were vilified. They were called anti-science idiots. Progressives put up lawn signs that said, "In this house we believe science is real," which was intended as a barb against Republicans or anyone who questioned the health authorities. Yet "the science" promoted by the CDC that the lawn-sign people believed in was half-baked. And if it was up to the CDC and the health establishment there would have been no way to prove them wrong.

In the face of the Massachusetts study's evidence the CDC finally relented and lowered its school distancing guidance from six feet on March 19, 2021. In numerous ways it was evident, very early, that six feet of distancing was not effective, yet this was ignored. It wasn't until nearly a full year later, after the Massachusetts study, that the guidance changed. And the only reason the CDC, and eventually New York, where my children live, changed their guidance was not because the CDC or NIH or state health authorities ran any studies. It was because people like Amy Falk, Tracy Høeg, Emily Oster, and Westyn Branch-Elliman took it upon themselves to do so. Because of their work, and because the Massachusetts governor chose not to follow the CDC, my kids and millions of others were finally able to go to school full time.

All of the remote learning they suffered through in their hybrid schedule, which forced them to lose more than half a year of school, did not achieve anything. Worse still, there was no evidence that full school closures imposed on millions of other children resulted in any fewer cases either. All of this was for naught.

The Massachusetts study was published in the journal *Clinical Infectious Diseases* on March 10, 2021. Within two weeks the CDC lowered its recommendation from a minimum of six feet to a minimum of three feet of distancing. It took a month after that until my district finally went full time in person, on April 19, more than a year after schools initially shut down.

It would take almost another entire year, until March 2022, before my kids didn't have to wear masks all day every day. But at least they were in school.

CONCLUSION

On March 20, 2020, Andrew Cuomo gave an impassioned speech in which he outlined his New York State on "PAUSE" (Policies Assure Uniform Safety for Everyone) executive order, which shut down much of society, including schools, in his state. "These actions will cause disruption," he said. "They will cause businesses to close. They'll cause employees to stay at home. They will cause much unhappiness. I understand that." Why was New York taking such dramatic action, he asked. "This is about saving lives," he answered. "And if everything we do saves just one life, I'll be happy."

As a policy position that lasted, to varying degrees, for three years, this was a terrible plan. Because in order to save one life another life, or multiple lives, might have to be sacrificed. A look at excess mortality—the number of deaths not just from COVID, but from *all causes*, including those as a result of pandemic policies, that exceed the expected number of deaths in a given place in a given period of time—is revealing.

Florida had a lower excess death rate than California, the model state for "taking the virus seriously." One state—that enforced strict social distancing, that required masks in nearly all social contexts, that shuttered businesses, that padlocked playgrounds, that isolated people from friends and family, that barred many of the activities that make life meaningful, and that kept many of its children out of school *for more than a year*—ended up with basically the same rate of excess deaths as another state that, after spring 2020, did almost none of these things.

Amazingly, even Florida's standardized *COVID* death rate—a rate adjusted for differences in age and other factors like prevalence of comorbidities—was lower than California's, despite the vast difference in interventions between the two states.

Cuomo's "if everything we do saves just one life" comment was manifestly stupid, yet it embodied the approach of the public health authorities in the US during the pandemic: a years-long fixation on trying to slow the rate of SARS-CoV-2 transmission without sufficiently understanding or acknowledging that every measure put in place to that end would necessitate a trade-off. Missed cancer screenings, delayed visits to the emergency room, interrupted treatments for chronic illnesses, deaths of despair (suicide, drug overdoses) from loneliness and isolation or job loss—all of these things that resulted from pandemic policies and a climate of fear add up.

Of course near-term death is not the only trade-off of salience. Studies found escalated rates of severe cases of appendicitis in kids, requiring surgery, because parents were too afraid to bring their children to the hospital—that is until the illness caused a degree of harm that could no longer be ignored. A 2021 National Survey of Children's Health found that an extraordinary 27 percent of children had delayed or missed preventative care due to the pandemic. Then there are the eating disorders and mental health issues that isolated kids and adolescents developed. And the lifelong effects for many kids from missed schooling. And the related lost sports seasons and athletics scholarships. It's not trivial to also note the canceled proms and graduation ceremonies and homecoming games. Given there was no benefit of keeping schools closed and canceling these events, it's hard to even call this a trade-off. It was just harm.

"If you're a public health person, you have this very narrow view of what the right decision is . . . you attach infinite value to stopping the disease. You attach a zero value to whether this actually totally disrupts people's lives, ruins the economy, and has many kids kept out of school in a way that they never quite recovered from. That was a mistake."

The above quote is not from Florida governor Ron DeSantis or the Swedish minister of health. It was spoken at a 2023 event by Francis Collins, the head of the NIH during the pandemic. With remarkable, almost unsettling candor, Collins went on:

What we did wrong is we failed to say every time there was a recommendation "guys, this is the best we can do right now, there's a good chance this is wrong." We didn't say that. We wanted to be sure people motivated themselves by what we said because we wanted change to happen in case it was right. But we did not admit our ignorance. That was a profound mistake.

Everything the philosophers Eric Winsberg and Jeremy Howick, and the infectious diseases specialist Westyn Branch-Elliman, and the epidemiologist Jennifer Nuzzo, and Great Barrington's Bhattacharya, Gupta, and Kulldorff, and others had predicted or observed, and in some instances tried to warn about, was encapsulated in these admissions by the man who oversaw America's public health establishment. Though many of the decisions were made with the best of intentions, the hubris and inanity of constructing an entire approach to the pandemic based on the projections of obviously flawed models, and then purposefully downplaying the lack of certainty about the effect of interventions in order to manipulate the public, left a large portion of the citizenry misinformed, afraid, and compliant with policies—chief among them, prolonged school closures—that lacked evidence of benefit but delivered guaranteed harms.

This doomed and foolish plan directed by the health authorities was greatly spurred along by a deeply politically divided populace, where tribalism on the Left fostered a medical establishment and influencer class that all but refused to veer from its team's position. And by a legacy media that failed at its most fundamental duties—to question those in power and report beyond a preconceived narrative. And entrenched teachers unions. And cowardly or cynical politicians. And afraid or feckless, or at least simply unfairly burdened school administrators, ill-suited for the task at hand.

One thing is clear: the school closures and broader harms unnecessarily and unfairly inflicted upon America's children were overdetermined.

* * *

There was a certain willful dishonesty and fantasy to the idea that making children sit alone, staring at screens, isolated in their homes, for hours each day, for weeks, and then month after month after month was going to be anything other than a tragedy for many children. Even those who apparently didn't suffer academically still lost something socially and psychologically.

In the latter years of the pandemic, and the immediate years following it, and surely for decades to come, researchers will continue to track academic scores and other measurable outcomes of school closures. This is important. But too much of a focus on academics and data misses something that's ineffable, though no less damaging of a harm from remote learning. As the sociologist William Bruce Cameron memorably once said, "Not everything that can be counted counts, and not everything that counts can be counted."

The psychologists Gabriel Radvansky and Jeff Zacks have written extensively about event cognition, and specifically about how people's experience of the world is defined by "event boundaries," that the physical places you pass through segment your awareness and memories. In a literal sense, for example, walking through a doorway creates an event boundary in people's minds. In essence, explained psychologist Fiona McPherson, event boundaries are beginnings and endings, and what we have always known is that beginnings and endings—the moments of transition, of movement, of new stimuli that spark our attention—are better remembered than middles. When, for weeks, and collectively for many months, for many kids totaling more than a year, children were kept home, parked in front of a screen, alone, for untold hours, instead of going to a physical place and interacting in person with peers and teachers, event boundaries—and the memories they engender—were never formed.

In spring 2023, I asked my son, who was finishing sixth grade, something about fourth grade and his year of hybrid and school closures. At first he said he had forgotten most of the particulars I had mentioned to him about remote learning. He marveled for a moment at his memory lapse. And then, as a vague wash of details and feelings came back to him about the frustrations, the unique and unfamiliar loneliness, and the profound, agonizing boredom, he paused for a long moment then shook his head. "Wow," he said, "I forgot how much that sucked."

In one regard, the lack of specificity of his recall—until nudged with a few details—would likely be cited by some people as evidence of resilience. And that view may very well be correct. After all, blocking out memories of unpleasant and especially uneventful tedium is a standard device of our minds, the former as a protective mechanism, the latter because why bother? But this resilience, if that is what we are to term it, is also evidence of what was lost. By keeping children in remote learning—a largely grim, solitary, and unstimulating affair that for most children took place without ever leaving their homes—they were cheated out of a year or more of childhood memories that they would have otherwise formed from experiences in the physical world by attending school (and athletic events, and plays, and orchestra concerts, and field trips). Remote learning was, at best, a year of middles.

"Events require clear demarcations to help us distinguish one from the other and form permanent memories of our experiences," wrote Christine Rosen, the chair of the Colloquy on Knowledge, Technology and Culture at the Institute for Advanced Studies at the University of Virginia. "During lockdown, our endless stream of Zoom business meetings and social meet-ups has had the effect of effacing those boundaries, flattening experience, and in the process altering the memories we will carry with us about this time of crisis—a small but not insignificant change."

Childhood is achingly brief, but we all retain images and scenes and sensations from those short years for the rest of our lives. For many kids, school closures have left them with indelible memories of trauma or hardship. For others, the lasting scar will be one of absence. Robbed of a physical experience—the sites, the smells, the feeling of laughing sitting next to a friend—the film scroll of youthhood memories for many children of the pandemic may likely suffer from a strange and conspicuous jump cut over a vast expanse of time in the early 2020s. Their lives left with an empty space of precious, missing scenes that never happened.

* * *

During the pandemic, public health officials' recommendations, and the policies that followed from them, were based on subjective *values* yet were presented to the public as objective science. It is my hope that during the next crisis the public possesses a heightened awareness of the difference between the two, and not only tolerates but demands a robust debate if the government aims to rescind a basic right, such as for a child to attend school.

ACKNOWLEDGMENTS

There are so many people who offered their time, expertise, wisdom, and friendship to me during the pandemic. All of those contributions, either directly or indirectly, helped make this book possible. I'd like to thank Daniel Engber, my editor at *Wired* and the *Atlantic*. Dan was the first, and for quite some time the only editor who believed what I was writing about schools, masks, and all other things COVID was important, well-researched, and deserving of an audience. Dan also had the acumen to regularly encourage me to turn the rage dial from a 10 to a 7. Similarly, I'd like to thank Jebediah Reed at *New York* for his enthusiastic support. Both Dan and Jeb had the courage to green-light articles that went against the accepted orthodoxy in the legacy media, and for that they deserve deepest praise. I could not ask for a wiser and more loyal agent than Eric Lupfer. Eric immediately understood and eagerly supported the thesis of this book, then tirelessly shopped it around until it found its home with Susan Buckley at MIT Press, to whom I am eternally grateful. Without Susan this book would be 1,000 pages, so anyone reading this owes her a thanks as well. Judith Feldmann, at MIT, also has my gratitude and praise. I want to thank and credit Jeff Tompkins for his work formatting the endnotes, copy editing, and fact checking. I'd also like to thank Karen Vaites, Natalya Murakhver, Erich Hartmann, Anish Koka, Ben Recht, Geneve Campbell, Kristin Gorman, Kristen Walsh, Daniele Lantagne, Alison Babb, Eli Klein (an art dealer who knows more about public health than most doctors and epidemiologists), Jeffrey Tucker, Douglas Rushkoff, Ari Wallach, Kelley Krohnert (who was an amazing resource for data acquisition and analysis), Matt Schiffman, Ramin Farzaneh, Maria Feldman, Renee Bailey, Christie Pesicka, Mark Herceg, Jenn Autuori, Nick Foy,

Michael Schlacter, Alex dal Piaz, Matthew Bring, Patrick Donohue, Sunetra Gupta, Martin Kulldorff, Jay Bhattacharya (a true mensch), Marty Makary, Monica Gandhi, Lucy McBride, Steve McConnell, Vinay Prasad, Eric Winsberg, Stephanie Harvard, Elissa Schecter-Perkins, Mark Gorelik, Sylvia Fogel, Wes Pegden, Emily Oster, and a huge thanks to Jennifer Nuzzo for sharing her experiences and insights. I am grateful to Westyn Branch-Elliman, who taught me more about medicine, public health, research methods, statistics, and how to read studies than any person has a right to learn without paying for a graduate degree. I'd like to thank Shira Doron, an incredible resource and friend. I'd like to thank Stefan Baral, Margery Smelkinson, Vladimir Kogan, Robert McNutt, Jake Scott, Ram Duriseti, Tracy Høeg (who was especially generous with her time), Amy Falk, Andy Bostom, Jonathan Ketcham, Jenin Younes, Alli Krug, Jen Reesman, Alex Washburne, Zeb Jamrozik, Anya Kamenetz, Joan Tronto, Louise-Ann McNutt, Daniel Sulmasy, Francois Balloux, Jeffrey Flier, Dimitri Christakis, Megyn Kelly, Jordan Peterson, Winston Marshall, and a huge thank you to Anthony LaMesa. I want to thank all the parents in Arlington and across the country who spoke with me for articles, this book, and mutual support. I also want to express my gratitude to Bari Weiss for allowing me to publish a number of great pieces with the Free Press, and especially for inviting me to take part in the Twitter Files. Zac Bissonnette was the first person I knew and trusted whom I saw tweet something skeptical about the narrative around COVID, back in April 2020. I'm grateful to have had Zac throughout the pandemic as a comrade in the questioning of experts and the media. I want to thank my mom and dad, and my sister, Susan. I want to thank my son, Zev, and my daughter, Eliana, for putting up with a dad who often worked late into the night and yelled more times than I can count "You're breaking my concentration!" when they came into my office. Lastly, with eternal love and gratitude, I want to thank my wife, Doreen, for her endless support, patience, tolerance, and for reading a thousand early drafts of my articles over the years.

NOTES

PREFACE

Page xi "primal scream": Tim Donahue, "My Coronavirus Routine: A Neighborhood Primal Scream," Opinion, *New York Times*, May 25, 2020, https://www.nytimes.com /2020/03/25/opinion/coronavirus-scream.html.

INTRODUCTION

Page 1 entire school system in America shut down: "Map: Coronavirus and School Closures in 2019–2020," *Education Week*, March 6, 2020, https://www.edweek.org /leadership/map-coronavirus-and-school-closures-in-2019-2020/2020/03.

Page 1 more than 50 million students: National Center for Education Statistics, "Fast Facts: Back-to-School Statistics," *Digest of Education Statistics*, "Table 203.45: Enrollment in public elementary and secondary schools, by level, grade, and state or jurisdiction: Fall 2020," https://nces.ed.gov/programs/digest/d22/tables/dt22_203.45.asp.

Page 1 school buses . . . : *American School & University*, March 1, 2009, https://www .asumag.com/facilities-management/transportation-parking/article/20846374/hop -on-the-bus; 479K school buses, 22.6 M kids transported: School Bus Fleet, *2021 Factbook* 66, no. 11, http://digital.schoolbusfleet.com/publication/?i=696373&p=1& pp=1&view=issueViewer.

Page 1 Free lunches: USDA Food and Nutrition Service, National School Lunch Program: https://fns-prod.azureedge.us/sites/default/files/resource-files/slsummar-3.pdf. In 2019 an average of 20.1 million free lunches were served. Disturbingly, during the height of school closures, in 2020, the number dropped to 15.9 million, and in 2021 it fell to just 10.9 million, though, according to the USDA, some portion of that drop was compensated for through the extension of summer meal programs.

Page 1 abandoned school playgrounds: National Center for Education Statistics, "Fast Facts: Educational Institutions," https://nces.ed.gov/fastfacts/display.asp?id=84. 2019–2020: 98,469 public schools (70,039 pre-K, elementary, middle; 4,901 "other" schools), 30,492 private schools, most of which presumably have playgrounds.

Page 3 Why were American schools, on average, and in particular in blue states, closed or disrupted longer than those in Europe: United Nations Educational, Scientific and

Cultural Organization (UNESCO), COVID-19 Recovery, "Education: From Disruption to Recovery," archived June 29, 2022, https://webarchive.unesco.org/web/2022 0629024039/https://en.unesco.org/covid19/educationresponse/.

Page 4 Gallup released the results of a poll: Sonal Desai, "On My Mind: They Blinded Us from Science," Franklin Templeton-Gallup Research Project, July 29, 2020, https://www.franklintempleton.com/articles/cio-views/on-my-mind-they-blinded -us-from-science.

Page 4 children under age fifteen accounted for an even more infinitesimal 0.04% of fatalities: 59 deaths out of 152,599 total. Data are through July 25, 2020, from the Centers for Disease Control and Prevention, National Center for Health Statistics. National Vital Statistics System, Provisional Mortality on CDC WONDER Online Database.

Page 5 In the fall of 2021: There were 2,179 deaths of people under age 25, and 620 deaths of people under age 18, out of a total of 726,389 deaths. Data are through September 2021, from the Centers for Disease Control and Prevention, National Center for Health Statistics. National Vital Statistics System, Provisional Mortality on CDC WONDER Online Database.

Page 5 suicides to drownings: In 2020, there were 199 COVID deaths of all children through age seventeen. By contrast, that year there were 767 drownings, and 1,679 suicides in that age group. In the following two years, when COVID deaths rose, they still were less than the number of kids who drowned and were multiples lower than the number who committed suicide.

It is also worth noting that these COVID mortality numbers are for COVID as simply a contributing cause of death, and some coroners listed Covid as a contributing cause of death even if there was not definitive evidence that was true. The mortality statistics for Covid as the "underlying" cause of death for people aged 0–17 are much lower: 2020: 141; 2021: 450; and 2022: 455.

The threat that COVID posed to children was also dwarfed by motor vehicle accidents and homicides, each of which led to the thousands of deaths in the 0–17 age bracket each year.

Data are from the Centers for Disease Control and Prevention, National Center for Health Statistics. National Vital Statistics System, Provisional Mortality on CDC WONDER Online Database. Accessed at http://wonder.cdc.gov/mcd-icd10-provisional .html on June 2, 2024.

Page 5 in many seasons, the flu: The comparison of COVID and flu deaths is fraught because of differences in how they were categorized, but based on official CDC estimates, more kids were hospitalized or died from influenza over multiple individual seasons in the decade before the pandemic, than from COVID in each of its first two years. In the 2012–2013 season, for example, the CDC estimates 1,160 children died from flu. In the 2014–2015 season, the estimate is 803. By comparison, the number of pediatric deaths with COVID in 2020 was 199, and in 2021 it was 612.

https://archive.cdc.gov/#/details?url=https://www.cdc.gov/flu/about/burden /2012-2013.html

https://archive.cdc.gov/#/details?url=https://www.cdc.gov/flu/about/burden
/2014-2015.html

https://www.cdc.gov/nchs/nvss/vsrr/covid_weekly/index.htm.

Page 5 average of one death a year in the US: Doyle Rice, *USA Today*, "Shark Attack Deaths: How Common Are They?" https://www.usatoday.com/story/news/nation /2015/06/15/shark-attacks/71251814/.

Page 5 vehicular accidents: https://crashstats.nhtsa.dot.gov/Api/Public/ViewPublica tion/813560#.

Page 6 "Remote schooling cannot even attempt": Alasdair Munro (@apsmunro), "All available evidence suggests 'remote schooling' failed even on the single function it is able to provide, which was education It cannot even attempt to provide," Twitter, August 6, 2022, 1:41 p.m., https://twitter.com/apsmunro/status/1555972391653752 833.

Page 7 World Health Organization: World Health Organization Regional Office for Europe, *Schooling during COVID-19: Recommendations from the European Technical Advisory Group for Schooling during COVID-19*, June 2021, https://apps.who.int/iris /bitstream/handle/10665/342075/WHO-EURO-2021-2151-41906-59077-eng.pdf. Thanks to Anthony LaMesa, whose writing about this report was my first exposure to it.

CHAPTER 1

Page 11 "Panic Shopping for Coronavirus Supplies, but Brunch Is Packed," Kimiko de Freytas-Tamura, *New York Times*, March 1, 2020.

Page 14 "Stay-at-home" order: New York State Governor's Press Office, "Video, Audio, Photos & Rush Transcript: Amid Ongoing COVID-19 Pandemic, Governor Cuomo Announces Statewide Public-Private Hospital Plan to Fight COVID-19," March 30, 2020, https://www.governor.ny.gov/news/video-audio-photos-rush-transcript-amid -ongoing-COVID-19-pandemic-governor-cuomo-announces-4.

Page 14 he repeatedly announced, with a metaphorical wave of the hand: Daniel Wolfe and Daniel Dale, "It's Going to Disappear': A Timeline of Trump's Claims that Covid-19 Will Vanish," CNN.com, October 31, 2020, https://www.cnn.com /interactive/2020/10/politics/covid-disappearing-trump-comment-tracker/.

Page 14 critical dearth of tests available: Suzy Khimm, Laura Strickler, and Brenda Breslauer, "Many Private Labs Want to Do Coronavirus Tests. But They're Still Facing Obstacles and Delays," NBC News, March 11, 2020, https://www.nbcnews.com /health/health-care/many-private-labs-want-do-coronavirus-tests-they-re-facing -n1156006. Ken Alltucker, "Feds Strive to Speed Up Coronavirus Testing after CDC's Slow Start: 'The Opportunity Was Missed,'" *USA Today*, March 3, 2020, Nation, https://www.usatoday.com/story/news/nation/2020/03/03/coronavirus-flawed-cdc -testing-kits-slowed-us-results/4930932002/.

Page 14 ventilators: Amy Feldman, "States Bidding Against Each Other Pushing Up Prices of Ventilators Needed to Fight Coronavirus, NY Governor Cuomo Says," *Forbes*,

March 28, 2020, https://www.forbes.com/sites/amyfeldman/2020/03/28/states-bidd
ing-against-each-other-pushing-up-prices-of-ventilators-needed-to-fight-coronavirus
-ny-governor-cuomo-says/.

Page 16 Thousandfold higher incidence: Cathrine Axfors et al., "Differential Covid-
19 Infection Rates in Children, Adults, and Elderly: Systemic Review and Meta-
analysis of 38 Pre-vaccination National Seroprevalence Studies," *Journal of Global
Health* 13 (2023).

Page 16 Michael Mulgrew: Adam Schrader, "Teacher's Union Escalates Fight with de
Blasio over NYC School Closures amid Coronavirus," *New York Post*, March 14, 2020,
https://nypost.com/2020/03/14/teachers-union-escalates-fight-with-de-blasio-over
-nyc-school-closures-amid-coronavirus/.

Page 16 The majority of COVID deaths in Italy, by early March: Margherita Stan-
cati, "Italy, with Aging Population, Has World's Highest Daily Deaths From Virus,"
Wall Street Journal, March 9, 2020, https://www.wsj.com/articles/italy-with-elderly
-population-has-worlds-highest-death-rate-from-virus-11583785086.

Page 16 Chinese Center for Disease Control and Prevention: Zunyou Wu and Jennifer M. McGoogan, "Characteristics of and Important Lessons from the Coronavirus
Disease 2019 (COVID-19) Outbreak in China: Summary of a Report of 72,314 Cases
from the Chinese Center for Disease Control and Prevention," *JAMA* 323, no. 13
(2020): 1239–1242.

Page 16 "Disease in children appears to be relatively rare and mild": "Report of the
WHO-China Joint Mission on Coronavirus Disease 2019 (COVID-19)," February 16–
24, 2020, https://acrobat.adobe.com/link/review/?pageNum=11&uri=urn%25253Aa
aid%25253Ascds%25253AUS%25253A5f509105-c8d1-4c1a-b7b6-054a98bdaf28.

CHAPTER 2

Page 19 Jennifer Nuzzo: Documentation related to the June 2006 meeting supplied
by Jennifer Nuzzo.

Page 19 D. A. Henderson: Donald G. McNeil Jr., "D.A. Henderson, Doctor Who
Helped End Smallpox Scourge, Dies at 87," *New York Times*, August 21, 2016; "In
Memoriam: Donald Ainslie Henderson MD, MPH '60," Johns Hopkins Bloomberg
School of Public Health, https://publichealth.jhu.edu/about/history/heroes-of-public
-health/donald-a-henderson; Pan American Health Organization, https://www.paho
.org/en/public-health-heroes/dr-donald-henderson.

Page 20 Carter Mecher: Institute of Medicine (US) Forum on Medical and Public
Health Preparedness for Catastrophic Events, *Dispensing Medical Countermeasures for
Public Health Emergencies: Workshop Summary* (Washington, DC: National Academies
Press, 2008), https://www.ncbi.nlm.nih.gov/books/NBK4102/; Michael Lewis, *The
Premonition: A Pandemic Story* (New York: W. W. Norton, 2021).

Page 20 "Interim Pre-pandemic Planning Guidance: Community Strategy for Pan-
demic Influenza Mitigation in the United States—Early, Targeted, Layered Use of
Nonpharmaceutical Interventions," US Department of Health and Human Services,
Centers for Disease Control and Prevention, February 2007.

Page 21 military computer programmers in 1957: "Work with New Electronic 'Brains' Opens Field for Army Math Experts," *Times* (Hammond, IN), November 10, 1957, https://www.newspapers.com/clip/50687334/the-times/. Amazingly, concerns about GIGO were even present in the 1860s. An English polymath named Charles Babbage had designed a mechanical computer, and, to his consternation, he was asked about it, "If you put into the machine wrong figures, will the right answers come out?" Babbage wrote of this: "I am not able rightly to apprehend the kind of confusion of ideas that could provoke such a question." Charles Babbage, *Passages from the Life of a Philosopher* (London, 1864; Project Gutenberg, 2018), ch. 5, https://www.gutenberg.org/files/57532/57532-h/57532-h.htm.

Page 21 A modeling study called "To Mask or Not to Mask": Steffen E. Eikenberry et al., "To Mask or Not to Mask: Modeling the Potential for Face Mask Use by the General Public to Curtail the COVID-19 Pandemic," *Infectious Disease Modelling* 5 (2020): 293–308.

Page 22 transmission in homes: Regarding transmission in school, it's important to understand that there are numerous studies that have found that most transmission occurs in the home. Therefore, a very low percentage of transmission in schools is not only possible, but likely. And, indeed, studies throughout the pandemic have consistently found school case rates to be lower, sometimes dramatically so, than community rates. Two examples: Alyssa LaFaro, "Household Deemed Most Common Place for COVID-19 Transmission," UNC Research (University of North Carolina at Chapel Hill), April 24, 2020, https://research.unc.edu/2020/04/24/household-deemed-most-common-place-for-covid-19-transmission/; Høeg et al., "COVID-19 Cases and Transmission in 17 K-12 Schools—Wood County, Wisconsin, August 31-November 29, 2020," *Morbidity and Mortality Weekly Report*, January 29, 2021.

Page 24 Glass got the idea: Lewis, *The Premonition: A Pandemic Story* (New York: W. W. Norton, 2021), 3.

Page 24 "form the backbone" and other Glass content: Robert J. Glass et al., "Targeted Social Distancing Design for Pandemic Influenza," *Emerging Infectious Diseases* 12, no. 11 (2006): 1671–1681, https://wwwnc.cdc.gov/eid/article/12/11/06-0255_article.

Page 24 "adults could continue to go to work" and other Glass content: Robert J. Glass, *Pandemic Influenza and Complex Adaptive System of Systems (CASoS) Engineering* (Albuquerque, NM: Sandia National Laboratory, 2009), https://proceedings.system dynamics.org/2009/proceed/papers/P1400.pdf.

Page 25 paper by the highly influential modeler Neil Ferguson: Neil M. Ferguson et al., "Strategies for Mitigating an Influenza Pandemic," *Nature* 442 (2006): 448–452.

Page 25 children and teens had closer contact with others: S. Cauchemez et al., "A Bayesian MCMC Approach to Study Transmission of Influenza: Application to Household Longitudinal Data," *Statistics in Medicine* 23, no. 22 (2004): 3469–3487.

Page 27 Transmission among children outside of school: David Zweig, "Hybrid Schooling May Be the Most Dangerous Option of All," *Wired*, August 6, 2020, https://www.wired.com/story/hybrid-schooling-is-the-most-dangerous-option-of-all/.

Page 28 one-third of US adults said they were deemed essential workers: Audrey Kearney and Cailey Muñana, "Taking Stock of Essential Workers," Henry J. Kaiser Family Foundation, May 1, 2020, https://www.kff.org/policy-watch/taking-stock-of-essential-workers/.

Page 28 Dr. Shira Doron: Westyn Branch-Elliman, Lloyd Fisher, and Shira Doron, "The Next 'Pandemic Playbook' Needs to Prioritize the Needs of Children—and a Clear Roadmap for Opening Schools," *Antimicrobial Stewardship & Healthcare Epidemiology* 3, no. 1 (2023): e82.

Page 29 termed "the honeymoon period" by researchers: Rafi Ahmed et al., "Protective Immunity and Susceptibility to Infectious Diseases: Lessons from the 1918 Influenza Pandemic," *Nature Immunology* 8 (2007): 1188–1193.

Page 29 2017 playbook: "Community Mitigation Guidelines to Prevent Pandemic Influenza—United States, 2017 Technical Report 1: Chapters 1–4," Centers for Disease Control and Prevention, *Morbidity and Mortality Weekly Report*, April 21, 2017.

Page 30 Case and hospitalization rates decline dramatically within six weeks of onset: Graphs from *New York Times*, https://www.nytimes.com/interactive/2021/us/new-york-covid-cases.html. The peak of cases in New York in spring 2020 was April 10. The peak of COVID hospitalizations was April 16.

Page 30 At the fastest, it was thought it might take around a year: Maegan Vazquez, "Task Force Health Expert Contradicts Trump about Coronavirus Vaccine Timing," CNN, March 3, 2020, https://www.cnn.com/2020/03/02/politics/donald-trump-coronavirus-vaccine-push-back/index.html.

Page 30 Incredibly, a nearly completely overlooked fact: Simonsen et al., "Pandemic versus Epidemic Influenza Mortality: A Pattern of Changing Age Distribution," *Journal of Infectious Diseases*, July 1998:178(1):53–60. And https://www.cdc.gov/mmwr/volumes/66/rr/rr6601a1.htm#T9_down–cited in the 2017 CDC report.

Page 31 In many seasons the flu posed a greater risk to children than COVID: See the note on the flu in the Introduction notes.

Page 31 identifying strategies for particular groups: https://www.cdc.gov/mmwr/volumes/66/rr/rr6601a1.htm#T2_down, table 2.

Page 31 Jennifer Nuzzo highlighted: Jennifer Nuzzo, "We Don't Need to Close Schools to Fight the Coronavirus," *New York Times*, March 10, 2020, https://www.nytimes.com/2020/03/10/opinion/coronavirus-school-closing.html.

CHAPTER 3

Page 33 Red Dawn: Eric Lipton, "The 'Red Dawn' Emails: 8 Key Exchanges on the Faltering Response to the Coronavirus," Covid-19 Guidance, *New York Times*, April 11, 2020, https://www.nytimes.com/2020/04/11/us/politics/coronavirus-red-dawn-emails-trump.html. https://int.nyt.com/data/documenthelper/6879-2020-covid-19-red-dawn-rising/66f590d5cd41e11bea0f/optimized/full.pdf; DocumentCloud, "Kings County, WA Emails—Covid Response, Select Pages," https://www.documentcloud.org/documents/6820644-AO-KCW-Covid-Emails1-3-27.html.

Page 34 kids at "the mall": This last point was a reference to a concern expressed by Robert Glass in a paper he published after his seminal paper on NPIs. Glass had written that his model showed if schools were closed and kids instead hung out at the mall that "closing schools actually made things worse." Robert J. Glass, "Pandemic Influenza and Complex Adaptive System of Systems (CASoS) Engineering," System Dynamics Society, 2009, https://proceedings.systemdynamics.org/2009/proceed/papers/P1400.pdf. Robert J. Glass et al., "Targeted Social Distancing Design for Pandemic Influenza," *Emerging Infectious Diseases* 12, no. 11 (2006): 1671–1681, https://www.ncbi.nlm.nih.gov/labs/pmc/articles/PMC3372334/.

Page 35 Governor Mike DeWine: Office of the Governor of the State of Ohio, "Governor DeWine Announces School Closures," news release, March 12, 2020, https://governor.ohio.gov/media/news-and-media/announces-school-closures. "DeWine closing bars and restaurants": Office of the Governor of the State of Ohio, "Governor DeWine Orders Ohio Bars & Restaurants to Close," news release, March 15, 2020, https://governor.ohio.gov/media/news-and-media/dewine-orders-ohio-bars-restaurants-to-close.

Page 35 sixteen states announced school closures: Andrew Ujifusa, "States Ordering Schools to Close in Response to Coronavirus," *Education Week*, March 12, 2020, https://www.edweek.org/education/states-ordering-schools-to-close-in-response-to-coronavirus/2020/03. Laura Meckler, "Seven States, D.C. Order All Schools Closed in Effort to Prevent Spread of Covid-19," *Washington Post*, March 13, 2020, https://www.washingtonpost.com/local/education/ohio-maryland-order-all-schools-closed-in-effort-to-prevent-spread-of-covid-19/2020/03/12/e4078b3a-6499-11ea-845d-e35b0234b136_story.html.

Page 35 Governor Andrew Cuomo of New York Office of the Governor of New York State, "Governor Cuomo Signs Executive Order Closing Schools Statewide for Two Weeks," news release, March 16, 2020, https://www.governor.ny.gov/news/governor-cuomo-signs-executive-order-closing-schools-statewide-two-weeks.

Page 35 exempting schools from the state's requirement of 180 days: Jon Campbell, "Cuomo Closes New York Schools Until April 15 as Coronavirus Spread Continues," *Democrat & Chronicle* (Albany), March 27, 2020, https://www.democratandchronicle.com/story/news/politics/albany/2020/03/27/new-york-closes-schools-through-least-april-14-coronavirus-spreads/2925758001/. Executive order 202.4, https://www.governor.ny.gov/sites/default/files/atoms/files/EO%20202.4.pdf. On canceling all gatherings, etc., see Office of the Governor of New York State, "Governor Cuomo Signs the 'New York State on PAUSE' Executive Order," news release, March 20, 2020, https://www.governor.ny.gov/news/governor-cuomo-signs-new-york-state-pause-executive-order.

CHAPTER 4

Page 37 Many thousands of flights were canceled: David Schaper, "Coronavirus Fears Lead to Canceled Flights and Concerns within the Travel Industry," NPR, March 4, 2020, https://www.npr.org/2020/03/04/812026357/coronavirus-fears-lead

-to-canceled-flights-and-concerns-within-the-travel-indust. Rani Molla, "Chart: How Coronavirus Is Devastating the Restaurant Business," *Vox*, March 16, 2020, https://www.vox.com/recode/2020/3/16/21181556/coronavirus-chart-restaurant-business-local. "Coronavirus: Airlines Cancel Thousands of Flights," BBC, March 10, 2020, https://www.bbc.com/news/business-51818492. Dawn Gilbertson and Chris Woodyard, "Delta Slashes Flight Capacity by 40%, Parks 300 Planes in Deepest Cuts in Company History," *USA Today*, March 10, 2020, https://www.usatoday.com/story/travel/airline-news/2020/03/10/coronavirus-american-airlines-flight-cuts-international-domestic-summer-travel/5005702002/.

Page 37 The models were in the ether: Denise Chow, "What We Know about the Coronavirus Model the White House Unveiled," NBC News, March 31, 2020, https://www.nbcnews.com/science/science-news/what-we-know-about-coronavirus-model-white-house-unveiled-n1173601. Nurith Aizenman, "5 Key Facts Not Explained In White House COVID-19 Projections," NPR, April 1, 2020, https://www.npr.org/sections/health-shots/2020/04/01/824744490/5-key-facts-the-white-house-isnt-saying-about-their-covid-19-projections.

Page 37 Imperial College pandemic models: Imperial College COVID-19 Response Team, "Report 9: Impact of Non-Pharmaceutical Interventions (NPIs) to Reduce COVID-19 Mortality and Healthcare Demand," March 16, 2020, https://www.imperial.ac.uk/media/imperial-college/medicine/mrc-gida/2020-03-16-COVID19-Report-9.pdf.

Page 38 the *Times* ran an entire feature: Sheri Fink, "White House Takes New Line after Dire Report on Death Toll," *New York Times*, March 16, 2020.

Page 38 Robert Glass: Robert J. Glass et al., "Targeted Social Distancing Design for Pandemic Influenza," *Emerging Infectious Diseases* 12, no. 11 (2006): 1671–1681, https://wwwnc.cdc.gov/eid/article/12/11/06-0255_article.

Page 38 "15 days" press conference: https://trumpwhitehouse.archives.gov/briefings-statements/remarks-president-trump-vice-president-pence-members-coronavirus-task-force-press-briefing-3/.

Page 39 Report 9, and how Ferguson and his team modeled the effect of school closures: Neil M. Ferguson et al., "Report 9: Impact of Non-Pharmaceutical Interventions (NPIs) to Reduce COVID-19 Mortality and Healthcare Demand," March 16, 2020, https://www.imperial.ac.uk/media/imperial-college/medicine/sph/ide/gida-fellowships/Imperial-College-COVID19-NPI-modelling-16-03-2020.pdf.

Page 39 Imperial College's modeled predictions: William Booth, "A Chilling Scientific Paper Helped Upend U.S. and U.K. Coronavirus Strategies," *Washington Post*, March 17, 2020, Europe, https://www.washingtonpost.com/world/europe/a-chilling-scientific-paper-helped-upend-us-and-uk-coronavirus-strategies/2020/03/17/aaa84116-6851-11ea-b199-3a9799c54512_story.html. Sheri Fink, "White House Takes New Line after Dire Report on Death Toll," *New York Times*, March 16, 2020.

Page 39 a 2005 modeling paper: Neil M. Ferguson et al., "Strategies for Containing an Emerging Influenza Pandemic in Southeast Asia," *Nature* 437 (2005): 209–214.

Page 39 *PLOS Medicine* paper: Joel Mossong et al., "Social Contacts and Mixing Patterns Relevant to the Spread of Infectious Diseases," *PLOS Medicine* 5, no. 3 (2008): e74.

The *PLOS Medicine* modeling paper elicits a long list of questions about its methodology, including as it relates to the claim about contact rates between children. To take but one of many examples of text that raises eyebrows, the paper states, "Children and adolescents were deliberately oversampled, because of their important role in the spread of infectious agents." (Remember, at the beginning of the pandemic children's role in transmission, unlike as it is with influenza, was found to be significantly weaker than that of adults. So this is a concerning data point as one of the building blocks for an assumption about the effect of school closures.)

Page 40 2008 paper coauthored by Ferguson: Simon Cauchemez et al., "Estimating the Impact of School Closure on Influenza Transmission from Sentinel Data," *Nature* 452 (2008): 750–754.

Page 41 Nancy Messonnier: Centers for Disease Control and Prevention, "Transcript for the CDC Telebriefing Update on COVID-19," February 26, 2020, https://stacks .cdc.gov/view/cdc/85310.

Page 42 disputed by Italian authorities: Craxi et al., "Rationing in a Pandemic: Lessons from Italy," *Asian Bioethics Review*, September 2020; 12(3): 325–330. "'Not a Wave, a Tsunami.' Italy Hospitals at Virus Limit," PBS, March 13, 2020, https://www .pbs.org/newshour/health/not-a-wave-a-tsunami-italy-hospitals-at-virus-limit.

Page 42 Dr. Stefan Baral: Stefan Baral et al., "The Public Health Response to COVID-19: Balancing Precaution and Unintended Consequences," *Annals of Epidemiology* 46 (2020): 12–13. They don't mention China by name, but Baral emailed me saying it was clear that's who they were referring to.

Page 42 "I can't imagine shutting down New York or Los Angeles": James Griffiths et al., CNN, January 24, 2020, "Coronavirus News," https://www.cnn.com/asia/live -news/coronavirus-outbreak-hnk-intl-01-24-20/index.html.

Page 43 Clifford Lane: Anthony Fauci deposition 11/23/2022, Missouri v. Biden, https://www.documentcloud.org/documents/23347988-fauci-deposition.

Page 43 Nicholas Thomas: "Covid Lockdowns Are Spreading a Year after China Shocked World," *Bloomberg*, January 17, 2021, https://www.bloomberg.com/news /articles/2021-01-17/from-the-bubonic-plague-to-2021-why-lockdowns-look-set-to -stay.

Page 43 Shigeru Omi: "China's Unproven Antiviral Solution: Quarantine of 40 Million," Lisa Du, *Bloomberg*, January 24, 2020, https://www.bloomberg.com/news/arti cles/2020-01-24/china-s-unproven-antiviral-solution-quarantine-of-40-million.

Page 44 Randi Weingarten: Dana Goldstein, "The Union Leader Who Says She Can Get Teachers Back in Schools," *New York Times*, February 8, 2021.

Page 45 Opinion pieces with titles like . . . : Michelle Goldberg, "Remote School Is a Nightmare. Few in Power Care," *New York Times*, Opinion, June 29, 2020.

Page 45 US Chamber of Commerce: Stephanie Ferguson and Isabella Lucy, "Data Deep Dive: A Decline of Women in the Workforce," US Chamber of Commerce,

April 27, 2022, https://www.uschamber.com/workforce/data-deep-dive-a-decline-of
-women-in-the-workforce.

Page 45 Kaitlyn Fontano: "Millions of Women Left Work during the Pandemic.
Where Are They Now?" *Wall Street Journal*, March 30, 2023, https://www.wsj.com
/podcasts/the-journal/millions-of-women-left-work-during-the-pandemic-where
-are-they-now/8e77b56c-65c2-4772-a0c0-f7fbdd42bdab.

Page 45 children without a home internet connection: Petula Dvorak, "When 'Back
to School' Means a Parking Lot and the Hunt for a Wi-Fi Signal," *Washington Post*,
Local, August 27, 2020, https://www.washingtonpost.com/local/when-back-to-school
-means-a-parking-lot-and-the-hunt-for-a-wifi-signal/2020/08/27/0f785d5a-e873
-11ea-970a-64c73a1c2392_story.html. "Kids using Taco Bell lot": Luis Alejo (@Super-
visorAlejo), "2 of our children trying to get WiFi for their classes outside a Taco Bell
in East Salinas," Twitter, August 26, 2020, https://twitter.com/SupervisorAlejo/status
/1298509984645279744. Bracey Harris, "Homework In A McDonald's Parking Lot,"
Huffington Post, June 27, 2020, https://www.huffpost.com/entry/mississippi-delta
-coronavirus_n_5ef5120cc5b612083c4ae75b.

Page 46 Exhibit A is a 2006 paper: "Disease Mitigation Measures in the Control
of Pandemic Influenza," Jennifer Nuzzo et al., *Biosecurity and Bioterrorism* 4, no. 4
(2006): 366–375.

Page 47 A 2011 paper by researchers from Georgetown: Tamar Klaiman et al., "Vari-
ability in School Closure Decisions in Response to 2009 H1N1: A Qualitative Systems
Improvement Analysis," *BMC Public Health* 11, article 73 (2011).

Page 48 "we're building the plane as we fly it": New Hampshire Department of Education Commissioner Frank Edelblut in Mary McIntyre, "As N.H. Schools Close for
the Year, Edelblut Outlines Remote Learning Efforts and Impacts," New Hampshire
Public Radio, April 17, 2020, https://www.nhpr.org/education/2020-04-17/as-n-h
-schools-close-for-the-year-edelblut-outlines-remote-learning-efforts-and-impacts.
New Jersey Governor Phil Murphy in "COVID-19 Leads to Burst of Info, but Some
Data Blocked in New Jersey," AP/CBS News Philadelphia, March 14, 2021, https://
www.cbsnews.com/philadelphia/news/covid-19-leads-to-burst-of-info-but-some
-data-blocked-in-new-jersey/.

CHAPTER 5

Page 49 Mike DeWine: DeWine St. Louis vs Philadelphia: NBC News, interview with
Ohio Governor Mike DeWine on *Meet the Press*, March 15, 2020, YouTube video,
47:31, https://www.youtube.com/watch?v=Mdlv0-AWTKQ. Transcript: https://www
.nbcnews.com/meet-the-press/meet-press-march-15-2020-n1159336.

Page 49 Philadelphia's folly versus St. Louis's wisdom: Sheri Fink, "Worst-Case Estimates for U.S. Coronavirus Deaths," *New York Times*, COVID-19 Guidance, March
13, 2020. Leah Asmelash, "Philadelphia Didn't Cancel a Parade during a 1918 Pandemic. The Results Were Devastating," CNN, March 15, 2020, https://www.cnn.com
/2020/03/15/us/philadelphia-1918-spanish-flu-trnd/index.html. Meagan Flynn, "What
Happens If Parades Aren't Canceled during Pandemics," *Washington Post*, March 12,

2020, Morning Mix, https://www.washingtonpost.com/nation/2020/03/12/pandemic -parade-flu-coronavirus/. Maria Godoy, "Flattening A Pandemic's Curve: Why Staying Home Now Can Save Lives," NPR, March 13, 2020, https://www.npr.org/sections /health-shots/2020/03/13/815502262/flattening-a-pandemics-curve-why-staying -home-now-can-save-lives.

Page 50 voltage drop: David A. Chambers et al., "The Dynamic Sustainability Framework: Addressing the Paradox of Sustainment amid Ongoing Change," *Implementation Science* 8, no. 117 (2013). Amy M. Kilbourne et al., "Implementing Evidence-Based Interventions in Health Care: Application of the Replicating Effective Programs Framework," *Implementation Science* 2, no. 42 (2007).

Page 50 as fidelity to interventions wanes: Christopher P. Reinders Folmer et al., "Social Distancing in America: Understanding Long-Term Adherence to COVID-19 Mitigation Recommendations," *PLOS ONE* 16, no. 9 (2021): e0257945.

Page 50 Robert Barro: Robert J. Barro, "Non-Pharmaceutical Interventions and Mortality in U.S. Cities during the Great Influenza Pandemic, 1918–1919," National Bureau of Economic Research Working Paper Series, April 2020 (revised August 2020), https://www.nber.org/system/files/working_papers/w27049/w27049.pdf.

Page 51 A 2009 World Health Organization report: Global Influenza Programme, World Health Organization, *Reducing Transmission of Pandemic (H1N1) 2009 in School Settings*, September 1, 2009, https://www.who.int/publications/i/item/reducing-trans mission-of-pandemic-(h1n1)-2009-in-school-settings.

Page 51 cases averted by school closures "remains uncertain": Gerardo Chowell et al., "Measuring the Benefits of School Closure Interventions to Mitigate Influenza," *Expert Review of Respiratory Medicine* 5, no. 5 (2011): 597–599.

Page 51 total number of people infected "may not be appreciably affected": Harpa Isfeld-Kiely and Seyed Moghadas, "Effectiveness of School Closure for the Control of Influenza: A Review of Recent Evidence," National Collaborating Centre for Infectious Diseases (Canada), March 2014, https://nccid.ca/publications/effectiveness-of -school-closure-for-the-control-of-influenza/.

Page 53 authors of a paper comparing the two pandemics: Harald Brüssow and Lutz Brüssow, "Clinical Evidence that the Pandemic from 1889 to 1891 Commonly Called the Russian Flu Might Have Been an Earlier Coronavirus Pandemic," *Microbial Biotechnology* 14, no. 5 (2021): 1860–1870.

Page 53 "molecular clock analysis": Leen Vijgen et al., "Complete Genomic Sequence of Human Coronavirus OC43: Molecular Clock Analysis Suggests a Relatively Recent Zoonotic Coronavirus Transmission Event," *Journal of Virology* 79, no. 3 (2005): 1595–1604.

Page 53 long-term care facility patients: David M. Patrick et al., "An Outbreak of Human Coronavirus OC43 Infection and Serological Cross-Reactivity with SARS Coronavirus," *Canadian Journal of Infectious Diseases & Medical Microbiology* 17, no. 6 (2006): 330–336; Ann R. Falsey et al., "Rhinovirus and Coronavirus Infection-Associated Hospitalizations among Older Adults," *Journal of Infectious Diseases* 185, no. 9 (2002): 1338–1341. Julie Hand et al., "Severe Respiratory Illness Outbreak

Associated with Human Coronavirus NL63 in a Long-Term Care Facility," *Emerging Infectious Diseases* 24, no. 10 (2018): 1964–1966; Infectious Disease Ethics (@ID_ethics), "Covid19 vs. 'common cold coronaviruses' Case Fatality Risks in Nursing Homes (Graph Below) Data:" Twitter, April 26, 2021, 12:52 a.m., https://twitter.com /ID_ethics/status/1386543801045381123.

Page 53 "The disease seems to be substantially less severe in children . . .": Nicola Principi et al., "Effects of Coronavirus Infections in Children," *Emerging Infectious Diseases* 16, no. 2 (2010): 183–188; Susanna Esposito et al., "Impact of Human Coronavirus Infections in Otherwise Healthy Children Who Attended an Emergency Department," *Journal of Medical Virology* 78 (2006): 1609–1615; M. Li and P. C. Ng, "Severe Acute Respiratory Syndrome (SARS) in Neonates and Children," *Archives of Disease in Childhood—Fetal and Neonatal Edition* 90 (2005): F461–F465; Lauren J. Stockman et al., "Severe Acute Respiratory Syndrome in Children," *Pediatric Infectious Disease Journal* 26, no. 1 (2007): 68–74, https://www.medscape.com/viewarticle /551274; US Department of Health and Human Services, Centers for Disease Control and Prevention, "In the Absence of SARS-CoV Transmission Worldwide: Guidance for Surveillance, Clinical and Laboratory Evaluation, and Reporting," Version 2, January 21, 2004, https://www.cdc.gov/sars/surveillance/absence.html.

Page 54 review published by the Italian Society of Medicine and Natural Sciences: Rosanna Iannarella et al., "Coronavirus Infections in Children: From SARS and MERS to COVID-19, a Narrative Review of Epidemiological and Clinical Features," *Acta Bio-Medica: Atenei Parmensis* 91, no. 3 (2020): e2020032.

Page 55 evidence that 1889 was a coronavirus: George S. Heriot and Euzebiusz Jamrozik, "Imagination and Remembrance: What Role Should Historical Epidemiology Play in a World Bewitched by Mathematical Modelling of COVID-19 and Other Epidemics?," *History and Philosophy of the Life Sciences* 43, article 81 (2021).

Page 55 One more devastating note: Estee Y. Cramer et al., "Evaluation of Individual and Ensemble Probabilistic Forecasts of COVID-19 Mortality in the United States," *PNAS* 119, no. 15 (2022): e2113561119.

Page 56 Oliver Wyman: "COVID-19 Pandemic Navigator," Oliver Wyman, https:// www.oliverwyman.com/our-expertise/insights/2020/apr/covid-19-pandemic-navi gator.html.

Page 56 Dean Karlen: The COVID-19 Scenario Modeling Hub, "The COVID-19 Scenario Modeling Hub Coordination Team," https://covid19scenariomodelinghub.org /team.html.

Page 57 IHME had received more than 400 million dollars: Sandi Doughton, "Historic Gift: Gates Foundation Gives $279 Million to University of Washington," *Seattle Times*, January 25, 2017, https://www.seattletimes.com/seattle-news/science /historic-gift-gates-foundation-gives-279-million-to-university-of-washington/; "About Us," Institute for Health Metrics and Evaluation, https://www.healthdata .org/about.

Page 57 Deborah Birx mentioned IHME's models: Institute for Health Metrics and Evaluation (IHME), "The Chris Murray Model," Facebook, April 2, 2020, video,

00:22, https://www.facebook.com/watch/?v=256957412004075; Institute for Health Metrics and Evaluation (IHME), "IHME Model Used By White House Coronavirus Taskforce," March 31, 2020, YouTube video, 00:40, https://www.youtube.com/watch?v=dC0cOKfe_Fs.

Page 57 CNN to *Politico* to PBS to the *Times*: Arman Azad, "Model Cited by White House says 82,000 People Could Die from Coronavirus by August, Even with Social Distancing," CNN, March 31, 2020, https://www.cnn.com/2020/03/30/health/coronavirus-us-ihme-model-us/index.html; Adam Cancryn, "How Overly Optimistic Modeling Distorted Trump Coronavirus Response," *Politico*, April 24, 2020, https://www.politico.com/news/2020/04/24/trump-coronavirus-model-207582; Ricardo Alonso-Zaldivar and Lauran Neergaard, "White House Turns to Statistical Models for Virus Forecast," *PBS NewsHour*, March 31, 2020, https://www.pbs.org/newshour/health/white-house-turns-to-statistical-models-for-virus-forecast; Quoctrung Bui, Josh Katz, Alicia Parlapiano, and Margot Sanger-Katz, "What 5 Coronavirus Models Say the Next Month Will Look Like," *New York Times*, April 22, 2020, https://www.nytimes.com/interactive/2020/04/22/upshot/coronavirus-models.html.

Page 57 Birx talked confidently and reassuringly: Kelsey Piper, "This Coronavirus Model Keeps Being Wrong. Why Are We Still Listening to It?," *Vox*, May 2, 2020, https://www.vox.com/future-perfect/2020/5/2/21241261/coronavirus-modeling-us-deaths-ihme-pandemic.

CHAPTER 6

Page 61 On March 31, Deborah Birx gave a joint press conference: White House Coronavirus Task Force, "Donald Trump Coronavirus Task Force Briefing Transcript March 31: 'Painful' Weeks Ahead," March 31, 2020, accessed via Rev.com, https://www.rev.com/blog/transcripts/donald-trump-coronavirus-task-force-briefing-transcript-march-31-painful-weeks-ahead.

Page 61 wearing an elegant silk scarf: US Department of State, "Members of the Coronavirus Task Force Hold a Press Briefing," YouTube (video), March 31, 2020, https://www.youtube.com/watch?v=e9v8ZZd1P0M; Lilah Ramzi, "Dr. Deborah Birx's Many Scarves Now Have Their Own Instagram Account," *Vogue*, April 9, 2020, https://www.vogue.com/article/dr-deborah-birx-scarves-instagram; Robin Givhan, "Of Course You've Noticed Deborah Birx's Style. That's Why It's So Reassuring," *Washington Post*, March 25, 2020, https://www.washingtonpost.com/lifestyle/2020/03/25/course-youve-noticed-deborah-birxs-style-thats-why-its-so-reassuring/.

Page 61 "15 days to slow the spread": Dan Mangan, "Trump Issues 'Coronavirus Guidelines' for Next 15 Days to Slow Pandemic," CNBC, March 16, 2020, https://www.cnbc.com/2020/03/16/trumps-coronavirus-guidelines-for-next-15-days-to-slow-pandemic.html; US Department of Justice, "15 Days to Slow the Spread," White House Coronavirus Task Force Official Guidelines, https://www.justice.gov/doj/page/file/1258511/download.

Page 62 giant foam sculpture dubbed "the mountain'": Jon Campbell, "Cuomo Unveils a Giant Foam Mountain Depicting COVID-19 Climb in NY. Social Media

Took Over," *Democrat & Chronicle*, June 29, 2020, https://www.democratandchroni
cle.com/story/news/politics/albany/2020/06/29/andrew-cuomo-unveils-foam
-mountain-visualize-nys-coivd-19-fight/3278852001/. March 1, first case, peaked 42
days later.

Page 63 By early May schools in the Netherlands: "Netherlands Wants to Fully Open
Primary Schools before the Summer," *Brussels Times* (Belgium), April 23, 2020,
https://www.brusselstimes.com/107722/netherlands-wants-to-fully-open-primary
-schools-before-the-summer.

Page 63 Germany saw certain areas open secondary schools: IAB-Forum, May 15,
2020, https://www.iab-forum.de/en/school-closings-during-the-covid-19-pandemic
-findings-from-german-high-school-students/.

Page 63 kids were permitted to hug their grandparents: Alix Culbertson, "Coronavirus: Swiss Children under 10 Allowed to Hug Grandparents as They 'Do Not Transmit COVID-19,'" *Sky News*, April 29, 2020, https://news.sky.com/story/coronavirus
-swiss-children-under-10-allowed-to-hug-grandparents-as-they-do-not-transmit
-covid-19-11980568.

Page 63 Montana and Wyoming : Zoe Kirsch, "As Covid-189 Keeps Most Schools
Shuttered the Rest of the Year, A Growing Number in Wyoming and Montana Partially Reopen," *The 74 Million*, May 6, 2020; https://www.the74million.org/article
/as-covid-keeps-most-schools-shuttered-for-the-rest-of-the-year-a-growing-number
-in-wyoming-and-montana-partially-reopen/.

Page 64 In early May, in Italy: Much of the reporting in this section is pulled from
my *Wired* article of May 11, 2020. David Zweig, "The Case for Reopening Schools,"
Wired, May 11, 2020, https://www.wired.com/story/the-case-for-reopening-schools/.

Page 64 Data from New York City at the same time showed seven deaths: New
York City Department of Health and Mental Hygiene, "Coronavirus Disease 2019
(COVID-19) Daily Data Summary," May 8, 2020, 6:00 p.m., https://www1.nyc.gov
/assets/doh/downloads/pdf/imm/covid-19-daily-data-summary-deaths-05092020-1
.pdf.

Page 64 underlying medical conditions: Even in January 2022, at a CDC advisory
committee meeting, when pediatric hospitalizations were presented, it was not
mentioned that roughly two-thirds of kids hospitalized with Covid had underlying
conditions.

Page 64 a remarkable document: Shikha Garg et al., "Hospitalization Rates and
Characteristics of Patients Hospitalized with Laboratory-Confirmed Coronavirus
Disease 2019—COVID-NET, 14 States, March 1–30, 2020," *Morbidity and Mortality
Weekly Report* 69 (April 17, 2020): 458–464.

Page 64 a week or so lag time from infection to hospitalization: Thomas Ward and
Alexander Johnsen, "Understanding an Evolving Pandemic: An Analysis of the
Clinical Time Delay Distributions of COVID-19 in the United Kingdom," *PLOS ONE*
16, no. 10 (2021): e0257978. ("Results for people under the age of 20 were discarded
because there were too few patients for a meaningful measurement of their epidemiological characteristics." But 20 to 29 was roughly 6.5–8.5 days.)

Page 65 Iceland: Daniel F. Gudbjartsson et al., "Spread of SARS-CoV-2 in the Icelandic Population," *New England Journal of Medicine* 82 (2020): 2302–2315.

Page 65 France: Kostas Danis et al., "Cluster of Coronavirus Disease 2019 (COVID-19) in the French Alps, February 2020," *Clinical Infectious Diseases* 71, no. 15 (August 2020): 825–832.

Page 65 Netherlands: RIVM (Dutch National Institute for Public Health and the Environment), "COVID-19," https://www.rivm.nl/en/coronavirus-covid-19/children-and-covid-19.

Page 65 Canada: Sarah Silverberg, MD, and Laura Sauvé, MD, MPH, FRCPC, "Caring for Children with COVID-19," British Columbia Centre for Disease Control, April 3, 2020, http://www.bccdc.ca/Health-Info-Site/Documents/Caring-for-children.pdf.

Page 65 Australia: National Centre for Immunisation Research and Surveillance (Australia), *COVID-19 in Schools—The Experience in NSW*, April 26, 2020, https://ncirs.org.au/sites/default/files/2020-04/NCIRS%20NSW%20Schools%20COVID_Summary_FINAL%20public_26%20April%202020.pdf.

Page 65 A joint press release in late April : David Zweig, "The Case for Reopening Schools," *Wired*, May 11, 2020, https://www.wired.com/story/the-case-for-reopening-schools/.

Page 66 An official from Denmark's disease control agency: Bojan Pancevski and Naja Dandanell, "Is It Safe to Reopen Schools? These Countries Say Yes," *Wall Street Journal*, World, May 31, 2020, https://www.wsj.com/articles/is-it-safe-to-reopen-schools-these-countries-say-yes-11590928949.

Page 66 education ministers: Council of the European Union, "Education, Youth, Culture and Sports Council" (video), May 17, 2020, https://video.consilium.europa.eu/event/en/24001?start_time=0.

Page 68 class size in Swedish lower schools: https://www.oecd-ilibrary.org/sites/b35a14e5-en/1/3/5/2/index.html?itemId=/content/publication/b35a14e5-en&_csp_=9689b83a12cab1f95b32a46f4225d1a5&itemIGO=oecd&itemContentType=book#tablegrp-d1e26913.

Page 68 report of just one "outbreak" at a school: Gretchen Vogel, "How Sweden Wasted a 'Rare Opportunity' to Study Coronavirus in Schools," *Science*, May 22, 2020, https://www.science.org/content/article/how-sweden-wasted-rare-opportunity-study-coronavirus-schools.

Page 68 out of 105,000 teachers employed by lower schools: Stefan Baral et al., "Leveraging Epidemiological Principles to Evaluate Sweden's COVID-19 Response," *Annals of Epidemiology* 54 (2021): 21–26; "Covid-19 in Schoolchildren: A Comparison between Finland and Sweden," Public Health Agency of Sweden, https://www.folkhalsomyndigheten.se/contentassets/c1b78bffbfde4a7899eb0d8ffdb57b09/covid-19-school-aged-children.pdf.

Page 68 This was not a small sample: A study, published in February 2021, found that teachers in upper secondary schools in Sweden, which were remote, had 3.25 cases per thousand, versus 5.91 cases per thousand for teachers in lower schools, which were in person. There are a couple things to note here. First, the preliminary results of the analysis came out in fall of 2020, so these data had no way of influencing policy in the spring. Second, although teachers in person had a higher rate of infection than those who were remote, one then has to ask: is 3.25 cases out of one thousand versus 5.91 cases out of one thousand worth keeping schools closed? "The Effects of School Closures on SARS-CoV-2 among Parents and Teachers," *PNAS*, February 11, 2021, 118 (9) e2020834118.

Page 69 Iceland: Thirty-two percent of students did not miss any school days in 2019/2020. https://www.statice.is/publications/news-archive/education/school-opera tion-in-compulsory-schools-2021-2023/. Also Carline Hall et al., "Schooling in the Nordic countries during the COVID-19 Pandemic," Institute for Evaluation of Labour Market and Education Policy.

DEEP DIVE: PEANUTS, LEMONS, AND EVIDENCE-BASED MEDICINE

Page 71 Official guidance from the American Academy of Pediatrics and the NIH: Committee on Nutrition, "Hypoallergenic Infant Formulas," *Pediatrics* 106, no. 2 (2000): 346–349.

Page 71 Israeli infants had been gobbling a snack: Viva Sarah Press, "Israel's Top Snack Bamba Prevents Peanut Allergy," ISRAEL21C (website), February 25, 2015, https://www.israel21c.org/israels-top-snack-bamba-prevents-allergy/.

Page 72 Benefits of early exposure: Megan Scudellari, "Cleaning up the Hygiene Hypothesis," *PNAS* 114, no. 7 (2017): 1433–1436; David P. Strachan, "Hay Fever, Hygiene, and Household Size," *BMJ* 299 (1989): 1259–1260, https://www.ncbi.nlm .nih.gov/pmc/articles/PMC1838109/pdf/bmj00259-0027.pdf.

Page 72 consumption of fish during infancy: I. Kull et al., "Fish Consumption during the First Year of Life and Development of Allergic Diseases during Childhood," *Allergy* 61, no. 8 (2006): 1009–1015; Bernt Alm et al., "Early Introduction of Fish Decreases the Risk of Eczema in Infants," *Archives of Disease in Childhood* 94, no. 1 (2008): 11–15.

Page 72 It took *seventeen years*: Scott H. Sicherer, "New Guidelines Detail Use of 'Infant-Safe' Peanut to Prevent Allergy," *AAP News*, January 5, 2017, https://publica tions.aap.org/aapnews/news/12250.

Page 72 actively harmed untold numbers of children: Edmond S. Chan et al., "Early Introduction of Foods to Prevent Food Allergy," *Allergy, Asthma, and Clinical Immunology: Official Journal of the Canadian Society of Allergy and Clinical Immunology* 14, no. 2 (2018): 94–101.

Page 73 James Lind: Iain Milne, "Who Was James Lind, and What Exactly Did He Achieve?" James Lind Library (website), 2012, https://www.jameslindlibrary.org /articles/who-was-james-lind-and-what-exactly-did-he-achieve/; Marcus White, "James Lind: The Man Who Helped to Cure Scurvy with Lemons," BBC News, October 4, 2016, https://www.bbc.com/news/uk-england-37320399; Ulrich Tröhler, "James Lind and Scurvy: 1747 to 1795," James Lind Library, 2003, https://www.jameslindli brary.org/articles/james-lind-and-scurvy-1747-to-1795/.

Page 74 expert opinion typically is near or at the very bottom: "Hierarchy of Evidence," Physiopedia (website), https://www.physio-pedia.com/Hierarchy_of_evidence.

Page 74 Spock advised parents: Jeremy Howick, *The Philosophy of Evidence-Based Medicine* (London: BMJ Books, 2011). Spock's advice for front sleeping began with the 1956 edition of his book.

Page 74 in countries where babies traditionally sleep on their backs: "Cot Death in Hong Kong" D. P. Davies, "Cot Death in Hong Kong: A Rare Problem?," *Lancet* 2, 8468 (1985): 1346–1349; "Sudden Infant Death Syndrome in Hong Kong": N. N. Lee et al., "Sudden Infant Death Syndrome in Hong Kong: Confirmation of Low Incidence," *BMJ* 298, no. 6675 (1989): 721.

Page 75 "School closures, sports closures, masking . . ." Tracy Beth Høeg quotation is from communication with Høeg, and is largely echoed here: Høeg, "Sacrificing Children's Health in the Name of Health," *Sensible Medicine* (Substack newsletter), August 12, 2022, https://www.sensible-med.com/p/sacrificing-childrens-health-in-the.

Page 76 financial conflicts of interest: Jeremy Howick, "Exploring the Asymmetrical Relationship between the Power of Finance Bias and Evidence," *Perspectives in Biology and Medicine* 62, no. 1 (Winter 2019): 159–187, https://philarchive.org/archive/HOWETA-4.

Page 76 "Power is knowledge": Bent Flyvbjerg, *Rationality and Power: Democracy in Practice* (Chicago: University of Chicago Press, 1998). Note: the actual translation of Bacon's words is "Knowledge itself is power."

Page 76 John Locke: http://www.rbjones.com/rbjpub/philos/classics/locke/ctb0epis.htm, part of *An Essay Concerning Human Understanding*. For those interested in philosophy, Locke's essay is powerful because, in part, it shows how this great thinker of the past is so relevant today. Back in the 1600s he was criticizing what we now would essentially call academese, scholars hiding behind big words and opaque language. http://www.rbjones.com/rbjpub/philos/classics/locke/ctb1c02.htm#24.

Page 77 evidence-based medicine (EBM): Neal Kohatsu et al., "Evidence-Based Public Health: An Evolving Concept," *American Journal of Preventive Medicine* 27, no. 5 (2004): 417–421.

CHAPTER 7

Page 79 to keep "children and students and educators safe": New York Governor Andrew M. Cuomo, "ASL: 05/01—NYS Schools and College Facilities Will Remain Closed for the Rest of the Academic Year," YouTube (video), May 1, 2020, https://www.youtube.com/watch?v=uoocI1ECZn8; Jason Slotkin, "New York Schools Will Stay Closed For Rest Of the School Year, Cuomo Says," NPR, May 1, 2020, https://www.npr.org/sections/coronavirus-live-updates/2020/05/01/849159856/new-york-schools-will-stay-closed-for-rest-of-the-school-year-cuomo-says; "New York Closes Schools through End of Academic Year," *New York Times*, May 1, 2020, New York, https://www.nytimes.com/2020/05/01/nyregion/coronavirus-new-york-update.html; Elizabeth Joseph and Jay Croft, "New York Schools Will Remain Closed For the Rest of the Academic Year, Gov. Cuomo Says," CNN, May 1, 2020, https://www.cnn .com/2020/05/01/us/ny-schools-closed-academic-year/index.html; Eyewitness News, "Coronavirus News: K-12, Colleges in NY State Closed for Rest of Academic Year," abc7ny.com, May 1, 2020, https://abc7ny.com/coronavirus-new-york-ny-cases-in -news/6142677/.

Page 79 "We must protect our children": Minyvonne Burke, "New York State Will Keep Schools, Colleges Closed for Rest of Academic Year," *NBC News*, May 1, 2020, https://www.nbcnews.com/news/us-news/new-york-state-will-keep-schools-colleges -closed-rest-academic-n1197791.

Page 80 proxy for prestige media: When not leading coverage, the *Times* is still generally reflective of the content and framing in other major media outlets, with the obvious exception of right-leaning FOX, and perhaps the *Wall Street Journal*. (It would be quite rare for NBC, CBS, CNN, and the *Washington Post* to cover a particular story, and from a certain viewpoint, for it to be absent in the *Times* or covered by the *Times* from an alternative angle.) I use "prestige" and "legacy" media interchangeably, referring to traditional TV and print outlets.

Page 80 a call Trump had with governors: "Texas and Ohio Push to Reopen; White House Promises to Help States Test," *New York Times*, April 27, 2020, https://www .nytimes.com/2020/04/27/us/coronavirus-live.html.

Page 80 "Schools Are Likely to Stay Shut for Months": Shawn Hubler, Erica L. Green, and Dana Goldstein, "Despite Trump's Nudging, Schools Are Likely to Stay Shut for Months," *New York Times*, April 28, 2020,

Page 81 "Cases Could Soar": Apoorva Mandivilli, "New Studies Add to Evidence that Children May Transmit the Coronavirus," *New York Times*, May 5, 2020.

Page 81 This article, tweeted approvingly: Eric Topol (@EricTopol), "Kids can transmit #COVID19. Despite @DFTBubbles last week suggesting children are 'immune' from spreading; it's just much less common and woefully understudied," Twitter, May 5, 2020, 3:38 p.m., https://twitter.com/EricTopol/status/1257756559142055936; Amesh Adalja (@AmeshAA), "'I think we have to take a holistic view of the impact of school closures on kids and our families. I do worry at some point, the accumulated harms from the virus—@JenniferNuzzo,'" Twitter, May 5, 2020, 6:00 p.m., https:// twitter.com/AmeshAA/status/1257792251834634241; Benjy Sarlin (@BenjySarlin), "Let's assume it turns out risk to kids is still relatively low. The next q is whether they contract coronavirus without symptoms then spread to teachers, staff," Twitter, May 13, 2020, 1:42 p.m., https://twitter.com/BenjySarlin/status/1260626521410 207745; Stephanie Armour (@StephArmour1), "New Studies Add to Evidence that Children May Transmit the Coronavirus—The New York Times," Twitter, May 9, 2020, 1:28 p.m., https://twitter.com/StephArmour1/status/1259173375253123073; Joseph Roy (@JosephRoy2023), "Wishing @RepTurzai would have read this before his tirade directed at educators and @pedroarivera2. Science matters now. Scoring political points with your base," Twitter, May 6, 2020, 6:57 p.m.; https://twitter.com /BASDSUPT/status/1258169115619057665. Sal Albanese (@SalAlbaneseNYC), "via

@nytimes insightful article with implications for NYC! Do we open schools in September? If they open is a strategy in place to protect children & staff (staggered days, part e learning & part in buildings)! A game plan is needed," Twitter, May 12, 2020, 9:53 p.m., https://twitter.com/SalAlbaneseNYC/status/1260387637665431559.

Page 81 The second study was not published: Christian Drosten et al., "An Analysis of SARS-CoV-2 Viral Load by Patient Age," *MedRxiv* (2020): 2020–2026; Munro criticism: Alasdair Munro (@apsmunro), "A German study claimed to find similar viral loads in children as adults, stating they're 'just as infectious,'" May 21, 2020, 11:33 a.m., https://twitter.com/apsmunro/status/1263493049142951936.

Page 82 *lower* viral loads than adults: Terry C. Jones et al., "Estimating Infectiousness throughout SARS-CoV-2 Infection Course," *Science* 373, no. 6551 (2021).

Page 82 "of course" outbreaks will happen: Alasdair Munro (@apsmunro), "Will outbreaks happen? Of course. But this is our new reality for the foreseeable future. We need to mitigate against the risks and ensure mechanisms for quick response (track/trace/isolate) are in place . . . ," May 21, 2020, 11:33 a.m., https://twitter.com /apsmunro/status/1263493054004187137. The notion that people were suggesting that children couldn't get infected at all or were incapable of spreading the virus was a canard; this was never a narrative that any legitimate expert or, as far as I saw, in any significant way regular people who advocated for opening schools were pushing. Nevertheless, health authorities and others repeatedly argued against this straw man.

Page 82 Iceland: Daniel F. Gudbjartsson et al., "Spread of SARS-CoV-2 in the Icelandic Population," *New England Journal of Medicine* 382, no. 24 (2020): 2302–2315;

Page 82 European Academy of Paediatrics: Valtýr Stefánsson Thors, "COVID-19 Series (#5): Iceland's Data on the Infectivity of Children Cross-Infection Risk," EAP Blog, April 2020, https://www.eapaediatrics.eu/eap-blog-covid-19-series-5-icelands -data-on-the-infectivity-of-children-cross-infection-risk/.

Page 82 a study of families in the Netherlands: David Zweig, "It's Ridiculous to Treat Schools Like Covid Hot Zones," *Wired*, June 24, 2020, https://www.wired.com/story /its-ridiculous-to-treat-schools-like-covid-hot-zones/.

Page 82 Australian study: National Centre for Immunisation Research and Surveillance (NCIRS), *COVID-19 in Schools—the Experience in NSW: 18 October 2021 to 17 December 2021*, February 18, 2022, https://www.ncirs.org.au/sites/default/files/2022 -02/NCIRS_NSW_Schools_COVID_Summary_Term_4_2021_Report%20-%2024-02 -2022_Final.pdf.

Page 82 French study: Kostas Danis et al., "Cluster of Coronavirus Disease 2019 (COVID-19) in the French Alps, February 2020," *Clinical Infectious Diseases* 71, no. 15 (August 2020): 825–832.

Page 82 Dutch study: RIVM (Dutch National Institute for Public Health and the Environment), "COVID-19," https://www.rivm.nl/en/coronavirus-covid-19/children

-and-covid-19 (cited by Nuzzo in Apoorva article, and cited by Munro). Additionally, Norwegian studies also suggested that there was no effect of school closure on spread, or it possibly made transmission worse. Alle Børn I Skole (@rniskole), "Også de norske sundhedsmyndigheder nåede tilbage i sommeren 2020 frem til at skolelukning ingen eller muligvis negativ effekt havde på smittespredningen" (translation: "The Norwegian health authorities also concluded back in the summer of 2020 that school closures had no or possibly a negative effect on the spread of infection"). February 1, 2021, 5:37 a.m., https://twitter.com/rniskole/status/1356189858881015808. Norwegian Institute of Public Health (Folkehelseinstituttet), *COVID-19-EPIDE-MIEN: Kunnskap, situasjon, prognose, risikoog respons i Norge etter uke 18*, May 5, 2020, https://www.fhi.no/contentassets/c9e459cd7cc24991810a0d28d7803bd0/vedlegg/notat-om-risiko-og-respons-2020-05-05.pdf.

Page 83 "Children are not substantially contributing to the spread": Kevin O'Sullivan, "No Evidence Children Are Covid-19 'Super SPpreaders,' says Hiqa," *Irish Times*, May 13, 2020, https://www.irishtimes.com/news/health/no-evidence-children-are-covid-19-super-spreaders-says-hiqa-1.4252521.

Page 83 Munro also coauthored a paper: Alasdair Munro and Saul N. Faust, "Children Are Not COVID-19 Super Spreaders: Time to Go Back to School," *Archives of Disease in Childhood* 105, no. 7 (2020): 618–619.

Page 84 far more negative in tone than coverage in non-US major sources: Bruce Sacerdote, Ranjan Sehgal, and Molly Cook, "Why Is All COVID-19 News Bad News?" National Bureau of Economic Research Working Paper Series, November 2020.

Page 84 a 1,700-word feature: Katrin Bennhold, "As Europe Reopens Schools, Relief Combines with Risk," *New York Times*, Europe, May 10, 2020 .

Page 84 Schools reopening in the UK: Ceylan Yeginsu, "If U.K. Schools Reopen, Will the Students Return?," *New York Times*, Europe, May 11, 2020.

Page 85 previously healthy fourteen-year-old boy: Pam Belluck, "'Straight-Up Fire' in His Veins: Teen Battles New Covid Syndrome," *New York Times*, Health, May 17, 2020.

Page 85 the *Times* ran an opinion piece: Chris Sommerfeldt, "'Still Too Early': Cuomo Bars Summer School in N.Y. amid Spike in Coronavirus-Linked Illness Afflicting Kids," *New York Daily News*, May 21, 2020, https://www.nydailynews.com/coronavirus/ny-coronavirus-cuomo-summer-school-20200521-7nelpchqbfbtjcvbt4wrrn5tri-story.html.

Page 85 another news piece about MIS-C: Joseph Goldstein and Jesse McKinley, "After 3 Children Die, a Race to Investigate a Baffling Virus Syndrome," *New York Times*, May 22, 2020.

Page 85 "One issue I don't believe is relevant": Russell Viner, "COVID-19—Message from the President, 22 May," Royal College of Paediatrics and Child Health (website), May 22, 2020, https://www.rcpch.ac.uk/news-events/news/covid-19-message-president-22-may.

Page 85 interview with the BBC: "Coronavirus: Children Affected by Rare Kawasaki-Like Disease," BBC, May 13, 2020, https://www.bbc.com/news/health-52648557.

Page 86 Northwell Health: "10 Things to Know About Northwell Health," Becker's Hospital Review (website), February 24, 2016, https://www.beckershospitalreview .com/hospital-management-administration/10-things-to-know-about-northwell -health.html.

Page 86 Cuomo gave a press conference: Cynthia Wachtell, "My Son Survived Terrifying Covid-19 Complications," *New York Times*, May 21, 2020.

Page 86 "Is Summer Camp Too Risky?": Sharon Otterman, "Parents Really Need a Break. But Is Summer Camp Too Risky?," *New York Times*, New York, May 22, 2020.

Page 87 Cuomo ultimately barred all overnight camps: Joseph Spector, "No Sleep-Away Camps This Summer, New York Says. Here's Why," *Democrat & Chronicle* (Albany), June 12, 2020, https://www.democratandchronicle.com/story/news/politics/albany /2020/06/12/no-sleep-away-camps-summer-new-york-says-heres-why/3178815001/.

Page 88 The same day as the *Times*'s news piece on MIS-C: Mark Landler, "Coronavirus Cases Fall in Europe's Capitals, but Fears Over Reopening Linger," *New York Times*, May 22, 2020.

Page 88 evidence of increased child abuse: See "Child abuse" and "Reporting of Child Maltreatment" in *"Deep Dive*: Harms of School Closures" endnotes.

Page 88 no longer getting a subsidized or free lunch: See "Free lunches" in the Introduction's endnotes.

Page 88 report from the US Government Accountability Office: GAO Report: "Pandemic Learning: Less Academic Progress Overall, Student and Teacher Strain, and Implications for the Future," June 8, 2022, https://www.gao.gov/products/gao-22 -105816.

Page 88 deemed essentially to be truants: Holly Kurtz, "National Survey Tracks Impact of Coronavirus on Schools: 10 Key Findings," *Education Week*, April 10, 2020, https://www.edweek.org/teaching-learning/national-survey-tracks-impact-of-coro navirus-on-schools-10-key-findings/2020/04.

Page 90 I found a sympathetic editor at *Wired*: David Zweig, "The Case for Reopening Schools," *Wired*, May 11, 2020, https://www.wired.com/story/the-case-for-reopening -schools/.

Page 90 notably, a piece in the *Wall Street Journal*: Jason Douglas, "Consensus Is Emerging That Children Are Less Vulnerable to Coronavirus," *Wall Street Journal*, April 27, 2020, https://www.wsj.com/articles/consensus-is-emerging-that-children -are-less-vulnerable-to-coronavirus-11587988688.

CHAPTER 8

Page 93 "conjures up a grim tableau of safety measures": David Zweig, "It's Ridiculous to Treat Schools Like Covid Hot Zones," *Wired*, June 24, 2020, https://www .wired.com/story/its-ridiculous-to-treat-schools-like-covid-hot-zones/.

Page 94 not beyond the risk for influenza: See "in many seasons, the flu" in the introduction endnotes.

Page 94 Nearly all of them ultimately got infected: Kristie E. N. Clarke et al., "Sero-prevalence of Infection-Induced SARS-CoV-2 Antibodies—United States, September 2021–February 2022," *Morbidity and Mortality Weekly Report* 71, no. 17 (April 29, 2022): 606–608.

Page 94 literature on community and school mask mandates: David Zweig, "The Science of Masking Kids at School Remains Uncertain," *New York*, August 20, 2021, https://nymag.com/intelligencer/2021/08/the-science-of-masking-kids-at-school-remains-uncertain.html; David Zweig, "The CDC's Flawed Cases for Wearing Masks in School," *Atlantic*, December 16, 2021, https://www.theatlantic.com/science/archive/2021/12/mask-guidelines-cdc-walensky/621035/.

Page 95 surgeon general: Huo Jingnan, "Why There Are So Many Different Guidelines for Face Masks for the Public," NPR, April 10, 2020, https://www.npr.org/sections/goatsandsoda/2020/04/10/829890635/why-there-so-many-different-guidelines-for-face-masks-for-the-public.

Page 95 Anthony Fauci: Arijeta Lajka, "Video Misleads on Fauci Emails," AP News, June 9, 2021, https://apnews.com/article/fact-checking-436900978804.

Page 95 April 1 CDC guidance: Tony McReynolds, "CDC: An About Face on Face Masks?," American Animal Hospital Association (website), April 1, 2020, https://www.aaha.org/publications/newstat/articles/2020-03/cdc-an-about-face-on-face-masks/. "How to Protect Yourself," Centers for Disease Control and Prevention (website), March 18, 2020, https://web.archive.org/web/20200331013336/https://www.cdc.gov/coronavirus/2019-ncov/prevent-getting-sick/prevention.html (accessed via Wayback Machine).

Page 95 "new information" had emerged: Jessica McDonald, D'Angelo Gore, and Eugene Kiely, "Video Wrong About Fauci, COVID-19," FactCheck.org, February 3, 2021, https://www.factcheck.org/2021/02/scicheck-video-wrong-about-fauci-covid-19/. Fauci quotes from *Washington Post* video: "Fauci on How His Thinking Has Evolved on Masks, Asymptomatic Transmission" (video), *Washington Post*, July 24, 2020, https://www.washingtonpost.com/video/washington-post-live/fauci-on-how-his-thinking-has-evolved-on-masks-asymptomatic-transmission/2020/07/24/799264e2-0f35-4862-aca2-2b4702650a8b_video.html.

Page 96 a research letter published in February: Yan Bai et al., "Presumed Asymptomatic Carrier Transmission of COVID-19," *Journal of the American Medical Association* 323, no. 14 (2020):1406–1407.

Page 96 study published in February in the *Journal of Infectious Diseases*: Ping Yu et al., "A Familial Cluster of Infection Associated with the 2019 Novel Coronavirus Indicating Possible Person-to-Person Transmission during the Incubation Period," *Journal of Infectious Diseases* 221, no. 11 (2020): 1757–1761.

Page 96 A letter in the *New England Journal of Medicine* on January 30: Camilla Rothe et al., "Transmission of 2019-nCoV Infection from an Asymptomatic Contact in Germany," *New England Journal of Medicine* 382 (2020): 970–971.

Page 96 "This evening I telephoned one of my colleagues in China": Kai Kupferschmidt, "Study Claiming New Coronavirus Can Be Transmitted by People without

Symptoms Was Flawed," *Science*, February 3, 2020 (updated June 2, 2020, and July 14, 2020), https://www.science.org/content/article/paper-non-symptomatic-patient-transmitting-coronavirus-wrong.

Page 96 Fauci himself even coauthored a paper: David M. Morens, Gregory K. Folkers, and Anthony S. Fauci, "The Concept of Classical Herd Immunity May Not Apply to COVID-19," *Journal of Infectious Diseases* 226, no. 2 (2022): 195–198.

Page 96 CDC knew asymptomatic transmission was not only possible but likely: At least as early as 2008 the CDC acknowledged "you may be able to pass on the flu to someone else before you know you are sick. Some persons can be infected with the flu virus but have no symptoms. During this time, those persons can still spread the virus to others." https://web.archive.org/web/20080116172122/https://www.cdc.gov/flu/about/disease/spread.htm.

Page 96 Dr. Maria Van Kerkhove: Will Feuer, "Asymptomatic Spread of Coronavirus Is 'Very Rare,' WHO says," CNBC, June 8, 2020, https://www.cnbc.com/2020/06/08/asymptomatic-coronavirus-patients-arent-spreading-new-infections-who-says.html.

Page 97 WHO officials walked back her statement: MaiRead McArdle, "WHO Clarifies Claim That Asymptomatic Transmission Is 'Very Rare,' Says It Was 'Misinterpreted,'" June 9, 2020, Yahoo!News, https://news.yahoo.com/walks-back-claim-asymptomatic-transmission-175455156.html.

Page 97 much-cited paper in *JAMA Network Open*: Michael Johansson et al., "SARS-CoV-2 Transmission from People without COVID-19 Symptoms," *JAMA Network Open*, January 7, 2021, 2021;4(1): e2035057.

Page 97 later statistics on asymptomatic index cases: Claude Muller, "Do Asymptomatic Carriers of SARS-COV-2 Transmit the Virus?" *Lancet Regional Health—Europe* 4, May 2021, 100082.

Page 97 minus strand PCR: Jessica Ferguson et al., "Use of a Severe Acute Respiratory Coronavirus Virus 2 (SARS-CoV-2) Strand-Specific Assay to Evaluate for Prolonged Viral Replication >20 Days from Illness Onset," *Infection Control and Hospital Epidemiology* 44, no. 12 (2023): 2078–2080.

Another study, out of the UK—in which volunteers were intentionally infected—found that just 7 percent of emissions into the air and environment from infected participants occurred before the first reported symptom. Taken together, the Stanford and UK studies call into question the entire pandemic response: forcing healthy kids to stay home from school, quarantining people without symptoms, mandating masks at the population level, limiting gatherings—all of these actions were based on the notion that anyone could be a "silent" unknowing spreader; therefore, interventions needed to be imposed not just on sick people, but on *everyone*, including people without symptoms. While it was technically true that people without symptoms could transmit the virus to others, these two tests—which were biological, rather than less-definitive epidemiological tests—showed that possibility was far, far less likely than what we were told. The implications of these findings are enormous, yet they are almost completely absent from public knowledge. David Zweig, *Silent Lunch*, "A Study's Bombshell Finding that Has Been Ignored," September 1, 2023, https://www.silentlunch.net/p/a-studys-bombshell-finding-that-has.

Page 97 Cochrane, the prestigious British review organization: Jingyi Xiao et al., "Nonpharmaceutical Measures for Pandemic Influenza in Nonhealthcare Settings—Personal Protective and Environmental Measures," *Emerging Infectious Diseases* 26, no. 5 (2020): 967–975; Tom Jefferson et al., "Physical Interventions to Interrupt or Reduce the Spread of Respiratory Viruses," *Cochrane Database of Systematic Reviews*, issue 1, art. no. CD006207 (2023).

Page 98 Fauci and other officials encouraged cloth masks: C. Raina MacIntyre et al., "A Cluster Randomised Trial of Cloth Masks Compared with Medical Masks in Healthcare Workers," *BMJ Open* 5, no. 4 (2015): e006577.

Page 99 "I don't think I'm going to be doing it": Lena H. Sun and Josh Dawsey, "New Face Mask Guidance Comes after Battle between White House and CDC," *Washington Post*, April 3, 2020, https://www.washingtonpost.com/health/2020/04 /03/white-house-cdc-turf-battle-over-guidance-broad-use-face-masks-fight-coro navirus/.

Page 100 masks only "work at the margins": David Wallace-Wells, "Dr. Fauci Looks Back: 'Something Clearly Went Wrong,'" *New York Times*, April 24, 2023.

Page 100 intervention bias: Andrew J. Foy and Edward J Filippone, "The Case for Intervention Bias in the Practice of Medicine," *Yale Journal of Biology and Medicine* 86, no. 2 (2013): 271–280, https://www.ncbi.nlm.nih.gov/pmc/articles/PMC3670446/.

Page 100 "a biological basis for the need for control": Lauren A. Leotti et al., "Born to Choose: The Origins and Value of the Need for Control," *Trends in Cognitive Sciences* 14, no. 10 (2010): 457–463.

Page 100 30 percent of antibiotic scrips unnecessary: US Department of Health and Human Services, Centers for Disease Control and Prevention, *Antibiotic Use in the United States, 2018 Update: Progress and Opportunities*, 2019, https://www.cdc.gov /antibiotic-use/stewardship-report/pdf/stewardship-report-2018-508.pdf.

Page 101 metal-on-metal hip replacements: Levin Papantonio Rafferty Law Firm (website), "FDA 510(k) Loophole to Be Closed? Don't Hold Your Breath," https:// www.levinlaw.com/news/fda-510k-loophole-be-closed-dont-hold-your-breath; Chris Elkins, "Hip Replacement Recall," DrugWatch, October 18, 2023, https:// www.drugwatch.com/hip-replacement/recalls/. https://dash.harvard.edu/bitstream /handle/1/11940233/ho_2012.pdf?sequence=1.

Page 101 prophylactic antibiotic use for surgeries: Branch-Elliman et al., "Association of Duration and Type of Surgical Prophylaxis with Antimicrobial-Associated Adverse Events," *JAMA Surgery*, April 24, 2019.

Page 101 "The Discordance between Evidence and Health Policy in the United States": Mohsen Malekinejad et al., "The Discordance between Evidence and Health Policy in the United States: The Science of Translational Research and the Critical Role of Diverse Stakeholders," *Health Research and Policy Systems* 16, article 81 (2018).

Page 101 programs continuing after they should have ended: Ross C. Brownson et al., "Understanding Mis-Implementation in Public Health Practice," *American Journal of Preventive Medicine* 48, no. 5 (2015): 543–551.

Page 101 A 2012 analysis: Adam G. Elshaug et al., "Over 150 Potentially Low-Value Health Care Practices: An Australian Study," *Medical Journal of Australia* 197, no. 10 (2012): 556–560.

Page 101 A 2019 study of misimplementation of public health measures: Karishma S. Furtado et al., "A Cross-Country Study of Mis-Implementation in Public Health Practice," *BMC Public Health* 19, article 270 (2019).

Page 102 Numerous studies at the time: R. R. Clayton et al., "DARE (Drug Abuse Resistance Education): Very Popular but Not Very Effective," US Department of Justice Office of Justice Programs, 1996, https://www.ojp.gov/ncjrs/virtual-library /abstracts/dare-drug-abuse-resistance-education-very-popular-not-very; Steven L. West and Keri K O'Neal, "Project D.A.R.E. Outcome Effectiveness Revisited," *American Journal of Public Health* 94, no. 6 (2004): 1027–1029.

Page 102 two programs of experimental curricula: W. B. Hansen and R. B. McNeal, "How D.A.R.E. Works: An Examination of Program Effects on Mediating Variables," *Health Education & Behavior* 24, no. 2 (1997), 165–176.

Page 102 "It's Good to Feel Like You're Doing Something": Stephanie Mazzucca et al., "It's Good to Feel Like You're Doing Something: A Qualitative Study Examining State Health Department Employees' Views on Why Ineffective Programs Continue to Be Implemented in the USA," *Implementation Science Communications* 3, article 4 (2022).

Page 103 Mere perception of control: Camille Amoura et al., "Desire for Control, Perception of Control: Their Impact on Autonomous Motivation and Psychological Adjustment," *Motivation and Emotion* 38, no. 3 (2014): 323–335.

Note that some people have a lower desire for control. But even for them, the public health authorities can function as their proxy. The authorities have control of the situation, and citizens need not take on any feelings of control but just have to follow orders dictated to them. Either way, some individuals—the citizens themselves or the authorities—are experiencing the benefits of a sense of control.

CHAPTER 9

Page 106 In an interview with the *Washington Post*: Laura Meckler and Lena H. Sun, "States Are Rushing to Close Schools. But What Does the Science on Closures Say?," *Washington Post*, March 16, 2020, Education, https://www.washingtonpost.com /local/education/states-are-rushing-to-close-schools-but-what-does-the-science-on -closures-say/2020/03/16/2cbb64da-6799-11ea-b313-df458622c2cc_story.html.

Page 107 The Report 9 model differentiated: Imperial College COVID-19 Response Team, "Report 9: Impact of Non-Pharmaceutical Interventions (NPIs) to Reduce COVID-19 Mortality and Healthcare Demand," March 16, 2020, https://www .imperial.ac.uk/media/imperial-college/medicine/mrc-gida/2020-03-16-COVID19 -Report-9.pdf.

Page 108 *"Remember without fail"*: Jean-Jacques Rousseau, "Emile, or On Education," 1762. Translation of quoted passage by Benedict Beckeld, quoted in *Western Self-Contempt* (Ithaca, NY: Cornell University Press, 2022), 232.

Page 109 "a map is not the territory": Alfred Korzybski, *Science and Sanity* (1933), 5th ed. (New York: Institute of General Semantics, 1995).

Page 112 Opposite of a cost-benefit calculation: Stephanie Harvard and Eric Winsberg, "Causal Inference, Moral Intuition, and Modeling in a Pandemic," *Philosophy of Medicine* 2, no. 2 (2021): 1–10.

Page 112 Fauci said, "If it looks like you're overreacting": "Transcript: Dr. Anthony Fauci Discusses Coronavirus on 'Face the Nation,' March 15, 2020," CBS News, March 15, 2020, https://www.cbsnews.com/news/transcript-dr-anthony-fauci-discusses -coronavirus-on-face-the-nation-march-15-2020/.

Page 112 UK behavioral scientists: Scientific Advisory Group for Emergencies (UK), "Options for Increasing Adherence to Social Distancing Measures 22nd March 2020," https://assets.publishing.service.gov.uk/government/uploads/system/uploads /attachment_data/file/882722/25-options-for-increasing-adherence-to-social-distancing -measures-22032020.pdf. I first learned of this through Laura Dodsworth's book *A State of Fear: How the UK Government Weaponised Fear During the Covid-19 Pandemic* (London: Pinter & Martin, 2021).

Page 112 The *Times* published a piece: Benedict Carey, "Complacency, Not Panic, Is the Real Danger," *New York Times*, Health, March 19, 2020.

Page 113 noninvasive testing of patients: Benjamin C. Sun and Rita F. Redberg, "Cardiac Testing after Emergency Department Evaluation for Chest Pain: Time for a Paradigm Shift?," *JAMA Internal Medicine* 177, no. 8 (2017): 1183–1184; Aniket A. Kawatkar et al., "Early Noninvasive Cardiac Testing After Emergency Department Evaluation for Suspected Acute Coronary Syndrome," *JAMA Internal Medicine* 180, no. 12 (2020): 1621–1629.

Page 114 abstinence-only programs: Kathrin F. Stanger-Hall and David W. Hall, "Abstinence-Only Education and Teen Pregnancy Rates: Why We Need Comprehensive Sex Education in the U.S.," *PLOS ONE* 6, no.10 (2011): e24658.

Page 114 peanut allergies: H. Eric Cannon, "The Economic Impact of Peanut Allergies," *American Journal of Managed Care* 24, no. 19 supplement (2018): S428-S433, https:// www.ajmc.com/view/the-economic-impact-of-peanut-allergies; Scott H. Sicherer et al., "U.S. Prevalence of Self-Reported Peanut, Tree Nut, and Sesame Allergy: 11-Year Follow-Up," *Journal of Allergy and Clinical Immunology* 125, no. 6 (2010): 1322–1326. Ruchi S. Gupta et al., "The Public Health Impact of Parent-Reported Childhood Food Allergies in the United States," *Pediatrics* 142, no. 6 (2018): e20181235.

Page 114 the phrase "risk benefit": Tammy C. Hoffmann and Chris Del Mar, "Discrepant Expectations about Benefits and Harms—Reply," *JAMA Internal Medicine* 177, no. 8 (2017): 1226–1227.

Page 116 facial recognition technology: P. Jonathon Philips et al, "An Other Race Effect for Face Recognition Algorithms," NIST, February 2010, https://nvlpubs.nist .gov/nistpubs/Legacy/IR/nistir7666.pdf.

Page 117 default thermostat setting: Ed Browne, "Office Aircon Is Sexist to Women, Study Finds," *Newsweek*, December 29, 2021, https://www.newsweek.com/office-aircon -temperature-sexist-unfair-women-overcooling-study-1663949.

Page 117 public infrastructure projects of Robert Moses: Robert A. Caro, *The Power Broker: Robert Moses and the Fall of New York* (New York: Alfred A. Knopf, 1974), *passim*.

Page 117 "knowledge translation": J. M. Grimshaw et al., "Knowledge Translation of Research Findings," *Implementation Science* 7, 50 (2012); Sharon E. Straus et al., "Defining Knowledge Translation," *CMAJ: Canadian Medical Association Journal* 181, nos. 3–4 (2009): 165–168; Pimjai Sudsawad, *Knowledge Translation: Introduction to Models, Strategies, and Measures* (National Center for the Dissemination of Disability Research, 2007), https://ktdrr.org/ktlibrary/articles_pubs/ktmodels/.

CHAPTER 10

Page 121 June news piece by NPR: Anya Kamenetz, "What Parents Can Learn From Child Care Centers That Stayed Open During Lockdowns," NPR, June 24, 2020, https://www.npr.org/2020/06/24/882316641/what-parents-can-learn-from-child-care-centers-that-stayed-open-during-lockdowns.

Page 122 Montana and Wyoming: "The Coronavirus Spring: The Historic Closing of U.S. Schools (A Timeline)," *Education Week*, July 1, 2020, https://www.edweek.org/leadership/the-coronavirus-spring-the-historic-closing-of-u-s-schools-a-timeline/2020/07. A small number of private schools in Idaho also reopened that spring.

Page 124 general direction of Oster's findings: Walter S. Gilliam et al., "COVID-19 Transmission in US Child Care Programs," *Pediatrics* 147, no. 1 (2021): e2020031971.

Page 124 More than 7 million American children: Susannah Howe, "Types of Care," New America, https://www.newamerica.org/in-depth/care-report/types-care/.

Page 125 More than 12 million kids: Jiashan Cui, Luke Natzke, and Sarah Grady, *Early Childhood Program Participation: 2019* (Washington, DC: National Center for Education Statistics, Institute of Education Sciences, 2020), https://files.eric.ed.gov/fulltext/ED607038.pdf.

Page 127 Swiss cheese model: Siobhan Roberts, "The Swiss Cheese Model of Pandemic Defense," *New York Times*, December 8, 2020.

CHAPTER 11

Page 129 Health commissioner of Nassau County: *New York Times*, "Flu Cases in City Continue to Rise," October 2, 1957, https://timesmachine.nytimes.com/timesmachine/1957/10/02/84981383.html?pageNumber=22.

Page 130 "The outbreaks were so explosive": D. A. Henderson et al., "Public Health and Medical Responses to the 1957–58 Influenza Pandemic," *Biosecurity and Bioterrorism: Biodefense Strategy, Practice, and Science* 7, no. 3 (2009): 265–273.

Page 130 29 percent of total enrollment . . . : Robert Alden, "Flu Up in Schools; State Aid Imperiled," *New York Times*, October 8, 1957, https://www.nytimes.com/1957/10/08/archives/flu-up-in-schools-state-aid-imperiled-29-out-of-school-in-flu.html.

Page 131 This daily performance earned him an Emmy: After Cuomo's sexual harassment scandal and subsequent resignation, his Emmy was rescinded, with his name and any reference to his receiving the award eliminated from International Academy materials.

Page 131 "The old model of everybody goes and sits in a classroom": "Andrew Cuomo, 'The old model'": Kevin Tampone, "Is Going to School in Person Obsolete? Cuomo Wonders Why 'Old Model' Persists," Syracuse.com, May 5, 2020, https://www.syracuse.com/coronavirus/2020/05/is-going-to-school-in-person-obsolete-cuomo-wonders-why-old-model-persists.html. Valerie Aguirre, "With an Additional 230 New Deaths, NY Gov. Cuomo Hosts Coronavirus Briefing (May 5)," WRAL News (Raleigh, NC), May 5, 2020 (transcript), https://www.wral.com/with-nearly-25-000-deaths-in-the-state-ny-gov-cuomo-hosts-coronavirus-briefing/19085282/.

As a side note, Gates may not be quite the visionary that Cuomo believed him to be. A nearly $1 billion education initiative related to teacher evaluations was found to be ineffective at improving student outcomes. This doesn't necessarily mean that Gates and his foundation don't implement other programs that are effective. But it's worth noting that, like everyone, he's capable of a colossal failure. And that this ten-digit failure was specifically in the realm of education is probably something Cuomo should have noted. Jeremy Berke, "A $1 Billion Gates Foundation-Backed Education Initiative Failed to Help Students, According to a New Report—Here's What Happened," *Business Insider*, June 27, 2018, https://www.businessinsider.com/bill-melinda-gates-foundation-education-initiative-failure-2018-6.

Page 132 Eric Schmidt: Office of the Governor of the State of New York, "Video, Audio, Photos & Rush Transcript: Amid Ongoing Covid-19 Pandemic, Governor Cuomo Announces Schmidt Futures Will Help Integrate NYS Practices and Systems with Best Advanced Technology Tools to Build Back Better," news release, May 6, 2020, https://www.governor.ny.gov/news/video-audio-photos-rush-transcript-amid-ongoing-covid-19-pandemic-governor-cuomo-announces-20.

Page 132 Naomi Klein: Naomi Klein, "Screen New Deal," Intercept, May 8, 2020, https://theintercept.com/2020/05/08/andrew-cuomo-eric-schmidt-coronavirus-tech-shock-doctrine/.

Page 133 broadband in their homes: Pew Research Center, "Internet/Broadband Fact Sheet," April 7, 2021, https://www.pewresearch.org/internet/fact-sheet/internet-broadband/.

Page 133 Google Classroom: Darrell Etherington, "Google Debuts Classroom, An Education Platform For Teacher-Student Communication," TechCrunch, May 6, 2014, https://techcrunch.com/2014/05/06/google-debuts-classroom-an-education-platform-for-teacher-student-communication/.

Page 133 Schmidt published an editorial: Eric Schmidt, "A Real Digital Infrastructure at Last," *Wall Street Journal*, March 27, 2020, https://www.wsj.com/articles/a-real-digital-infrastructure-at-last-11585313825.

Page 136 In 1922 Edison said: Associated Press, "Edison Predicts Film Will Replace Teacher, Books," *Recorder* (Monterey, VA), May 18, 1923, via *Virginia Chronicle*: Digi-

tal Newspaper Archive, https://virginiachronicle.com/?a=d&d=HR19230518.2.11&e
=-------en-20--1--txt-txIN---------.

Page 136 Harry Arthur Wise was skeptical: Todd Oppenheimer, *The Flickering Mind: Saving Education from the False Promise of Technology* (New York: Random House, 2003), excerpted via *New York Times*, January 4, 2004, https://www.nytimes.com /2004/01/04/books/chapters/the-flickering-mind.html.

Page 137 In the 1990s, Bill Clinton: President William J. Clinton, "Remarks Accepting the Presidential Nomination at the Democratic National Convention in Chicago," August 29, 1996, American Presidency Project, https://www.presidency.ucsb .edu/node/222870.

Page 138 "equivocal at best": Natalie Wexler, "How Classroom Technology Is Holding Students Back," *MIT Technology Review*, December 19, 2019, https://www.tech nologyreview.com/2019/12/19/131155/classroom-technology-holding-students -back-edtech-kids-education/.

Page 139 Jeb Bush: Jeb Bush, "It's Time to Embrace Distance Learning—and Not Just Because of the Coronavirus," *Washington Post*, May 3, 2020, Opinions, https://www .washingtonpost.com/opinions/2020/05/03/jeb-bush-its-time-embrace-distance -learning-not-just-because-coronavirus/.

Page 139 spring closures in the Netherlands: Per Engzell et al., "Learning Loss Due to School Closures during the COVID-19 Pandemic," *PNAS* 118, no. 17 (2021): e2022376118.

Page 140 Blunt headlines: Tawnell D. Hobbs and Lee Hawkins, "The Results Are In for Remote Learning: It Didn't Work," *Wall Street Journal*, June 5, 2020, https://www .wsj.com/articles/schools-coronavirus-remote-learning-lockdown-tech-11591375078.

Page 140 "Why Zoom Is Terrible": Kate Murphy, "Why Zoom Is Terrible," *New York Times*, April 29, 2020.

Page 141 meme surfaced on Reddit: Kevin Owdziej (r/facepalm), "I understand the need for this (I really really do) but this sucks so much," Reddit, August 18, 2020, accessed January 4, 2024, https://www.reddit.com/r/facepalm/comments/iccp6w/i _understand_the_need_for_this_i_really_really_do/.

CHAPTER 12

Page 145 meeting of the EU education ministers: Education, Youth, Culture and Sports Council, "Press Conference Following the Video Conference of Ministers of Education," Council of the EU and the European Council, June 22, 2020, video, 16:40, https://video.consilium.europa.eu/event/en/24040?start_time=0.

Page 146 Michelle Goldberg: Michelle Goldberg, "Remote School Is a Nightmare. Few in Power Care," *New York Times*, June 29, 2020.

Page 147 A few days after Goldberg's piece: Jennifer B. Nuzzo and Joshua M. Sharfstein, "We Have to Focus on Opening Schools, Not Bars," *New York Times*, July 1, 2020.

Page 147 American Academy of Pediatrics released guidance: Lauren Camera, "Pediatric Group Calls for Children to Return to Schools Despite Coronavirus," *U.S. News & World Report*, June 29, 2020, https://www.usnews.com/news/education-news /articles/2020-06-29/pediatric-group-calls-for-children-to-return-to-schools-despite -coronavirus; Dana Goldstein, "Why a Pediatric Group Is Pushing to Reopen Schools This Fall," *New York Times*, June 30, 2020.

Page 149 President Trump tweeted: Trump Twitter Archive v2, https://www.thet rumparchive.com/. Some of Trump's tweets I refer to were retweets.

Page 150 official White House Twitter account: The White House 45 Archived (@ WhiteHouse45), "Dr. Atlas: 'The President's priority is to open the schools and open them safely,'" Twitter, August 12, 2020, 7:32 p.m., https://twitter.com/WhiteHouse 45/status/1293691767913668608; "America's children are a top priority. President Trump joined teachers, parents, & physicians to discuss how to get our kids safely back to school. We've put forth," Twitter, August 15, 2020, 9:02 p.m., https://twitter .com/WhiteHouse45/status/1294801658279604225; "Janie, a mother from South Carolina: 'Schools not only provide the academics for students with special needs, but it also provides the much-needed therapies and,'" Twitter, 1:44 p.m., https:// twitter.com/WhiteHouse45/status/1294691383807287301.

Page 150 his constant calls for the economy to reopen: Jennifer Rubin, "Trump Cares More about the Stock Market than Humans," *Washington Post*, March 23, 2020, https://www.washingtonpost.com/opinions/2020/03/23/trump-cares-more -about-stock-market-than-humans/; Maegan Vazquez, "Trump Mostly Focuses on Economy—Rather than Health—for Minority Groups Hit Hardest by Covid-19," CNN, May 21, 2020, https://www.cnn.com/2020/05/21/politics/donald-trump-mino rities-coronavirus-economy/index.html; Susan Milligan, "Trump's Choice: The Economy or Human Lives," *U.S. News & World Report*, March 24, 2020, https://www .usnews.com/news/national-news/articles/2020-03-24/trumps-choice-on-coronavi rus-the-economy-or-human-lives.

Page 151 "Georgia's Experiment in Human Sacrifice": Amanda Mull, "Georgia's Experiment in Human Sacrifice," *Atlantic*, April 29, 2020, https://www.theatlantic .com/health/archive/2020/04/why-georgia-reopening-coronavirus-pandemic /610882/.

Page 151 the virus would just "go away": Daniel Wolfe and Daniel Dale, "It's Going to Disappear': A Timeline of Trump's Claims that Covid-19 Will Vanish," CNN, October 31, 2020, https://www.cnn.com/interactive/2020/10/politics/covid-disappearing -trump-comment-tracker/.

Page 151 Trump announced plans to withdraw troops: Joshua Keating, "Are Democrats Hypocrites for Criticizing Trump's Troop Withdrawals?," *Slate*, December 21, 2018, https://slate.com/news-and-politics/2018/12/democrats-and-trumps-troop-with drawals-is-the-criticism-hypocritical.html.

Page 151 numerous high-profile Democrats: Caroline Kelly, "'I Will Not Take His Word for It': Kamala Harris Says She Would Not Trust Trump Alone on a Coronavirus

Vaccine," CNN, September 9, 2020, https://www.cnn.com/2020/09/05/politics/kamala
-harris-not-trust-trump-vaccine-cnntv/index.html.

Page 152 "someone with a big megaphone": Rick Hess, quoted in Eliza Shapiro,
"How Trump's Push to Reopen Schools Backfired," *New York Times*, August 13,
2020.

Page 152 A 2017 survey: "Educator Political Perceptions, a National Survey," Education Week Research Center, 2017.

Page 153 Randi Weingarten: David A. Graham, "How Trump Closed Down the
Schools," *Atlantic*, July 17, 2020, https://www.theatlantic.com/ideas/archive/2020
/07/why-schools-cant-fully-reopen-fall/614353/.

Page 153 Lily Eskelsen García: Peter Baker and Erica L. Green, "Trump Leans on
Schools to Reopen as Virus Continues Its Spread," *New York Times*, July 7, 2020;
Anita Kumar and Nicole Gaudiano, "Trump Wants to Reopen Schools. Hint: It's
Not Just About Education," *Politico*, July 8, 2020, https://www.politico.com/news
/2020/07/08/trump-reopen-schools-353245.

Page 153 Seth Meyers: @LateNightSeth, "Donald Trump Is the Last Person We Can
Trust to Safely Reopen Schools: A Closer Look," *Late Night with Seth Meyers*, July 13,
2020, video (via YouTube), 14:29, https://www.youtube.com/watch?v=9Lv3l9zU6dU.

Page 153 Neera Tanden: Anthony LaMesa (@ajlamesa), "While European governments were working during summer 2020 to safely reopen schools in the fall, @
neeratanden politicized the issue, Tanden put presidential politics," Twitter, December 26, 2021, 6:53 p.m., https://twitter.com/ajlamesa/status/1475253435381518340.

Page 153 Trump's advocacy for schools: Stephen Collinson, "Trump Ignores
Recent Calamities in His Push to Open Schools," CNN, July 8, 2020, https://www
.cnn.com/2020/07/08/politics/donald-trump-schools-coronavirus-education/index
.html.

CHAPTER 13

Page 157 American Academy of Pediatrics (AAP): American Academy of Pediatrics
(website), "Pediatricians, Educators and Superintendents Urge a Safe Return to
School This Fall," news release, July 10, 2020, https://www.aap.org/en/news-room
/news-releases/aap/2020/pediatricians-educators-and-superintendents-urge-a-safe
-return-to-school-this-fall/.

Page 157 its new statement seemed to contradict that goal: Anya Kamenetz,
"Nation's Pediatricians Walk Back Support For In-Person School," NPR, July 10, 2020,
https://www.npr.org/sections/coronavirus-live-updates/2020/07/10/889848834
/nations-pediatricians-walk-back-support-for-in-person-school.

Page 158 organizations remained in relative lockstep: One of the most egregious
examples of what can only be described as collusion between multiple ostensibly
independent groups in the American public health establishment was the messaging
around the pediatric vaccine and myocarditis. See: David Zweig, "The CDC Owes

Parents Better Messaging on the Vaccine for Kids," *Wired*, July 16, 2021, https://www
.wired.com/story/the-cdc-owes-parents-better-messaging-on-the-vaccine-for-kids/.

Page 160 Physicians in general overrepresent as liberal: Janet Adamy and Paul Over-
berg, "Doctors, Once GOP Stalwarts, Now More Likely to Be Democrats," *Wall Street
Journal*, October 6, 2019, https://www.wsj.com/articles/doctors-once-gop-stalwarts
-now-more-likely-to-be-democrats-11570383523.

Page 160 infectious diseases and pediatrics ranked: Margot Sanger-Katz, "Your Surgeon Is Probably a Republican, Your Psychiatrist Probably a Democrat," *New York
Times*, October 6, 2016, https://www.nytimes.com/2016/10/07/upshot/your-surgeon
-is-probably-a-republican-your-psychiatrist-probably-a-democrat.html.

Page 160 Just 12 percent of faculty: Samuel J. Abrams and Amna Khalid, "Are
Colleges and Universities Too Liberal? What the Research Says About the Political
Composition of Campuses and Campus Climate," American Enterprise Institute, October 21, 2020, https://www.aei.org/articles/are-colleges-and-universities-too-liberal
-what-the-research-says-about-the-political-composition-of-campuses-and-campus
-climate/.

Page 160 Stanford political scientist Adam Bonica: Adam Bonica et al., "Ideological Sorting of Physicians in Both Geography and the Workplace," *Journal of Health
Politics, Policy and Law* 45, no. 6 (2020): 1023–1057.

Page 160 just 4.4 percent of epidemiologists: Elizabeth A DeVilbiss et al., "Assessing
Representation and Perceived Inclusion Among Members of the Society for Epidemiologic Research," *American Journal of Epidemiology* 189, no. 10 (2020): 998–1010.

Page 162 wildly overestimated the likelihood of hospitalization: Jonathan Rothwell
and Sonal Desai, "How Misinformation Is Distorting COVID Policies and Behaviors,"
Brookings Institution, December 22, 2020, https://www.brookings.edu/research/how
-misinformation-is-distorting-covid-policies-and-behaviors/. Jordan Boyd, "Study:
Majority Of Americans Grossly Overestimated COVID-19 Hospitalization Rates,"
Federalist, March 22, 2021, https://thefederalist.com/2021/03/22/study-majority-of
-americans-grossly-overestimated-covid-19-hospitalization-rates/; Wändi Bruine de
Bruin et al., "Political Polarization in US Residents' COVID-19 Risk Perceptions,
Policy Preferences, and Protective Behaviors," *Journal of Risk and Uncertainty* 61, no. 2
(2020): 177–194.

"News bias on perception of Covid risk": Kenneth A. Lachlan et al., "COVID-19
Echo Chambers: Examining the Impact of Conservative and Liberal News Sources
on Risk Perception and Response," *Health Security* 19, no. 1 (2021): 21–30.

"Systematic review of risk perceptions": Sabrina Cipolletta et al., "Risk Perception
towards COVID-19: A Systematic Review and Qualitative Synthesis," *International
Journal of Environmental Research and Public Health* 19, no. 8 (2022): 4649.

Page 163 victimhood culture: Bradley Campbell and Jason Manning, "Microaggression and Moral Cultures," "Microaggression and Moral Cultures," *Comparative
Sociology* 13, no. 6 (2014): 692–726; Conor Friedersdorf, "The Rise of Victimhood
Culture," *Atlantic*, September 11, 2015, https://www.theatlantic.com/politics/archive
/2015/09/the-rise-of-victimhood-culture/404794/.

Page 164 "protective care": Berenice Fisher and Joan Tronto, "Toward a Feminist Theory of Caring," in Emily K. Abel and Margaret K. Nelson, eds., *Circles of Care: Work and Identity in Women's Lives* (Albany: State University of New York Press, 1990), 35–62; Ethics of Care (website), interview with Joan Tronto, October 16, 2009, https://ethicsofcare.org/joan-tronto/.

CHAPTER 14

Page 165 Reuters ran a story: Dan Whitcomb and Rich McKay, "Trump Calls COVID School Closures a 'Terrible Decision' as Cases and Deaths Rise," Reuters, July 14, 2020, https://www.reuters.com/article/us-health-coronavirus-usa-idCAKCN24F1Y9.

Page 165 *LA Times* ran a piece: Los Angeles Times Editorial Board, "Trump Has Zero Understanding of What It Will Take to Safely RU.S. Schools," *Los Angeles Times*, Opinion, July 8, 2020, https://www.latimes.com/opinion/story/2020-07-08 /editorial-trump-trivializes-the-challenge-facing-u-s-schools.

Page 166 July interview with the *Atlantic*: David A. Graham, "How Trump Closed Down the Schools," *Atlantic*, July 17, 2020, https://www.theatlantic.com/ideas /archive/2020/07/why-schools-cant-fully-reopen-fall/614353/.

Page 166 July 8, CNBC article: Christina Wilkie, "Trump Threatens to Cut Funding for Schools, Slams CDC Reopening Guidelines as Too Tough and Expensive," CNBC, July 8, 2020, https://www.cnbc.com/2020/07/08/coronavirus-trump-threatens-to-cut -school-funding-slams-cdc-reopening-guidelines.html.

Page 166 *Washington Post* ran a story that quoted Senator Patty Murray: Laura Meckler, "Trump Pushes and Threatens in Bid to Fully Reopen Schools," Education, *Washington Post*, July 8, 2020, https://www.washingtonpost.com/education/trump -schools-cdc-pence/2020/07/08/8a52d400-c14b-11ea-b4f6-cb39cd8940fb_story .html.

Page 166 ""President Donald Trump's new push to open schools": Stephen Collinson, "Trump Ignores Recent Calamities in His Push to Open Schools," CNN, July 8, 2020, https://www.cnn.com/2020/07/08/politics/donald-trump-schools-coronavirus -education/index.html.

Page 166 Opening schools in the fall "could be dangerous": Eric Lutz, "Trump Tries to Bully Schools into Reopening in Pandemic He's Made Worse," *Vanity Fair*, July 8, 2020, https://www.vanityfair.com/news/2020/07/trump-tries-to-bully-schools-into -reopening-in-pandemic-hes-made-worse.

Page 167 Lily Eskelsen Garcia: CBS Evening News (@CBSEveningNews), "Pres. Trump insists schools must open in the fall, saying local officials who keep them closed are doing so for political reasons," Twitter, July 7, 2020, 6:43 p.m., https://twitter.com /CBSEveningNews/status/1280633681271566338.

Page 167 too many schools are in older buildings: Cindy Long, "School Ventilation Must Be Addressed in Reopening Plans," National Education Association, August 20, 2020, https://www.nea.org/advocating-for-change/new-from-nea/school-ventilation -must-be-addressed-reopening-plans.

Page 167 Government Accountability Office report: Valerie Strauss, "More Than Half of America's Public Schools Need Major Repairs: U.S. Report," *Washington Post*, June 4, 2020, https://www.washingtonpost.com/education/2020/06/04/more-than-half -americas-public-schools-need-major-repairs-us-report/.

Page 167 *Politico* piece on July 10: Michael Stratford, Nicole Gaudiano, and Juan Perez Jr., "Trump's Campaign to Open Schools Provokes Mounting Backlash Even from GOP," *Politico*, July 10, 2020, https://www.politico.com/news/2020/07/10 /trump-schools-backlash-coronavirus-356721.

Page 167 centered on teachers' fears: Steven Greenhouse, "Teachers Across the Country Worry About a Rush to Reopen Schools," *New Yorker*, August 10, 2020, https://www.newyorker.com/news/news-desk/teachers-across-the-country-worry -about-a-rush-to-reopen-schools.

Page 167 "rush" to open schools in the South: Yaryna Serkez and Stuart A. Thompson, "Should Schools in Your County Be Open?," *New York Times*, August 14, 2020, https://www.nytimes.com/interactive/2020/08/14/opinion/politics/covid-school -reopening-guidelines.html.

Page 167 July piece in the online magazine *Vox*: Anna North, "The Debate over Reopening America's K–12 Schools, Explained," *Vox*, July 10, 2020, https://www.vox .com/2020/7/10/21310099/schools-reopen-open-reopening-trump-public-covid.

Page 167 Gavin Newsom . . . tweeted: Gavin Newsom (@GavinNewsom), "In CA, science will determine when a school can be physically open—and when it must close. But learning must be non-negotiable. Schools must provide meaningful learning," Twitter, July 17, 2020, 3:48 p.m., https://twitter.com/gavinnewsom/status /1284213443457806337.

Page 168 Coverage of Newsom's policies: Jill Cowan, "Newsom Order Would Keep Most California Schools Online," *New York Times*, July 17, 2020; Lyanne Melendez and Alix Martichoux, "Gov. Newsom Announces which California School Districts Can Reopen in the Fall amid Coronavirus Crisis," ABC7 News (San Francisco), July 17, 2020, https://abc7news.com/gov-newsom-update-today-schools-california-reopen ing-covid/6321087/.

Page 168 triple-byline 2,200-word feature: Pam Belluck, Apoorva Mandavilli, and Benedict Carey, "How to Reopen Schools: What Science and Other Countries Teach Us," *New York Times*, July 11, 2020.

Page 169 Megan Ranney: Megan Ranney, MD (@meganranney), "But . . . What does it mean for the rest of us? Once #COVID19 infections start to rise, it would be foolhardy to keep schools open IRL. And we should be planning NOW," Twitter, July 31, 2020, 9:35 a.m., https://twitter.com/meganranney/status/1289192862563749889.

Page 170 from motor vehicles to drownings: There are more child deaths from drowning each year, and roughly *three times* the number of children die from motor vehicle related deaths than from Covid in a year. There were 1,184 traffic fatalities for kids age fourteen and younger in 2021: https://crashstats.nhtsa.dot.gov/Api /Public/ViewPublication/813456. Nine hundred forty-five children die each year

from drowning: https://www.childrenssafetynetwork.org/infographics/facts-childhood
-drowning. (Also see note in the introduction endnotes.)

Page 170 teachers in Sweden: The relative risk was average for teachers. Taxi and
pizza baker, page 7: Public Health Agency of Sweden, *Förekomst av covid-19 i olika
yrkesgrupper*, 2020, https://www.folkhalsomyndigheten.se/contentassets/5e248b82cc
284971a1c5fd922e7770f8/forekomst-covid-19-olika-yrkesgrupper.pdf.

Page 171 Sweden was the world's "cautionary tale": Peter S. Goodman, "Sweden Has
Become the World's Cautionary Tale," *New York Times*, Covid-19 Guidance, July 7,
2020, https://www.nytimes.com/2020/07/07/business/sweden-economy-coronavirus
.html.

Page 171 It was a "pariah": Isabella Kwai, "E.U.–China Talks, Sweden, Working From
Home: Your Tuesday Briefing," *New York Times*, June 23, 2020, https://www.nytimes
.com/2020/06/23/briefing/european-union-china-sweden-working-from-home
.html.

Page 171 "Sweden Took Its Own Path": "As Coronavirus Cases Top 3 Million, Fauci
Warns Against Misreading a Falling Death Rate," *New York Times*, July 7, 2020, https://
www.nytimes.com/2020/07/07/world/coronavirus-updates.html.

  There were two brief mentions of the Swedish data in the *Times*, both in pieces by
outside writers. One was by me, in an article on the emergence of "pod" homeschool
programs, and the other was in an opinion piece by Emily Oster, coaching people
that there will be cases in schools and that that's okay. David Zweig, "$25,000 Pod
Schools: How Well-to-Do Children Will Weather the Pandemic," *New York Times*,
New York, July 30, 2020; Emily Oster, Sweden: Emily Oster, "What Will Schools Do
When a Teacher Gets Covid-19?" *New York Times*, July 28, 2020.

Page 171 Whether schools were open or not "had no measurable direct impact":
Helena Soderpalm, "Sweden's Health Agency Says Open Schools Did Not Spur
Pandemic Spread among Children," Reuters, July 15, 2020, https://www.reuters.com
/article/us-health-coronavirus-sweden-schools/swedens-health-agency-says-open
-schools-did-not-spur-pandemic-spread-among-children-idUSKCN24G2IS; Public
Health Agency of Sweden, *Covid-19 in Schoolchildren: A Comparison between Finland
and Sweden*, 2020, https://www.folkhalsomyndigheten.se/contentassets/c1b78bffbf
de4a7899eb0d8ffdb57b09/covid-19-school-aged-children.pdf.

Page 172 Dr. Monica Gandhi: Tracy Beth Høeg, Dr. Monica Gandhi, and Lillian
Brown, "Widespread Coronavirus Testing at Schools Is a Bad Idea," *Washington Post*,
April 19, 2021, https://www.washingtonpost.com/outlook/2021/04/19/schools-covid
-testing-cost/. Ninety percent of positive results could be incorrect.

Page 174 Robert Barro's analysis of the 1918 pandemic: Robert J. Barro, "Non-
Pharmaceutical Interventions and Mortality in U.S. Cities during the Great Influenza Pandemic, 1918–1919," National Bureau of Economic Research Working Paper
Series, April 2020 (revised August 2020), https://www.nber.org/system/files/working
_papers/w27049/w27049.pdf.

Page 174 mobility data: Edouard Mathieu et al., "Coronavirus Pandemic (COVID-19)"
(2020), retrieved from https://ourworldindata.org/covid-google-mobility-trends.

Page 174 other observational studies: Amy Falk et al., "COVID-19 Cases and Transmission in 17 K–12 Schools—Wood County, Wisconsin, August 31–November 29, 2020," *Morbidity and Mortality Weekly Report* 70, no. 4 (2021): 136–140.

Page 174 he got busted for trysts: Anna Mikhailova et al., "Exclusive: Government Scientist Neil Ferguson Resigns after Breaking Lockdown Rules to Meet His Married Lover," *Telegraph*, May 5, 2020, https://www.telegraph.co.uk/news/2020/05/05/exclusive-government-scientist-neil-ferguson-resigns-breaking/.

Page 174 On the day after Thanksgiving: Aamer Madhani, "Birx Travels, Family Visits Highlight Pandemic Safety Perils," Associated Press, December 20, 2020, https://apnews.com/article/travel-pandemics-only-on-ap-delaware-thanksgiving-52810c224 88fff7e6bb70746bdc9bc61. Matthew Dessem, "Deborah Birx Traveled to Delaware to Gather with Family over Thanksgiving, Despite Her Own Guidelines," *Slate*, December 20, 2020, https://slate.com/news-and-politics/2020/12/birx-thanksgiving -delaware-gathering-guidelines-against-holiday-travel.html.

Page 175 "How 132 Epidemiologists Are Deciding": Claire Cain Miller and Margot Sanger-Katz, "How 132 Epidemiologists Are Deciding When to Send Their Children to School," *New York Times*, June 12, 2020, https://www.nytimes.com/2020/06/12 /upshot/epidemiologists-decisions-children-school-coronavirus.html.

Page 177 epidemiologists described themselves as risk averse: Claire Cain Miller, Kevin Quealy, and Margot Sanger-Katz, "Hundreds of Epidemiologists Expected Mask-Wearing in Public for at Least a Year," *New York Times*, May 13, 2021, https:// www.nytimes.com/2021/05/13/upshot/epidemiologists-coronavirus-masks.html.

Page 177 Perencevich wrote a strange and detailed post: Eli Perencevich, "Preventing Norovirus Transmission in Your Home," Controversies in Hospital Infection Prevention (blog), April 10, 2013, https://haicontroversies.blogspot.com/2013/04 /preventing-norovirus-transmission-in.html.

Page 177 Eleanor Murray: Dr. Ellie Murray, ScD (@EpiEllie), "I am so so worried for all the young children in my life." Twitter, August 15, 2021, 10:24a.m., https://twitter .com/EpiEllie/status/1426912674584178693; Dr. Ellie Murray, ScD (@EpiEllie), "Boston-area friends: If you live in Boston, Brookline, or Chelsea, your local health department director could really use a call or email from you encouraging them to have schools keep masks on till summer," Twitter, June 12, 2022, 4:34 p.m., https:// twitter.com/EpiEllie/status/1536084495845232643?s=20; Dr. Ellie Murray, ScD (@ EpiEllie), "Genuine q for ppl more concerned about schools being closed than covid: are you aware mandatory schooling is barely a century old in this country?" Twitter, August 21, 2021, 2:59 p.m., https://twitter.com/EpiEllie/status/1429156161614405 634?s=20.

DEEP DIVE: IT'S "BASIC PHYSICS"—MITIGATION MISINFORMATION AND THE CASE OF HEPA FILTERS

Page 180 Claims about mask mandates being necessary and beneficial: The evidence base on school masking is highly contentious. The one indisputable claim is that the evidence is—*at best*—mixed. There were zero randomized trials of school masking. And of the remaining lower- quality studies, for every one that purported to show a benefit there was another that showed no benefit. When the evidence is this weak, it is impossible to claim, as so many officials and health professionals did, with any honesty that school mask mandates were clearly beneficial. David Zweig, "The Science of Masking Kids at School Remains Uncertain," *New York*, August 20, 2021, https://nymag.com/intelligencer/2021/08/the-science-of-masking-kids-at-school-remains-uncertain.html. "The Case Against Masks at School," Smelkinson et al., *Atlantic*, January 26, 2022, https://www.theatlantic.com/ideas/archive/2022/01/kids-masks-schools-weak-science/621133/.

Page 183 on German kindergartens: Falkenberg et al., "Effect of portable HEPA filters on COVID-19 period prevalence: an observational quasi-interventional study in German kindergartens," *BMJ Open* 13 (2023): e072284.

Page 183 the other study, published by the CDC: Jenna Gettings et al., "Mask Use and Ventilation Improvements to Reduce COVID-19 Incidence in Elementary Schools —Georgia, November 16–December 11, 2020," *Morbidity and Mortality Weekly Report* 70, no. 21 (2021): 779–784.

Page 183 convalescent plasma failed to yield any benefits: Nick Paul Taylor, "Convalescent Plasma Fails Phase 2 in Moderate COVID-19 Patients," Fierce Biotech (website), October 23, 2020, https://www.fiercebiotech.com/biotech/convalescent-plasma-fails-phase-2-moderate-covid-19-patients.

"Failed in high-risk outpatients": US Department of Health and Human Services, National Institutes of Health, "NIH Study Shows No Significant Benefit of Convalescent Plasma for COVID-19 Outpatients with Early Symptoms," news release, August 18, 2021, https://www.nih.gov/news-events/news-releases/nih-study-shows-no-significant-benefit-convalescent-plasma-covid-19-outpatients-early-symptoms.

"Failed to reduce mortality": "Trial Finds Limited Effectiveness of Convalescent Plasma for Covid-19 Patients," *BMJ*, October 23, 2020, https://www.bmj.com/company/newsroom/trial-finds-limited-effectiveness-of-convalescent-plasma-for-covid-19-patients/.

"Risks": US Food & Drug Administration, "Emergency Use Authorization (Eua) of Covid-19 Convalescent Plasma for Treatment of Coronavirus Disease 2019 (Covid-19)," EUA Fact Sheet for Patients, December 28, 2021, https://www.fda.gov/media/141479/download.

"May help some people": NYU Langone Health (website), "New Study Validates Benefits of Convalescent Plasma for Some Patients with COVID-19," press release, January 25, 2022, https://nyulangone.org/news/new-study-validates-benefits-convalescent-plasma-some-patients-covid-19.

Page 184 Dr. H. Clifford Lane: Rita Rubin, "Testing an Old Therapy Against a New Disease: Convalescent Plasma for COVID-19," *JAMA* 323, no. 21 (2020): 2114–2117.

Page 185 Dr. Vinay Prasad: Vinay Prasad, "What Happens When Cases Go Up?" February 10, 2022, Vinay Prasad's Observations and Thoughts (Substack newsletter), https://vinayprasadmdmph.substack.com/p/what-happens-when-cases-go-up. Vinay Prasad, "It's the Compulsion that Needs to Be Restricted," Brownstone Institute

(website), February 26, 2022, https://brownstone.org/articles/its-the-compulsion-that
-needs-to-be-restricted/.

Page 186 windows that didn't open or no windows: Valerie Strauss, "Congress Urged
to Provide Billions of Dollars to Fix Crumbling School Buildings that Pose Threat to
Safety," *Washington Post*, Answer Sheet, July 22, 2020, https://www.washingtonpost
.com/education/2020/07/22/congress-urged-provide-billions-dollars-fix-crumbling
-school-buildings-that-pose-threat-safety/; Andrea Michelson, "A Simulation of
Coronavirus Spread in a Classroom Found Kids in the Back Corners Were Safest.
Here's Why," *Business Insider*, October 20, 2020, https://www.businessinsider.com
/classroom-covid-simulation-kids-back-corner-safest-exposure-2020-10. Alvin Powell,
"Is Go-Slow Schools' Reopening Failing kKids?" *Harvard Gazette*, October 14, 2020,
https://news.harvard.edu/gazette/story/2020/10/is-the-slow-approach-to-reopening
-schools-failing-kids/; Dale Mezzacappa, Emily Rizzo, and Neena Hagen, "Just One-
Third of Elementary Classrooms in Philly Meet Minimum Ventilation Standards,"
WHYY/NPR (Philadelphia, PA), October 29, 2020, https://whyy.org/articles/philly
-parents-asked-to-make-school-return-decision-with-incomplete-confusing-info/; Zoë
Kirsch, "Exclusive: NYC Teachers Union Launches Its Own Investigation of School
Building Air Quality amid COVID Threat, UFT President Says," The 74 (website),
August 5, 2020, https://www.the74million.org/article/exclusive-nyc-teachers-union
-launches-its-own-investigation-of-school-building-air-quality-amid-covid-threat
-uft-president-says/; Sydney Leahy and Ashika Srivastava, "DeKalb's Reopening Plan:
Is It Worth the Risk?," *Blue & Gold* (official newspaper of Chamblee High School,
Chamblee, GA) October 18, 2020, https://chambleeblueandgold.com/8719/news
/dekalbs-reopening-plan-is-it-worth-the-risk/.

Page 186 Randi Weingarten: Randi Weingarten (@rweingarten), "And what if you're
in a classroom without windows? What if the windows aren't able to be opened?
This is why schools need the resources to update their ventilation," Twitter, February
27, 2021, 6:50 p.m., https://twitter.com/rweingarten/status/1365811525466935304;
Randi Weingarten (@rweingarten), "In some schools the windows are painted shut,
they don't have ventilation, they don't have money for soap. We have to make
sure those are safe, with the safeguards," Twitter, February 15, 2021, 9:42 a.m.,
https://twitter.com/rweingarten/status/1361325031645667329; Randi Weingarten
(@rweingarten), "This is unacceptable. 'Our rooms are tiny, the windows, there's
ventilation issues. Also just with our bathroom situation, there are older bathrooms,
not a lot,'" Twitter, July 15, 2020, 11:21 p.m., https://twitter.com/rweingarten
/status/1283602728921575424.

Page 186 state and local laws typically require . . . ventilation: New York City Department of Education (website), "School Building Ventilation Status," accessed April
26, 2024, https://www.schools.nyc.gov/school-life/space-and-facilities/space-and
-facilities-reports/building-ventilation-status.

Page 186 In New York City . . . if a classroom does not have windows: Annalise
Knudson, "Coronavirus: How to Find Ventilation Inspection Results for Your Child's
School," SILive.com, September 9, 2020, https://www.silive.com/coronavirus/2020

/09/coronavirus-how-to-find-ventilation-inspection-results-for-your-childs-school
.html.

Page 187 96 percent of its classrooms: NBC New York, "96% of NYC School Buildings Pass Ventilation Inspection; See the Ones That Haven't," September 7, 2020,
https://www.nbcnewyork.com/news/local/doe-identifies-10-school-buildings-lack
ing-proper-ventilation-ahead-of-start-date/2605169/.

Page 187 Johns Hopkins School Ventilation Report: Paula J. Olsiewski et al., *School
Ventilation: A Vital Tool to Reduce COVID-19 Spread* (Baltimore, MD: Johns Hopkins
Center for Health Security, 2021), https://centerforhealthsecurity.org/sites/default
/files/2023-02/20210526-school-ventilation.pdf.

Page 188 Government Accountability Office report: "School Districts Frequently
Identified Multiple Building Systems Needing Updates or Replacement," June 2020.

Page 189 a systematic review of studies of air filtration: Mousavi et al., "COVID-19
Outbreak and Hospital Air Quality: A Systematic Review of Evidence on Air Filtration and Recirculation," *Environmental Science & Technology* 55, no. 7 (2020).

Page 190 The MMWR study: Jenna Gettings et al., "Mask Use and Ventilation
Improvements to Reduce COVID-19 Incidence in Elementary Schools—Georgia,
November 16–December 11, 2020," *Morbidity and Mortality Weekly Report* 70, no. 21
(2021): 779–784.

Page 190 a study in the *Lancet*: Lotte Jonker et al., "SARS-CoV-2 Incidence in Secondary Schools; the Role of National and School-Initiated COVID-19 Measures," *BMC
Public Health* 23, 1243 (2023).

Page 190 "School systems should use . . . ultraviolet": US National Institute for
Occupational Safety and Health, *Environmental Control for Tuberculosis: Basic Upper-
Room Ultraviolet Germicidal Irradiation Guidelines for Healthcare Settings*, March 2009,
https://www.cdc.gov/niosh/docs/2009-105/default.html.

Page 191 take a daily low-dose aspirin: Allison Aubrey and Will Stone, "Older Adults
Shouldn't Start a Routine of Daily Aspirin, Task Force Says," NPR, April 26, 2022,
https://www.npr.org/sections/health-shots/2022/04/26/1094881056/older-adults
-shouldnt-start-a-routine-of-daily-aspirin-task-force-says.

Page 192 what about peer review: Julia Belluz and Steven Hoffman, "Let's Stop Pre-
tending Peer Review Works," *Vox*, December 7, 2015, https://www.vox.com/2015/12
/7/9865086/peer-review-science-problems; Adam Mastroianni, "The Rise and Fall of
Peer Review," *Experimental History*, December 13, 2022, https://www.experimental
-history.com/p/the-rise-and-fall-of-peer-review; Richard Smith, "Peer Review: A
Flawed Process at the Heart of Science and Journals," *Journal of the Royal Society of
Medicine* 99, no. 4 (2006): 178–182, https://www.ncbi.nlm.nih.gov/pmc/articles
/PMC1420798/.

CHAPTER 15

Page 195 open schools in Sweden: Stefan Baral, Rebecca Chandler, Ruth Gil Prieto,
Sunetra Gupta, Sharmistha Mishra, and Martin Kulldorff, "Leveraging Epidemiological

Principles to Evaluate Sweden's COVID-19 Response," *Annals of Epidemiology*, February 2021 (online November 2020).

Page 196 *Emmaus* was a fake: Edward Dolnick, *The Forger's Spell: A True Story of Vermeer, Nazis, and the Greatest Art Hoax of the Twentieth Century* (New York: Harper/ HarperCollins Publishers, 2008). I'd like to thank Zac Bissonnette for bringing the Vermeer forgeries story to my attention.

Page 197 Dr. Bernard Fisher questioned: Jo Cavallo, "Dr. Bernard Fisher's Breast Cancer Research Left a Lasting Legacy of Improved Therapeutic Efficacy and Survival," *ASCO Post*, May 15, 2013, https://ascopost.com/issues/may-15-2013/dr-bernard -fishers-breast-cancer-research-left-a-lasting-legacy-of-improved-therapeutic-efficacy -and-survival.aspx.

Page 197 Fisher forged ahead: Susan Okie, "Treating Breast Cancer," *Washington Post*, Politics, October 29, 1979, https://www.washingtonpost.com/archive/politics /1979/10/29/treating-breast-cancer/4a2cf642-ffe9-438c-ae05-12e34db634da/.

Page 199 Collective delusions are as old as time: Emile Durkheim, *The Elementary Forms of the Religious Life*, trans. Joseph Ward Swain (London: George Allen & Unwin, 1915; Project Gutenberg, 2012).

Page 199 effect on in-group cohesion: James Brooks et al., "Uniting against a Common Enemy: Perceived Outgroup Threat Elicits Ingroup Cohesion in Chimpanzees," *PLOS ONE* 16, no. 2 (2021): e0246869.

Page 199 Jonathan Haidt: Coleman Hughes host, "The Death of Conversation with Jonathan Haidt," *Conversations with Coleman* (podcast), June 25, 2022.

Page 200 "Dr. Mehmet Oz": Frank Bruni, "The Unholy Alliance of Trump and Dr. Oz," *New York Times*, Opinion, April 8, 2020, https://www.nytimes.com/2020/04/08 /opinion/coronavirus-trump-dr-oz.html; Noah Weiland and Maggie Haberman, "Oracle Providing White House with Software to Study Unproven Coronavirus Drugs," *New York Times*, United States, Covid-19 Guidance, March 24, 2020, https://www .nytimes.com/2020/03/24/us/politics/trump-oracle-coronavirus-chloroquine.html.

Page 200 "April 15 interview on FOX": Paul Rudnick (@PaulRudnickNY), "On Fox Dr. Oz called re-opening schools 'an appetizing opportunity' with a death rate of only '2 to 3 percent.' He was later seen hanging upside down from a tree," Twitter, April 16, 2020, 12:21 p.m., https://twitter.com/PaulRudnickNY/status/125082171543909 5808; Randi Weingarten (@rweingarten), "I am wondering if Dr Oz would say this if it was his own kids were part of the 2–3%. . . . How morally outrageous of someone who says he is a doctor. . . . ," Twitter, April 16, 2020, 4:48 p.m., https://twitter .com/rweingarten/status/1250888941047287810; Soledad O'Brien (@soledadobrien), "Well, holy shit. This clip from Dr. Oz is insane: 'Schools are a very appetizing opportunity . . . the opening of schools might only cost us 2-to-3 percent. . . .'" Twitter, April 16, 2020, 11:34 a.m., https://twitter.com/soledadobrien/status/125080 9759382544386.

Page 201 nice piece in the *Lancet*: Russell M. Viner et al., "School Closure and Management Practices during Coronavirus Outbreaks including COVID-19: A Rapid Systematic Review," *Lancet* 4, no. 5 (2020): 397–404.

Page 201 Report 9 from Imperial College London: Neil M. Ferguson et al., "Report 9: Impact of Non-Pharmaceutical Interventions (NPIs) to Reduce COVID-19 Mortality and Healthcare Demand," Imperial College London, March 16, 2020.

Page 202 "Betsy DeVos today said 'only' .02% of kids are likely to die": James Scott #TeamOrca (@LongerTables), "So, Betsy Devos today said 'only' .02% of kids are likely to die when they go back to school. That's 14,740 children. Welcome back!" Twitter, July 11, 2020, 9:20 p.m., https://twitter.com/Jscott1145/status/1282122 551481774081. 14,740Kim LaCapria, "Did Betsy DeVos Say 'Only .02 Percent' of Students Would Die if Schools Reopened?," Truth Or Fiction? (website), July 13, 2020, https://www.truthorfiction.com/did-betsy-devos-say-only-02-percent-of-students -would-die-if-schools-reopened/; Kurt Eichenwald (@kurteichenwald), "See these kids & teachers murdered at Sandy Hook? Multiply that by 500. That number— 14,000 children—is the number @BetsyDeVosED said was acceptable loss," Twitter, July 12, 2020, 6:07 p.m., https://twitter.com/kurteichenwald/status/1282436547707 654146.

Page 202 "We know the mortality rate in [people] under 25": @tiyenin, "Dr. Birx Claims 0.1% Coronavirus Mortality among Youth," July 12, 2020, YouTube video, 0:36, https://www.youtube.com/watch?v=kQJjnvp-Fwg.

Page 202 What the title didn't explain: Eileen Sullivan and Erica L. Green, "As Trump Demanded Schools Reopen, His Experts Warned of 'Highest Risk,'" New York Times, July 10, 2020. Centers for Disease Control and Prevention Community Interventions and Critical Populations Task Force, CRAFT Schools Briefing Packet, July 8, 2019, accessed via New York Times, January 2, 2024, https://int.nyt.com/data /documenthelper/7072-school-reopening-packet/b70172f2cc13c9cf0e6a/optimized /full.pdf#page=1.

Page 203 Nancy Pelosi said on CNN: CNN Politics (@CNNPolitics), "House Speaker Nancy Pelosi says the Trump administration's push to restart in-person learning in schools is 'messing with the health of our children,'" Twitter, July 12, 2020, 9:47 a.m., https://twitter.com/cnnpolitics/status/1282310493361905664?s=21.

Page 203 Biden campaign ran numerous ads: Democratic National Committee, @ TheDemocrats, "This Is Not a Test," YouTube, July 27, 2020, video, 00:58, https:// www.youtube.com/watch?v=I8FuY1RbfD4.

Page 204 "We must protect our children": MeidasTouch (@MeidasTouch), "NEW VIDEO Trump is pushing to reopen our schools. Who is pushing to protect our children? The only ones that are coming to save us are us. We need 4,300 retweets," Twitter, July 17, 2020, 8:00 p.m., https://twitter.com/MeidasTouch/status/128427690 5894502401.

CHAPTER 16

Page 206 Leana Wen: Leana Wen (@DrLeanaWen), "This is an important study as we think about how to safely reopen schools. Children <10 years old were about half as likely as adults to spread #covid19," Twitter, July 20, 2020, 10:32 a.m., https:// twitter.com/DrLeanaWen/status/1285221109923749888.

Page 206 Randi Weingarten . . . tweeted the article: Randi Weingarten (@rweingar-ten), "We cannot afford for state leaders to act like school age kids are not getting sick themselves or that they cannot be super spreaders," Twitter, July 20, 2020, 6:08 p.m., https://twitter.com/rweingarten/status/1285335855406686208.

Page 206 At least one school district: Nick Foy (@TheNickFoy), "It wasn't just par-ents. Our school board had initially approved some in-person teaching, but shifted to all remote after that @apoorva_nyc article. Of course," Twitter, August 11, 2020, 8:26 a.m., https://twitter.com/TheNickFoy/status/1293161745889075205. Emails from Foy also confirm this.

Page 206 South Korea study: Apoorva Mandavilli, "Older Children Spread the Coronavirus Just as Much as Adults, Large Study Finds," *New York Times*, July 18, 2020.

Page 206 Yet the study came under immediate criticism: Zeynep Tufekci (@zeynep), "I'm aware of similar: kids as young as 10 that were set to have in-person interaction with resources and protections (including outdoors) are now online-only," Twitter, August 11, 2020, 8:37 a.m., https://twitter.com/zeynep/status/129316466215929 8562; Jonas Ludvigsson (@ludvigsson), "1/7. A South Korean study of 65,000 people is said to show that Children (aged 10–19 years) spread the #coronavirus #COVID19 just as Much as adults. This is," Twitter, July 21, 2020, 12:25 p.m., https://twitter .com/ludvigsson/status/1285611882603253763; Jieun Kim, et al., "Role of Children in Household Transmission of COVID-19," *Archives of Disease in Childhood* 106, no. 7 (2021): 709–711.

Page 206 Dr. Alasdair Munro: Alasdair Munro (@apsmunro), "A very interesting study here from South Korea, doing widespread contact tracing to give us a huge data set on secondary attack rates (SAR) for #COVID19 from," Twitter, July 19, 2020, 6:17 a.m., https://twitter.com/apsmunro/status/1284794506265722881. "A few weeks ago a study from SK got lots of attention for reportedly showed children aged 10–19 were just as, or more infectious than adults with #COVID19 But that was not the whole story," Twitter, August 10, 2020, 11:55 a.m., https://twitter.com/apsmunro /status/1292852036720091136.

Page 207 "Joseph Allen": Joseph Allen (@j_g_allen), "THREAD This study is going around top scientists. I have diff interpretation: The 2nd col in Table 2 is 'non-household' contacts, which would be the data to apply," Twitter, July 19, 2020, 5:44 a.m., https://twitter.com/j_g_allen/status/1284786278094053378.

Page 207 Zeynep Tufekci: Zeynep Tufekci (@zeynep), "A really important thread on that South Korea/kids study that got widespread coverage that, in my view, was not warranted because even without extra info, its statistics," Twitter, August 11, 2020, 7:49 a.m., https://twitter.com/zeynep/status/1293152552012349441.

Page 207 "widespread coverage": The *Times* coverage, along with other news stories on the South Korea study, was posted multiple times in my small town's parent Facebook group, eliciting panicked comments. It was one of many instances in which I observed national patterns personally, on the local level.

Page 207 Dr. Muge Cevik: Muge Cevik (@mugecevik), "I hope some scientists will give up citing this paper to support their preconceived opinions about children. This nyt article sadly created a lot of social media traction," Twitter, August 15, 2020, 11:12 a.m., https://twitter.com/mugecevik/status/1294653076243132417.

Page 207 "the rushed, sensational reporting around it": Zeynep Tufekci (@zeynep), "This study, and the rushed, sensational reporting around it, more than almost any other, single-handedly caused so many schools who were equipped and ready to shut," Twitter, August 15, 2020, 11:52 a.m., https://twitter.com/zeynep/status/1294 663269085577216.

Page 208 dead bodies lying in the streets of Wuhan: Agence France-Presse, "A Man Lies Dead in the Street: The Image that Captures the Wuhan Coronavirus Crisis," *Guardian*, January 31, 2020, https://www.theguardian.com/world/2020/jan/31/a -man-lies-dead-in-the-street-the-image-that-captures-the-wuhan-coronavirus-crisis.

Page 209 Georgia summer camp: Christine M. Szablewski et al., "SARS-CoV-2 Transmission and Infection among Attendees of an Overnight Camp—Georgia, June 2020," *Morbidity and Mortality Weekly Report* 69, no. 31 (2020): 1023–1025; Roni Caryn Rabin, "The Coronavirus Infected Hundreds at a Georgia Summer Camp," *New York Times*, July 31, 2020, https://www.nytimes.com/2020/07/31/health/coro navirus-children-camp.html; Chelsea Janes, "Report: Coronavirus Infected Scores of Children and Staff at Georgia Sleep-Away Camp," *Washington Post*, July 31, 2020, https://www.washingtonpost.com/health/2020/07/31/georgia-children-covid-out break/; Ally Mauch, "260 Kids and Staff Test Positive for Coronavirus at Georgia Overnight Camp, CDC Says," *People*, August 1, 2020, https://people.com/health/260 -kids-staff-test-positive-coronavirus-at-georgia-overnight-camp-cdc/; Marsha Vivi-nate (@marsha_vivinate), "260 Children and Staff Test Positive for COVID at Georgia Overnight Camp. 231 under 17 years old. Dr. Blackstock advises that children shouldn't return to school," Twitter, July 31, 2020, 7:33 p.m., https://twitter.com /marsha_vivinate/status/1289343503756009472; The ReidOut (@thereidout), "Right now, going to school shouldn't be an option for students and families. @uche_black-stock on #TheReidOut," Twitter, July 31, 2020, 7:10 p.m., https://twitter.com/there idout/status/1289337717395005448; CNN (@CNN), "A coronavirus outbreak at a Georgia sleep-away camp this June could have implications for school reopening, the US Centers for Disease Control and Prevention says," Twitter, July 31, 2020, 7:45 p.m., https://twitter.com/CNN/status/1289346507611742209; Chris Lu (@ ChrisLu44), "This is an ominous sign for schools in the fall: 597 children and staff attended an overnight camp in Georgia. 76% of the attendees who were tested came back," Twitter, July 31, 2020, 5:10 p.m., https://twitter.com/ChrisLu44/status/1289 307551142572032.

Page 210 "case of the missing denominator": Karen Vaites, a prominent activist for opening schools, may have been the first person to start using this phrase. Alexan-der Russo (@alexanderrusso), "Where's the context in this NYT survey? Where are the denominators? There's precious little provided. It's little more than raw numbers and seems designed to fan," Twitter, August 26, 2020, 11:37 a.m., https://twitter

.com/alexanderrusso/status/1298645809978892290; Karen Vaites (@karenvaites), "Today's Case of the Missing Denominator comes to us care of @SusanBEdelman and @MelissaKleinNYP, with this piece on the 'significant spike' in NYC schools," Twitter, October 10, 2020, 8:17 p.m., https://twitter.com/karenvaites/status/13150 84134247735298. "Friends, we have another Case of the Missing Denominator! In @ FeliciaGans's @BostonGlobe story on cases in MA schools—a story which is otherwise quite good," Twitter, October 12, 2020, 6:37 p.m., https://twitter.com/karen vaites/status/1315783705336705024.

Page 210 Emily Oster: https://docs.google.com/spreadsheets/d/1e4RGnqt5j7dOqn2 uo7lsf97g-8UP0-Z-fLTSngBwvRs/edit#gid=1949603537.

Page 211 The trend of these articles: Isabel Kershner and Pam Belluck, "When Covid Subsided, Israel Reopened Its Schools. It Didn't Go Well.," *New York Times*, August 4, 2020. Noga Tarnopolsky, "Israeli Data Show School Openings Were a Disaster That Wiped Out Lockdown Gains," *Daily Beast*, July 14, 2020, https://www.thedailybeast .com/israeli-data-show-school-openings-were-a-disaster-that-wiped-out-lockdown -gains.

Page 211 politicians, a torrent of journalists, and . . . Weingarten: Randi Weingarten (@rweingarten), "Israel thought it beat #covid, (unlike in the US) then it opened schools the way Trump wants. It failed, the virus spread & now they are starting slow," Twitter, August 4, 2020, 6:29 p.m., https://twitter.com/rweingarten/status /1290776893982220288; Steve Glazer (@Steve_Glazer), "Important lesson via @NY Times https://t.co/flzwiwxhl7," Twitter, August 4, 2020, 8:10 p.m., https://twitter .com/Steve_Glazer/status/1290802342086893568.

Page 211 3 million children under the age of eighteen: State of Israel, Central Bureau of Statistics, "Selected Data for the International Child Day 2020," media release, November 18, 2020, https://www.cbs.gov.il/en/mediarelease/Pages/2020/Selected -Data-for-the-International-Child-Day-2020.aspx.

Page 211 261 students and faculty were infected: Dov Lieber, "Israel Shuts Some Schools as Coronavirus Cases Jump After Reopening," *Wall Street Journal*, June 3, 2020.

Page 212 Malls, markets, restaurants, bars, and beauty parlors all opened: TOI Staff, "Let's Shop! Israelis Head to Malls, Markets and Gyms after Six Weeks of Closure," *Times of Israel*, May 7, 2020, https://www.timesofisrael.com/israelis-head-to-malls -markets-and-gyms-after-six-weeks-of-closure/.

Page 212 "Israelis Fear Schools Reopened Too Soon": Felicia Schwartz, "Israelis Fear Schools Reopened Too Soon as Covid-19 Cases Climb," *Wall Street Journal*, July 14, 2020.

Page 212 Paul Krugman: Paul Krugman (@paulkrugman), "One of the defining features of the US Covid debacle has been refusal to learn from other countries. Now, as much of the country prepares to open schools, we should," August 1, 2020, 7:01 a.m., https://twitter.com/paulkrugman/status/1289516593374875650.

Page 214 Florida, . . . like the rest of America: Worldometer (website), "California," accessed January 4, 2024, https://www.worldometers.info/coronavirus/usa

/california/; "Florida," accessed January 4, 2024, https://www.worldometers.info /coronavirus/usa/florida/.

Page 215 "argument from authority": Philosopher Gary Curtis explains that Locke did not overtly call *ad verecundiam* a fallacy, but that Locke wrote that only *ad judicium*, "of all the four, brings true instruction with it, and advances us in our way to knowledge." "Thus, at the very least, *ad verecundiam* and the other two were viewed by Locke as inferior types of argument," Curtis writes. "*Argumentum Ad Verecundiam* (Argument from Authority)," Lander University (Greenwood, SC) Philosophy Department, https://philosophy.lander.edu/logic/authority.html. Jean Goodwin, "Forms of Authority and the Real Argumentum Ad Verecundiam," OSSA Conference Archive (1997).

Page 216 their skepticism all but vanished: Over time, questioning of statements and policies from Fauci et al. and public health institutions increased among the legacy media, particularly on matters in which emerging facts overtly conflicted with the authorities' stance, making the discordance impossible to ignore. (One example was reports from the FBI and Department of Energy that called into question Fauci's generally dismissive position on the possibility that the pandemic may have begun as a lab leak.)

Page 216 Georgia as the vilified failure: Richard Fausset, "1,193 Quarantined for Covid. Is This a Successful School Reopening?," *New York Times*, August 12, 2020.

Page 217 other counties . . . had not opened schools: Georgia Department of Audits and Accounts, Performance Audit Division, "COVID-19's Impact on K–12 Education," Performance Audit–Report No. 21-03, November 2021, https://www.audits.ga .gov/ReportSearch/download/27408.

Page 217 story that journalists wanted to tell: Katie Shepherd, "Teachers Returned to a Georgia School District Last Week. 260 Employees Have Already Gone Home to Quarantine," *Washington Post*, August 4, 2020, https://www.washingtonpost.com /nation/2020/08/04/school-outbreaks-reopening-georgia/.

Page 218 Mull doubled down: Amanda Mull, "America's Authoritarian Governor," *Atlantic*, August 8, 2020, https://www.theatlantic.com/health/archive/2020/08 /georgia-brian-kemp-authoritarian/615010/.

Page 219 Donald Campbell: Donald T. Campbell, "Assessing the Impact of Planned Social Change," *Evaluation and Program Planning* 2 (1979): 67–90; Wikipedia, "Campbell's Law," last edited September 8, 2023 (accessed January 2, 2024), https:// en.wikipedia.org/wiki/Campbell%27s_law; Explified (@Explified), "Campbell's Law Explained," July 4, 2020, YouTube video, 5:15, https://youtu.be/xlm_cQwc-9M.

Page 219 surrogate "endpoint": Thomas R. Fleming, "Surrogate Endpoints in Clinical Trials," *Drug Information Journal* 30, no. 2 (1996): 315–591. Surrogate endpoints do not "provide compelling or definitive evidence about the treatment's effect on clinical efficacy measures."

More on surrogate endpoints: Thomas Robert Weihrauch and Pierre Demol, "The Value of Surrogate Endpoints for Evaluation of Therapeutic Efficacy," *Drug Information Journal* 32, no. 3 (1998): 737–743.

Page 220 Georgia Department of Health data: Covid-19 in Georgia (website), "Covid Positive Hospitalizations (regardless of reason for admission)" (graph), accessed January 2, 2024, https://www.covid-georgia.com/state-data/hospitalizations/.

Page 220 The outbreak did not result in one hospitalization: Chen Stein-Zamir et al., "A Large COVID-19 Outbreak in a High School 10 Days after Schools' Reopening, Israel, May 2020," *Eurosurveillance* 25, no. 29 (2020): pii=2001352.

The *Times* piece said that, according to the principal, a few teachers were hospitalized. But this contradicts the official report on the outbreak published in the medical journal.

One final point about the Israeli school outbreak: It appeared that some students attended school while they were symptomatic. On Twitter, Dr. Muge Cevik, a specialist in infectious diseases and virology at the University of St. Andrews, in Scotland, flagged this detail before the *Times* piece ran. This suggested that a portion of the outbreak, perhaps significantly so, was because people went to school with symptoms. There was no basis to suggest that it was a lack of masks, rather than symptomatically ill people gathering together, that was the prime driver of the outbreak. The classic advice, "if you're sick stay home," which Swedish schools followed, very well may be the most effective mitigation of all. (This doesn't mean people without symptoms can't also transmit the virus, but keeping symptomatic people at home may have far more impact than other interventions. See endnote in chapter 8 on this point.) Rather than the absence of a mask requirement as the emphasized takeaway from the story, the fact that kids attended school with symptoms would have been the more instructive lesson to use as the lede.

Page 221 A quarter of adult New York City residents: Preeti Pathela et al., "Seroprevalence of Severe Acute Respiratory Syndrome Coronavirus 2 Following the Largest Initial Epidemic Wave in the United States: Findings From New York City, 13 May to 21 July 2020," *Journal of Infectious Diseases* 224, no. 2 (2021): 196–206.

Page 221 Black and Hispanic adults were at greater than a 30 percent infection rate: See fig. 1c in Jefferson M. Jones et al., "Updated US Infection- and Vaccine-Induced SARS-CoV-2 Seroprevalence Estimates Based on Blood Donations, July 2020-December 2021," *JAMA* 328, no. 3 (2022): 298–301.

CHAPTER 17

Page 223 5% or lower: CNBC Television, "N.Y. Gov. Andrew Cuomo on Reopening Schools: We're Not Going to Use Our Children as Guinea Pigs," July 13, 2020, YouTube video, 7:52, https://www.youtube.com/watch?v=pIkQpHpMElg; Roni Caryn Rabin and Apoorva Mandavilli, "New York Is Positioned to Reopen Schools Safely, Health Experts Say," *New York Times*, August 7, 2020; Johns Hopkins University of Medicine, Coronavirus Resource Center (website), "Which U.S. States Meet WHO Recommended Testing Criteria?" last updated September 14, 2022, https://coronavirus.jhu.edu/testing/testing-positivity.

On May 12, 2020, WHO advised that before reopening, rates of positivity in testing should be 5 percent or lower for at least 14 days.

Page 224 5 percent threshold: David Dowdy and Gypsyamber D'Souza, "COVID-19 Testing: Understanding the 'Percent Positive,'" Johns Hopkins Bloomberg School of Public Health (website), August 10, 2020, https://publichealth.jhu.edu/2020/covid -19-testing-understanding-the-percent-positive.

Page 224 "infection rate": Steven J. Phipps et al., "Robust Estimates of the True (Population) Infection Rate for COVID-19: A Backcasting Approach," *Royal Society Open Science* 7, no. 11 (2020): 200909; Charles F. Manski and Francesca Molinari, "Estimating the COVID-19 Infection Rate: Anatomy of an Inference Problem," *Journal of Econometrics* 220, no. 1 (2021): 181–192; "States Ranked by COVID-19 Test Positivity Rates," Becker's Clinical Leadership (website), last updated December 15, 2022, https://www.beckershospitalreview.com/public-health/states-ranked-by-covid -19-test-positivity-rates-july-14.html.

Page 224 Jerome Adams: David K. Li and Caitlin Fichtel, "NYC Schools to Close as City Reaches 3 Percent Test Positivity Threshold," *NBC News*, November 18, 2020, https://www.nbcnews.com/news/us-news/nyc-schools-close-city-reaches-3-percent -test-positivity-threshhold-n1247899; Eliza Shapiro and Dana Rubinstein, "Did It Hit 3%? Why Parents and Teachers Are Fixated on One Number," *New York Times*, November 15, 2020. Jerome Adams, U.S. Surgeon General (@Surgeon_General), "There is no hard cutoff right now, but in general, we like to see positivity rates less than 10% in a community. There are also a number of other factors to consider," Twitter, July 24, 2020, 12:29 p.m., https://twitter.com/Surgeon_General/status/1286 700155769675776.

To make matters worse, New York State and New York City each calculated the city's percentage differently, with results more than half a percentage point apart.: Joseph Goldstein and Jesse McKinley, "New York City Hit a 3% Positive Test Rate. Or Did It?," *New York Times*, November 22, 2020.

Page 225 In Arizona the magic formula: Lauren Camera, "School Reopening Thresholds Vary Widely across the Country," *U.S. News & World Report*, August 13, 2020, https://www.usnews.com/news/education-news/articles/2020-08-13/school-reopen ing-thresholds-vary-widely-across-the-country.

Page 225 Michael Kearney: Michael Kearney, "Persuading Audiences with Statistical Evidence," ResearchGate, January 2014, https://www.researchgate.net/publication /322819700_Persuading_Audiences_with_Statistical_Evidence.

On statistical evidence being more persuasive, see E. J. Baesler and J. K. Burgoon, "The Temporal Effects of Story and Statistical Evidence on Belief Change," *Communication Research* 21, no. 5 (1994): 582–602.

Page 226 "when feasible": Centers for Disease Control and Prevention, "Considerations for Schools," updated May 19, 2020, https://web.archive.org/web/202005211 21021/https://www.cdc.gov/coronavirus/2019-ncov/community/schools-childcare /schools.html.

Page 227 the origin of six feet: Carl Flügge: Ben Guarino, "Six Feet May Not Be Enough to Protect against Coronavirus, Experts Warn," *Washington Post*, August 27, 2020, https://www.washingtonpost.com/health/2020/08/27/coronavirus-social

-distancing-6-feet/. I. Eames et al., "Airborne Transmission of Disease in Hospitals," *Journal of the Royal Society, Interface* 6, Suppl. 6 (2009): S697–702.

Page 227 Albert Ko: Sarah Qari and Pat Walters, "Dispatch 4: Six Feet," Radiolab, April 11, 2020, audio, 22:18, https://radiolab.org/episodes/dispatch-4-six-feet.

Page 227 studies of transmission on airplanes: Sonja J. Olsen et al., "Transmission of the Severe Acute Respiratory Syndrome on Aircraft," *New England Journal of Medicine* 349, no. 25 (2003): 2416–2422.

To make matters worse, even the authors of the first airplane study made a dubious claim about most transmission occurring within three rows. They wrote "the distance covered by three economy-class rows on a Boeing 737–300 is 2.3 m (90 in.)"—in other words 7.5 feet—and that "The risk to passengers was greatest if they were seated in the same row as the index patient or within three rows in front of him." However, if you look at the diagram of the plane they included in the paper, which shows the index patient and probable SARS positive cases, the distribution was very dispersed, with infected people as far as seven rows away across the aisle. There were just three probable cases in the three rows in front of the index, yet there were *four cases* clustered four and five rows in front of the index patient, and the rest were spread throughout the cabin. The data in their own paper contradicts their conclusion.

Sarah Qari, the producer on the public radio program who interviewed Albert Ko, the Yale scientist quoted in the episode, apparently did not fact-check Ko's statement. When I emailed with Ko he would only correspond with me off the record, although he indicated that his comments in the radio interview weren't just related to that one study, and he sent me a second airplane transmission study. The second study was actually a modeling paper. It contained one line related to "two rows" in front or behind an index case being the most likely zone of transmission. No data in the paper were provided to support this claim; however it had two citations of WHO documents. One document I was unable to find, and the other one, "WHO Technical Advice for Case Management of Influenza A(H1N1) in Air Transport," from 2009, said that a "close contact" was someone within two rows in front of or behind the index case. But, once again, no evidence was provided to support this metric of two rows. And, more importantly, for the purposes of this discussion, remember, two rows is not six feet. I recognize these details may seem tedious to some people, but the details matter because this supposedly is what the policy that kept tens of millions of American children out of school was based on.

Page 228 I corresponded with Ko: Modeling paper Ko sent me: Vicki Stover Hertzberg, "Behaviors, Movements, and Transmission of Droplet-Mediated Respiratory Diseases during Transcontinental Airline Flights," *PNAS* 115, no. 14 (2018): 3623–3627. WHO paper cited by the paper Ko sent: World Health Organization, "WHO Technical Advice for Case Management of Influenza A(H1N1) in Air Transport," May 13, 2009, https://infektologie.cz/Docasne/AirTransport.pdf.

Additional WHO document mentioning two rows, but with no evidence: World Health Organization, "WHO Recommended Measures for Persons Undertaking

International Travel from Areas Affected by Severe Acute Respiratory Syndrome (SARS)," *Weekly Epidemiological Record*, no. 14, April 4, 2003, 97–99.

Page 228 Scott Gottlieb: Olafimihan Oshin, "Gottlieb: 'Nobody Knows' Origins of Six-Foot Social-Distancing Recommendation," *The Hill*, September 19, 2021, https://thehill.com/homenews/sunday-talk-shows/572926-gottlieb-nobody-knows-where-six-foot-distancing-recommendation/.

"Gottlieb 'inoperable,' compromise": Graison Dangor, "CDC's Six-Foot Social Distancing Rule Was 'Arbitrary', Says Former FDA Commissioner," *Forbes*, September 19, 2021, https://www.forbes.com/sites/graisondangor/2021/09/19/cdcs-six-foot-social-distancing-rule-was-arbitrary-says-former-fda-commissioner/?sh=726598d3e8e6.

Page 228 Fauci . . . admitted: Judy Woodruff, "What Dr. Fauci Wants You to Know about Face Masks and Staying Home as Virus Spreads," PBS, April 3, 2020, https://www.pbs.org/newshour/show/what-dr-fauci-wants-you-to-know-about-face-masks-and-staying-home-as-virus-spreads#transcript. "It just sort of appeared": Select Subcommittee on the Coronavirus Pandemic (@COVIDSelect), Twitter, January 10, 2024, https://twitter.com/COVIDSelect/status/1745048323852005634. Michael Merschel, "Fauci Offers a Covid 19 Lesson and Looks to the Future," *American Heart Association News*, November 17, 2020, https://www.heart.org/en/news/2020/11/17/fauci-offers-a-covid-19-lesson-and-looks-to-the-future.

Page 228 Francis Collins: Committee on Oversight and Accountability, Select Subcommittee on the Coronavirus Pandemic, Interview of Francis Collins, MD, Friday, January 12, 2024, https://oversight.house.gov/wp-content/uploads/2024/05/Collins-Transcript-5.16-Release.pdf.

Page 228 six-foot guidance: Centers for Disease Control and Prevention, "Reopening Guidelines," https://cdn.cnn.com/cnn/2020/images/04/30/reopening.guidelines.pdf, accessed via Jacqueline Howard, Kevin Liptak, and Nick Valencia, "CDC's Draft Guidance for Reopening amid Coronavirus Includes Spaced-Out Seating in Schools, Disposable Menus in Restaurants," CNN, April 30, 2020, https://www.cnn.com/2020/04/30/health/coronavirus-usa-cdc-reopening-bn-wellness/index.html; Centers for Disease Control and Prevention, "CDC Activities and Initiatives Supporting the COVID-19 Response and the President's Plan for Opening America Up Again," May 2020, https://web.archive.org/web/20200601062531/https://www.cdc.gov/coronavirus/2019-ncov/downloads/php/CDC-Activities-Initiatives-for-COVID-19-Response.pdf; CDC, "Activities and Initiatives," May 2020.

Page 228 CDC refused to provide answers to me: In a response to my request for evidence behind the six feet of distancing guidance overall, and specifically the agency's six-foot guidance for schools, a public affairs specialist at the CDC would not answer my query and instead told me I would have to submit a public records request. So I submitted a formal Freedom of Information Act request to find out what, exactly, was discussed at the CDC in relation to its six foot guidance. I asked for records during January and February 2020 around the general six foot guidance; records from April 15 through June 1, 2020, around six feet of spacing for desks in schools; and records from May 1 to June 1, 2020 around the inclusion of the term "when feasible" for six feet of distancing to the school guidance. Six and a half weeks later I received eighty pages of internal emails, nearly all of which were redacted. One has to wonder: why did the CDC black out entire pages supposedly related to a discussion of six feet of distancing?

The only emails in the tranche that weren't redacted contained no content related to the origins of the CDC's decision to use six feet as its distancing benchmark.

Page 230 six feet . . . conferred no benefit: Joseph G. Allen and Sara Bleich, "Why Three Feet of Social Distancing Should Be Enough in Schools," *Washington Post*, November 12, 2020, https://www.washingtonpost.com/opinions/2020/11/12/three -feet-social-distancing-schools-coronavirus/.

Page 231 William Hanage: Joe Mathieu, "Harvard Epidemiologist: 'Hybrid' Model For Reopening Schools Is 'Probably Among The Worst' Options," Boston Public Radio (WGBH), July 30, 2020, https://www.wgbh.org/news/local/2020-07-30/harvard -epidemiologist-hybrid-model-for-reopening-schools-is-probably-among-the-worst -options.

Page 231 all echoed that view: David Zweig, "Hybrid Schooling May Be the Most Dangerous Option of All," *Wired*, August 6, 2020, https://www.wired.com/story /hybrid-schooling-is-the-most-dangerous-option-of-all/.

Page 231 forced to close for ten days: Melanie Grayce West, "New York City to End Rule That Closed Schools After Two Covid-19 Cases," *Wall Street Journal*, April 5, 2021.

Page 233 44 square feet rule: David Zweig, "44 Square Feet: A School-Reopening Detective Story," *Wired*, September 10, 2020, https://www.wired.com/story/44-square -feet-a-school-reopening-detective-story/.

Page 235 popularity of outdoor classes: Ginia Bellafante, "Schools Beat Earlier Plagues with Outdoor Classes. We Should, Too," *New York Times*, July 17, 2020.

Page 235 being outdoors had other long-observed benefits: North American Association for Environmental Education (website), https://naaee.org/eepro/research /library/outdoor-education-and-science-0; Andrew Bauld, "Make Outdoor Learning Your Plan A," August 18, 2021, Harvard Graduate School of Education, https://www .gse.harvard.edu/ideas/usable-knowledge/21/08/make-outdoor-learning-your-plan.

Page 237 a phenomenon I wrote about: David Zweig, "$25,000 Pod Schools: How Well-to-Do Children Will Weather the Pandemic," *New York Times*, July 30, 2020. This article initially included multiple paragraphs detailing evidence that schools did not drive transmission, including quotes from doctors, who authored a study on transmission in the journal *Pediatrics*, saying things such as "I would not want to close schools or operate at decreased capacity" just to try to maintain six feet of distancing. It will not surprise readers that the *Times* editors cut all of that content before publication.

Page 237 petition advocating for schools to open: Hastings-on-Hudson Parents, "Petition to Reopen Hastings-on-Hudson Schools Full Time," Change.org, August 19, 2020, https://www.change.org/p/superintendent-valerie-henning-piedmonte-and-boe -petition-to-reopen-hastings-on-hudson-schools-full-time.

CHAPTER 18

Page 242 August 2020 letter: Hastings Teachers Association, "Open Letter to Community about Re-Entry," August 14, 2020, https://www.hastingsta.org/single-post/2020/08/14/open-letter-to-community-about-re-entry. (It was also surprising and odd to see my *Wired* article that warned about hybrid schedules cited in the letter. The article explicitly made the case that hybrid's questionable advantage over, and even possible worse outcome than full-time school meant that choosing the latter was the sensible course of action, which undermined the letter's position that schools should be closed.)

Page 242 Megan Ranney: Megan Ranney (@meganranney), "Oh and ps. Masks aren't harmful. (Screenshot from article, with citations.)," Twitter, January 27, 2022, 10:39 p.m., https://twitter.com/meganranney/status/1486906706483417092; Ashley L. Ruba and Seth D. Pollak, "Children's Emotion Inferences from Masked Faces: Implications for Social Interactions during COVID-19," *PLOS ONE* 15, no. 12 (2020): e0243708.

As evidence for the claims that masks hurt no one, Ranney cited a study where the authors wrote, "We are unaware of published research on the long-term effects, if any, on intermittent masking." Never mind that before the pandemic no researcher ever would have gotten institutional approval, let alone found willing participants to study the effects of masking little kids for eight hours a day for more than a year since doing so obviously would have been considered unethical. As the saying goes, the absence of evidence is not evidence of absence.

Page 242 widely scorned opinion piece: Judith Danovitch, "Actually, Wearing a Mask Can Help Your Child Learn," *New York Times*, August 18, 2020; Vinay Prasad (@VPrasadMDMPH), "Wow, it is a uniquely American idea that making 2 year olds wear a mask for 6+ hrs in day care (but not the 2 hours when they sleep side by side) & adults mask," Twitter, August 18, 2021, 10:39 a.m., https://twitter.com/VPrasadMDMPH/status/1428003593227968514; Sarah Haider (@SarahTheHaider), "A horrendously bad piece. Almost propaganda," Twitter, August 18, 2021, 8:42 p.m., https://twitter.com/SarahTheHaider/status/1428155470922067969.

Page 242 "friend of the court" brief: American Academy of Pediatrics (@AmerAcadPeds), "Babies and young children study faces, so you may worry that having masked caregivers would harm children's language development. There are no studies to support," Twitter, August 12, 2021, 12:29 p.m., https://twitter.com/AmerAcadPeds/status/1425857041457942542; Erich Hartmann (@erichhartmann), Screens for those that have asked: [screenshots]," Twitter, August 18, 2021, 5:19 p.m., https://twitter.com/erichhartmann/status/1428104312237006849.

Page 242 More on this unusual brief:

The governor of Texas signed an order barring mask mandates in schools. A group of parents sued, claiming the ban on mandates disadvantaged their children, who had special needs. The case landed in the 5th Circuit, federal court [No. 21–51083]. Outside organizations that are interested in a court case can file what's known as an "amicus brief," conversationally known as a "friend of the court" brief, offering expert opinion to aid the court in understanding the issue at hand. The AAP, in partnership with the Texas Pediatric Society, filed such a brief in this case.

Supporting the plaintiffs' view, the AAP brief argued that it was *"beyond any doubt"* that 1) Covid poses "grave risks to children" 2) school mask mandates "significantly reduce the spread of Covid-19," and 3) mask aren't harmful to children. (My book extensively addresses points 1 and 2 so I won't do so here.) To support the third claim, the brief cited a study that compared emotional inferences made by children with adults wearing masks versus adults wearing sunglasses versus adults with their faces uncovered. Referring to the study, the brief noted "it appears that masks do not negatively impact children's emotional inferences to a greater degree than sunglasses," and that "children may reasonably infer whether someone wearing a mask is sad or angry."

The bar of "harm" set by the AAP—whether a child could reasonably infer if a masked adult was sad or angry—was so preposterous it was hard to believe it was real. Obviously students and teachers don't wear sunglasses all day every day in class, so to compare mask mandates to sunglasses made no sense. Further, I can tell through a computer screen if someone is sad or angry, but that doesn't mean seeing them through a screen is not a diminishment relative to seeing them in person. Worse still, the study the AAP cited concluded that wearing masks, while in some ways similar to sunglasses, nevertheless *diminished children's ability to detect and decipher emotions*. This was hardly an endorsement for the idea that masks don't have costs. Rather, it explicitly showed the opposite.

Moreover, there was no evidence that school mask mandates meaningfully reduced Covid transmission. All in, there is a reason why the World Health Organization did not recommend masks on any child under aged 6, and the ECDC recommended against children in primary school wearing masks. It is remarkable that the AAP was so confident in its position, *in opposition to the WHO and ECDC*, that it joined a court case brief to assert that a lack of a mask mandate on kids caused a net harm.

In July of 2022, the court ruled in favor of Texas, and dismissed the plaintiff's suit.

Page 242 "no such thing as learning loss": Jason McGahan, "Exclusive: Cecily Myart-Cruz's Hostile Takeover of L.A.'s Public Schools," *Los Angeles* magazine, August 26, 2021, https://www.lamag.com/citythinkblog/cecily-myart-cruz-teachers-union/.

A professor of education: Diane Ravitch, "Don't Believe the 'Learning Loss' Hoax," Diane Ravitch's Blog, March 17, 2021, https://dianeravitch.net/2021/03/17/dont-believe-the-learning-loss-hoax/.

More on the myth of learning loss: Peter Greene, "A Learning Loss Debunkery Reader," Curmudgucation (blog), March 14, 2021, https://curmudgucation.blogspot.com/2021/03/a-learning-loss-debunkery-reader.html.

Online teaching resource hub: TeachWire (UK), accessed January 5, 2024, https://www.teachwire.net/.

A poem: Rae Pica, "Should We Be Worried About Learning Loss in Early Childhood?," (personal website), August 2020, https://www.raepica.com/2020/08/learning-loss-in-early-childhood/.

Rae Pica, the education consultant, wrote about the myth of "learning loss" specifically for early childhood, for which she rightly criticized a pedagogy of young children being evaluated with standardized tests and doing worksheets, and instead argued that at that age a more holistic approach to education is better, focusing on play and imagination. But Pica assumed that all young children would have an enriching experience while locked out of school, that the alternative to "sit in your chair and memorize stuff" would be a carefree existence of creativity and wonder, rather than one spent viewing garbage on an iPad for endless hours, or being stuck in a chaotic or even dangerous home. Like many others had done, Pica raises some legitimate critiques of the education system in America, but conflates that critique with a defense of school closures.

Page 243 teachers union for the LA unified school district: United Teachers Los Angeles (website), "We Are UTLA," accessed January 5, 2024, https://utla.net/about -us/; 600,000 students: Michael Burke and Daniel J. Willis, "Los Angeles Unified Enrollment Dips below 600,000, a First in More Than Three Decades," *EdSource*, April 21, 2020, https://edsource.org/2020/los-angeles-unified-enrollment-dips-below -600000-a-first-in-more-than-three-decades/629378.

Page 244 Public schools in Los Angeles did not open until April of 2021: Kyle Stokes, "Everything We Know About LAUSD's Plan to Reopen Schools," *LAist*, April 19, 2021, https://laist.com/news/education/guide-everything-we-know-about-lausds-plan-to -reopen-schools-in-april.

Page 244 a coalition of teachers unions: Demand Safe Schools (website), "Demands," July 29, 2020, https://web.archive.org/web/20200729040138/https://www.demand safeschools.org/demands/. "About," July 29, 2020, https://web.archive.org/web/2020 0729042546/https://www.demandsafeschools.org/about/.

Page 244 Randi Weingarten . . . criticism was false: Victor Nava, "Randi Weingarten Fact-Checked by Twitter After Claiming She Tried to Reopen Schools During COVID," *New York Post*, May 9, 2023, https://nypost.com/2023/05/09/randi-wein garten-fact-checked-by-twitter-after-claiming-she-advocated-to-reopen-schools-during -covid/.

Page 245 In Washington, DC, teachers piled body bags: Madeline Peltzer, "DC Teachers Line Up Body Bags to Protest School Reopening," *Townhall*, July 29, 2020, https://townhall.com/tipsheet/madelinepeltzer/2020/07/29/dc-teachers-line-up -body-bags-to-protest-school-reopening-n2573377.

Page 245 In Milwaukee, the teachers union tweeted: Paul Blest, "Teachers Are Making Their Own Gravestones and Coffins to Protest Going Back to School," *Vice*, August 4, 2020, https://www.vice.com/en/article/y3zxp5/teachers-are-making-their -own-gravestones-and-coffins-to-protest-going-back-to-school.

Page 245 In Haverhill, Massachusetts: Allison Corneau, "Haverhill School Tensions: Teachers Stage COVID-19 Death Display; Mayor Eyes State Data to Support Reopening," *Eagle-Tribune* (Andover, MA), August 13, 2020, https://www.eagletribune.com /news/haverhill/haverhill-school-tensions-teachers-stage-covid-19-death-display

-mayor-eyes-state-data-to-support/article_65e66486-4a79-5f57-9e4b-b8da406a2e6f
.html.

Page 245 An Arizona union created a template: Corey A. DeAngelis, "Fund Students Instead of Systems," Cato Institute, August 10, 2020, https://www.cato.org
/commentary/fund-students-instead-systems.

Page 245 rally in New York City: Jeffrey Kopp, Madeleine Stix, Natalia V. Osipova, and Eric Levenson, "NYC Teachers Protest School Reopenings with Mock Caskets and Skeletons," CNN, March 3, 2021, https://www.cnn.com/2020/08/26/us/nyc-teachers
-protest-covid.

Page 245 Prince William Education Association: Associated Press, "Teachers' Union Apologizes for Using Coffin Props at Protest," *12 On Your Side* (WWBT, Richmond, VA), October 9, 2020, https://www.nbc12.com/2020/10/09/teachers-union-apologizes
-using-coffin-props-protest/.

Page 245 child-sized coffins: "Child-Sized Coffins in Prince William Teachers' Protest Caravan Spark Outrage," *InsideNoVa* (Woodbridge, VA), October 8, 2020, https://
www.insidenova.com/headlines/child-sized-coffins-in-prince-william-teachers
-protest-caravan-spark-outrage/article_3ceeef7c-0986-11eb-9e3d-bbb4f4044b3a.html.

Page 245 teachers getting end-of-life affairs in order: Theresa Waldrop, "Teachers Are So Worried About Returning to School That They're Preparing Wills," CNN, July 16, 2020, https://www.cnn.com/2020/07/16/us/coronavirus-teachers-preparing-wills/index
.html.

Similar sentiments: Gretty Garcia, "Teachers Are Writing Their Wills," The Cut (blog), July 20, 2020, https://www.thecut.com/2020/07/teachers-are-writing-wills-as
-schools-reopen-amid-covid.html. Nicholas Ferroni (@NicholasFerroni), "Going back to school in 2019 . . . TEACHERS: I need your help paying for school supplies because we are so underfunded. Going back to school in 2020 . . . TEACHERS: I need . . . ," Twitter, July 15, 2020, 1:15 p.m., https://twitter.com/NicholasFerroni
/status/1283450231057768448. Weingarten, free wills: Randi Weingarten (@rwein-garten), "Florida law firm offering free living wills for teachers returning to school amid coronavirus surge," Twitter, July 15, 2020, 6:04 p.m., https://twitter.com
/rweingarten/status/1283522873223720963. Florida teacher: Emily Bloch, "Teachers Are Drafting Wills Along with Lesson Plans; One Even Wrote Her Own Obituary," *USA Today*, August 13, 2020, https://www.usatoday.com/story/news/education
/2020/08/13/florida-teachers-writing-wills-obituaries-school-reopening-coronavirus
/3362679001/. Duval Schools Pandemic Solutions Team, post by Whitney Leigh, "School Board Meeting Tomorrow 8/4/2020: I will be there with my obituary, ready to read," Facebook, August 4, 2020, https://www.facebook.com/groups/572642573
643740/permalink/600084054232925/.

Page 246 Taking a bullet: Rebecca Martinson, "I Won't Return to the Classroom, and You Shouldn't Ask Me To," *New York Times*, July 18, 2020, Sunday Opinion.

Page 246 the two largest teachers unions in the country: American Federation of Teachers (website), "Reopening School Buildings Safely," accessed January 5, 2024, https://www.aft.org/our-community/reopen-schools/reopening-school-buildings

-safely. Mary Ellen Flannery, "Educators Prepare for Reopening with Living Wills and Life Insurance," neaToday (website of the National Education Association), July 22, 2020, https://www.nea.org/advocating-for-change/new-from-nea/educators -prepare-reopening-living-wills-and-life-insurance.

Page 246 AFT said it would support: Collin Binkley, "National Teacher Union Supports Strikes Over Reopening Plans," AP, July 28, 2020, https://apnews.com/article /virus-outbreak-ma-state-wire-politics-strikes-oh-state-wire-4e8a446186df3c1962137 dbe9faf7f38.

Page 246 Chicago Teachers Union: Nader Issa and Fran Spielman, "Chicago Teachers Union to call for strike vote at meeting next week," *Sun-Times* (Chicago), Augugst 4, 2020, https://chicago.suntimes.com/education/2020/8/4/21354570/chicago-teachers -union-strike-vote-cps-public-schools-pandemic-remote-learning-hybrid.

Page 246 Lori Lightfoot: Issa and Spielman, "Chicago Public Schools Will Go Fully Remote to Start the Fall," *Sun-Times*, August 4, 2020, https://chicago.suntimes.com /education/2020/8/4/21354898/chicago-public-schools-remote-fall-no-classes-coro navirus-covid.

Page 246 following "the science": Issa and Spielman, "Chicago Public Schools Staying Closed due to Worsening COVID-19 Conditions, Lightfoot Says," *Sun-Times*, August 5, 2020, https://chicago.suntimes.com/education/2020/8/5/21355448/chicago -public-schools-remote-learning-coronavirus.

Page 247 at its essence, political: Open Secrets, "Teachers Union Summary," accessed January 5, 2024, https://www.opensecrets.org/industries/indus.php?ind=l1300.

"Teachers Union Background," accessed January 5, 2024, https://www.opensecrets .org/industries/background.php?cycle=2022&ind=l1300. "Who are the Biggest Organization Donors?" accessed January 5, 2024, https://www.opensecrets.org/elections -overview/top-organizations. "What are the biggest political action committees?" accessed January 5, 2024, https://www.opensecrets.org/elections-overview/top-pacs.

Page 248 Jill Biden's first official event: Julian Peeples, "First Lady Meets with Educators on Day One," *California Educator*, January 22, 2021, https://www.cta.org /educator/posts/first-lady-meets-with-educators-on-day-one.

Page 248 A paper analyzing public schools' responses to COVID: Michael T. Hartney and Leslie K. Finger, "Politics, Markets, and Pandemics: Public Education's Response to COVID-19," *Perspectives on Politics* 20, no. 2 (2022): 457–473.

Page 248 top ten states with the highest in-person school percentage . . . : "Burbio's K-12 School Opening Tracker," Burbio (website), accessed January 5, 2024, https:// about.burbio.com/school-opening-tracker.

By "heavily Democratic" or Republican I mean the party affiliation of residents of those states; in most, but not all, instances this also meant the governorship, and state level offices aligned politically with opening percentages.

Page 249 structural protection: This same hot potato dynamic played out again later in the pandemic regarding pediatric Covid vaccine mandates. At various stages, the CDC and its advisory committee recommended different pediatric age groups get vaccinated for Covid and, after boosters were authorized, be "up to date" on doses. Members of the CDC and FDA advisory committees specifically said their authorization approval votes for the vaccines should not be taken as an endorsement to mandate them (in part because the vaccines did not stop infection, they did not stop transmission, and many children already had a degree of immunity from prior infection). Nevertheless, museums, theaters, concert venues, restaurants and, most devastatingly, youth sports leagues, after school programs, and summer camps, along with a number of private schools, mandated vaccination or boosters for children to attend or participate. When questioned about these mandates the answer often given by those who made the requirement was that they were following CDC guidance. The CDC in turn said it merely made recommendations and that the agency wasn't responsible for local mandates.

Page 250 return to the security consultants: Altaris Consulting Group (website), "Who We Are," accessed January 6, 2024, http://altarisgroup.com/about-us/.

Page 250 44 square feet of space: David Zweig, "44 Square Feet: A School-Reopening Detective Story," *Wired*, September 10, 2020, https://www.wired.com/story/44 -square-feet-a-school-reopening-detective-story/.

Page 253 Black-owned small businesses: Robert Fairlie, "The Impact of COVID-19 on Small Business Owners: Evidence from the First Three Months After Widespread Social-Distancing Restrictions," *Journal of Economics and Management Strategy* 29, no. 4 (Winter 2020): 727–740.

More on small business harms: Alexander W. Bartik, "The Impact of COVID-19 on Small Business Outcomes and Expectations," *PNAS* 117, no. 30 (2020): 17656– 17666; Robert Fairlie, "The Impact of Covid-19 Restrictions on Small Businesses in the US," IZA World of Labor, October 26, 2020, https://wol.iza.org/opinions /impact-of-covid-19-restrictions-on-small-businesses-in-us.

Page 253 Fauci explicitly advocated for school closures: "Dr. Fauci Press Briefing on Coronavirus Outbreak," *C-SPAN*, March 12, 2020, https://www.c-span.org/video /?470338-1/dr-fauci-press-briefing-coronavirus-outbreak.

Page 254 Fauci . . . gave de Blasio "his blessing": Jesse McKinley, "De Blasio Used Last-Minute Text to Tell Cuomo Schools Would Stay Shut," *New York Times*, April 13, 2020.

Page 254 Fauci warned that we "really better be very careful": Alex Rogers, "Fauci Responds to Rand Paul: 'I Have Never Made Myself Out to Be the End-All,'" CNN, May 12, 2020, https://www.cnn.com/2020/05/12/politics/rand-paul-fauci-testimony /index.html.

Page 254 35% of working mothers: Misty L. Heggeness et al., "Tracking Job Losses for Mothers of School-Age Children During a Health Crisis," US Census Bureau, March 3, 2021, https://www.census.gov/library/stories/2021/03/moms-work-and-the -pandemic.html.

Page 254 one in three moms: Misty L. Heggeness and Jason M. Fields, "Working Moms Bear Brunt of Home Schooling While Working During COVID-19," US Census

Bureau, August 18, 2020, https://www.census.gov/library/stories/2020/08/parents -juggle-work-and-child-care-during-pandemic.html.

Page 254 one million working women were still missing: Stephanie Ferguson and Isabella Lucy, "Data Deep Dive: A Decline of Women in the Workforce," US Chamber of Commerce, April 27, 2022, https://www.uschamber.com/workforce /data-deep-dive-a-decline-of-women-in-the-workforce.

Page 255 "I don't give advice about economic things": Alex Rogers, "Fauci responds to Rand Paul: 'I have never made myself out to be the end-all'," CNN, May 12, 2020, https://www.cnn.com/2020/05/12/politics/rand-paul-fauci-testimony/index.html.

Page 255 Low-income mothers: Steven H. Woolf et al., *How Are Income and Wealth Linked to Health and Longevity?* (Richmond, VA: Urban Institute and Virginia Commonwealth University, 2015).

Page 255 home nurse visits: Margaret A. McConnell et al., "Effect of an Intensive Nurse Home Visiting Program on Adverse Birth Outcomes in a Medicaid-Eligible Population: A Randomized Clinical Trial," *JAMA* 328, no. 1 (2020): 27–37.

Page 256 disappointing news: Maggie McConnell (@maggiemcconnell), "While it is hard to deliver disappointing news, I hope this evidence underscores the urgent need to better understand drivers of adverse birth outcomes and," Twitter, July 5, 2022, 12:31 p.m., https://twitter.com/maggiemcconnell/status/1544358280490897 408?s=20.

The author did note that future analyses would look at other outcomes. So it's possible this study will find that the intervention will ultimately yield some later benefits. But all of the initial outcomes that were studied failed to improve outcomes. Heather H. Burris (@hhburris), "I'm so sorry. Must be disappointing. Highlights that we still don't understand the pathophysiology enough to intervene to prevent outcomes like PTB. @DocElovitz," Twitter, July 5, 2022, 1:53 p.m., https:// twitter.com/hhburris/status/1544378881372733445?s=20.

Page 256 Michael Barnett: Michael L. Barnett (@ml_barnett), "Why didn't this common sense intervention work?? Perhaps those who declined to be in the trial would have benefitted more. But the results emphasize that the health," Twitter, December 30, 2022, 1:43 p.m., https://twitter.com/ml_barnett/status/16088966838 36051457?s=20.

Harvard T. H. Chan School of Public Health (website), "New research on intensive nurse home visiting program shows no impact on birth outcomes; study is ongoing," news release, July 5, 2022, https://www.hsph.harvard.edu/news/press-releases /new-research-on-intensive-nurse-home-visiting-program-shows-no-impact-on -birth-outcomes-study-is-ongoing/. Chan School, "South Carolina Nurse-Family Partnership Study," https://www.hsph.harvard.edu/sc-nfp-study/.

Page 256 2021 "megastudy": Katherine L. Milkman et al, "Megastudies Improve the Impact of Applied Behavioural Science," *Nature* 600 (2021): 478–483.

Page 257 "Fauci Blames Virus Surge on U.S. Not Shutting Down Completely," Reuters, July 13, 2020, https://www.reuters.com/article/us-heatlh-coronavirus-fauci /fauci-blames-virus-surge-on-u-s-not-shutting-down-completely-idUKKCN24E2JI.

Page 257 "It's that simple": Office of the Governor of the State of New York, "Video, Audio, Photos & Rush Transcript: Amid Ongoing COVID-19 Pandemic, Governor Cuomo Announces Collaboration with Gates Foundation to Develop a Blueprint to Reimagine Education in the New Normal," May 5, 2020, https://www.governor .ny.gov/news/video-audio-photos-rush-transcript-amid-ongoing-covid-19-pandemic -governor-cuomo-announces-19.

Cuomo's replacement in the governor's mansion perpetuated the same fake cause and effect. On December 10, 2021, in anticipation of a "winter surge," New York governor Kathy Hochul announced a statewide mask mandate, to go into effect two days later, to "help protect New Yorkers." Yet by January 9 the weekly daily average of cases had risen more than *seven times*, from 10,144 to 74,182. On January 31, 2022, cases had fallen to a weekly daily average of 12,951, and Hochul declared "thanks to our efforts, including mask regulations, cases are declining." The attribution to masks for the falling cases numbers, when they had exploded in the weeks following the mandate, was demonstrably absurd.

Page 260 Chris Licht: Tim Alberta, "Inside the Meltdown at CNN," *Atlantic*, June 2, 2023, https://www.theatlantic.com/politics/archive/2023/06/cnn-ratings-chris-licht -trump/674255/.

Page 261 swings chained together: CBC News, "A Swing Set Is Chained Up and Wrapped in Caution Tape in a Toronto Park. (Photo: Turgut Yeter, CBC)," Facebook, April 6, 2020, https://www.facebook.com/cbcnews/photos/a.10150640531594604 /10158513533994604/?type=3; Rochelle Staab, "Child Playing in an Empty Play-ground with Roped Off Swing Set" (photo), May 10, 2020, COVID-19 Community Archive, TESSA Digital Collections of the Los Angeles Public Library, https://tessa2 .lapl.org/digital/collection/COVID-19/id/147.

Page 261 Skate parks were shut down: "Coronavirus: San Clemente Fills Skatepark with 37 Tons of Sand After Skaters Ignore 'No Trespassing' Signs," CBS Los Angeles, April 17, 2020, https://www.cbsnews.com/losangeles/news/coronavirus-san-clemente -skatepark-37-tons-sand-social-distancing/.

Page 261 elementary schoolchildren in the New York City winter: Jon Fredericks (@ fredericks44), "Currently at PS 321 in Park Slope @UFT @NYCMayor how can you look yourselves in the mirror!! It's 32 degrees outside!! How!!," Twitter, December 20, 2021, 11:44 a.m., https://twitter.com/fredericks44/status/1472971134190727176.

CHAPTER 19

Page 265 Wealthy Virginia county: US Census Bureau, QuickFacts: Arlington County, Virginia (accessed January 6, 2024), https://www.census.gov/quickfacts /arlingtoncountyvirginia.

Page 265 Francisco Durán: Arlington Public Schools (website), "Dr. Francisco Durán," public profile page accessed January 7, 2024, https://www.apsva.us/departments /superintendents-office/dr-duran-bio/.

Page 266 first day of school arrived: Arlington Public Schools, Department of School & Community Relations, "Superintendent Announcements and Updates," September

10, 2020, accessed January 7, 2024, https://go.boarddocs.com/vsba/arlington/Board
.nsf/files/BTBTVS74FFA6.

Page 266 APE launched a postcard campaign: Arlington Parents for Education
(Arlington, VA), "Who We Are," accessed January 7, 2024, https://www.arlington
parentsforeducation.org/who-we-are.

Page 266 "Zoom in a room": Amy Zimmer, "Tensions Rise at Some of NYC's Top
High Schools Over 'Zoom in a Room' for On-Campus Students," *Chalkbeat New York*,
April 23, 2021, https://ny.chalkbeat.org/2021/4/23/22400166/ny-high-school-zoom
-remote-learning-teacher-accommodations; Jocelyn Gecker, Janie Har, and Amy
Taxin, "'Zoom in a Room'? California's Schools Lag in Reopening Push," AP, April
14, 2021, https://apnews.com/article/los-angeles-san-francisco-distance-learning-coro
navirus-pandemic-california-46766e48d1a26f77cca1e3b712186d39; Eric Spillman,
"LAUSD's 'Zoom in a Room' Format for In-Person Learning Fails to Draw Back Vast
Majority of High Schoolers," KTLA (Los Angeles, CA), May 10, 2021, https://ktla
.com/news/local-news/lausds-zoom-in-a-room-format-for-in-person-learning-fails
-to-draw-back-vast-majority-of-high-schoolers/; Anya Kamenetz and Aubri Juhasz,
"'Learning Hubs' Offer Free Child Care and Learning—But Only for a Lucky Few,"
NPR, September 1, 2020, https://www.npr.org/2020/09/01/906663624/-learning
-hubs-offer-free-child-care-and-learning-but-only-for-the-lucky-few.

Page 266 "remote learning hub": Meredith Stutz, "Guilford County Schools opens
'Internet Hubs' to Help Close Connectivity Gap," WX11 (Winston-Salem, NC), September. 12, 2020, https://www.wxii12.com/article/guilford-county-schools-internet
-hubs-to-help-close-connectivity-gap-students-greensboro-covid19/34000756.

Page 267 exact dates "TBD": Arlington Public Schools, "2020–21 School Year Moni-
toring Report," November 17, 2020 update, https://go.boarddocs.com/vsba/arlington
/Board.nsf/files/BVFT3C6E04EA/$file/D-1%20School%20Year%202020-21%20
Update%20111720%20-%203%20PM.pdf; National Center for Education Statistics,
"Fast Facts: Educational Institutions," accessed January 7, 2024, https://nces.ed.gov
/fastfacts/display.asp?id=84.

Page 268 "All classrooms . . . have outside air ventilation": Arlington Public Schools,
"2020–21 School Year Monitoring Report," September 10, 2020, https://go.boarddocs
.com/vsba/arlington/Board.nsf/files/BTBV3L7BE2D2 School Year 2020–2021 Update
Presentation 091020.pdf.

Page 269 Montgomery County, Maryland: Caitlynn Peetz, "MCPS Will Open Schools
March 1 for Some Small Groups of Students," MoCo360, February 9, 2021, https://
moco360.media/2021/02/09/mcps-will-open-schools-march-1-for-some-small-groups
-of-students/.

Page 270 Burbio School Opening Tracker: Burbio, "Burbio's K–12 School Opening
Tracker," online dataset accessed January 7, 2024, https://about.burbio.com/school
-opening-tracker.

Page 270 *Washington Post* piece: Valerie Strauss, "The racist effects of school reopening during the pandemic—by a teacher," *Washington Post*, July 23, 2020, https://www

.washingtonpost.com/education/2020/07/23/racist-effects-school-reopening-during
-pandemic-by-teacher/.

Page 271 Chicago Teachers Union tweeted: The CTU tweet was deleted at some
point after it posted. (It is worth noting that the CTU has innumerable tweets with
charges of racism, including accusing Lori Lightfoot, then-mayor of Chicago, who is
Black, of racism for firing some teachers.)

Page 271 Devon Horton: "Evanston Superintendent Accused Parents of 'White
Supremacist Thinking' for Asking to Put Children Back in School," *North Cook News*,
January 14, 2021, https://northcooknews.com/stories/572349932-evanston-superin
tendent-accused-parents-of-white-supremacist-thinking-for-asking-to-put-children
-back-in-school.

Page 271 school reopening plan in Cambridge, Massachusetts: Statement by the
Cambridge, MA Educators of Color Coalition, January 9, 2021, https://drive.google
.com/file/d/1wcUc9oGpes9-SmDPtefSz2iqiXMGcwch/view; Marc Levy, "No Confidence' Voted for School District Officials; Educators Want Say in Hiring Next
Superintendent," *Cambridge Day*, January 22, 2021, https://www.cambridgeday
.com/2021/01/22/no-confidence-voted-for-school-district-officials-educators-want
-say-in-hiring-next-superintendent/.

Page 271 Pasco, Washington: Jason Rantz, "Rantz: Union head says opening schools
is 'white supremacy,' suicide concern 'white privilege'," KTTH (Seattle, WA), January
13, 2021, https://mynorthwest.com/2452577/rantz-union-head-says-opening-schools
-is-white-supremacy-suicide-concern-white-privilege/. John McKay, "Pasco Teacher's
Union Pushing Remote Learning Petition," KFLD (Pasco, WA), January 5, 2021,
https://newstalk870.am/pasco-teachers-union-pushing-remote-learning-petition/.
Pasco Association of Educators, "For Safety and Equity, Return Pasco Students to
Remote Learning," petition on Change.org, December 15, 2020, https://www.change
.org/p/aphillips-psd1-org-for-safety-and-equity-return-pasco-students-to-remote
-learning.

Page 271 Megan Ranney: Megan Ranney (@meganranney), "I also acknowledge that
much of the school reopening debate has ignored the lived experience of BIPOC who
are both at higher risk for #COVID19, and higher risk of," Twitter, January 26, 2021,
10:47 pm, https://x.com/meganranney/status/1354274727683125251; Rashelle Chase,
"The 'Reopen Schools Now!' Debate Is Rooted in Racism," Scary Mommy (website),
January 6, 2021, https://www.scarymommy.com/movement-reopen-schools-racist.

Page 272 actually protective for adults: David Zweig, "Why Spending Time with
Kids Might Actually Help Protect You from COVID," *New York*, December 9, 2022.
https://nymag.com/intelligencer/2022/12/spending-time-with-kids-might-help-protect
-adults-from-covid.html.

Page 273 "recipe for propagating structural racism": Mackenzie Mays, "LA Teachers
Union Slams California Schools' Plan as 'Propagating Structural Racism,'" *Politico*,
March 2, 2021, https://www.politico.com/states/california/story/2021/03/02/la-teachers
-union-slams-state-plan-as-propagating-structural-racism-1366367.

Page 273 San Diego County school district: Tori Richards, "Opening Schools Is White Supremacy and Slavery, California School Board Member Charges," *Washington Examiner*, February 25, 2021, https://www.washingtonexaminer.com/news/opening-schools-racist-trustee-says; Spring Ruckle, "So this is how the board meeting went last night, the woman talking chose to not have her camera on but she is the VP of the school board. She's making decisions," Facebook, February 24, 2021, video, 4:50, https://www.facebook.com/spring.vick/posts/10222260093345705; La Mesa-Spring Valley Schools (@lmsvschools), "LMSV Board Meeting, February 23, 2021," YouTube video, February 24, 2021, 2:02:04, https://youtu.be/mb_nAVtNCBU.

Page 273 parents in New York City held a rally: Ginia Bellafante, "Restaurants and Broadway Are Coming Back. What About Our Schools?," *New York Times*, May 7, 2021.

Page 276 Cecily Myart-Cruz: Emily Crane, "LA Teacher's Union Leader Blames 'White Wealthy Parents' for the Rush to Reopen Schools after Gov. Newsom Reveals Plan to Pay Districts to Get Students Back in Classrooms Quicker," *Daily Mail* (UK), March 2, 2021, https://www.dailymail.co.uk/news/article-9318333/LA-teachers-union-leader-blames-white-wealthy-parents-rush-reopen-schools.html.

Page 276 Maryam Qudrat: Lauren Fruen and Emily Crane, "Afghan-American Mom Slams 'Racist' LA Teachers Union for Asking Her Ethnicity When She Pushed to Reopen Schools—After They Said Only 'White Wealthy Parents' Want Children to Return to Classrooms," *Daily Mail* (UK), March 4, 2021, https://www.dailymail.co.uk/news/article-9325897/Mom-called-schools-reopen-says-racially-profiled-LA-teachers-union.html; Maryam Qudrat, "Teachers Union Prefers Parents Remain Silent: Maryam Qudrat," *Los Angeles Daily News*, March 14, 2021, https://www.dailynews.com/2021/03/14/teachers-union-prefers-parents-to-remain-silent-maryam-qudrat/.

Page 277 Lamar Freeman: Bill Melugin, "South LA Parents Say They Want Schools to Reopen, Disagree with UTLA President's Remarks," FOX11 Los Angeles, March 2, 2021, https://www.foxla.com/news/south-la-families-say-minorities-want-schools-to-reopen-disagree-with-utla-presidents-remarks.

CHAPTER 20

Page 280 Gavin Newsom's four children: Lara Korte, "Fact Check: Are Gavin Newsom's Kids 'Living through Zoom School'?," *Sacramento Bee*, March 22, 2021, https://www.sacbee.com/news/politics-government/capitol-alert/article250067849.html.

Page 280 opportunity for a free public education: *The Consequences of School Closures: Intended and Unintended: Testimony before the Select Subcommittee on the Coronavirus Pandemic Hearing*, 118th Congress, 1st sess., March 28, 2023 (statement of David Zweig, journalist and author).

Institute of Education Sciences at the U.S. Department of Education, runs ERIC (Educational Resources Information Center)

Page 280 Massachusetts Bay Colony: "The Old Deluder Act (1647), From *Records of the Governor and Company of the Massachusetts Bay in New England* (1853) II: 203,"

The Elizabeth Murray Project: A Resource Site for Early American History, accessed January 7, 2024, https://web.csulb.edu/colleges/cla/projects/EM/smdeluder.html.

Page 281 act of 1647: David Carleton, "Old Deluder Satan Act of 1647 (1647)," Free Speech Center at Middle Tennessee State University, first published 2009, updated December 15, 2023, https://www.mtsu.edu/first-amendment/article/1032/old-deluder -satan-act-of-1647. The option for a young person to continue their education was so valued by the government that every family "able and willing" in New England was asked to give "college corn"—a peck of grain or equivalent value in wam- pum—to support Harvard. Samuel Eliot Morison, "Dunster Struggles On, 1650– 1654," in *Harvard College in the Seventeenth Century, Part I* (Cambridge, MA: Harvard University Press, 1936), 26–39.

Page 281 "rare as a comet": John Adams, "A Dissertation on the Canon and the Feudal Law," No. 3, 30 September 1765. https://founders.archives.gov/documents /Adams/06-01-02-0052-0006#PJA01d068n2; Anthony Brandt, "Do We Care If Johnny Can Read?," *American Heritage* 31, no. 5, August/September 1980, https:// www.americanheritage.com/do-we-care-if-johnny-can-read.

Page 281 American Revolution . . . free local schools: Center on Education Policy, *History and Evolution of Public Education in the US* (Washington, DC: The George Washington University Graduate School of Education and Human Development, 2020), https://files.eric.ed.gov/fulltext/ED606970.pdf.

Page 282 Horace Mann: Stephen V. Monsma and J. Christopher Soper, *The Chal- lenge of Pluralism: Church and State in Five Democracies* (Lanham, MD: Rowman and Littlefield, 2009).

Page 282 1918 compulsory education every state: Michael S. Katz, *A History of Com- pulsory Education Laws* (Bloomington, IN: Phi Delta Kappa, 1976), via Institute of Education Sciences, https://eric.ed.gov/?id=ED119389.

Early schooling text derived from multiple sources, including: Center on Edu- cation Policy, History and Evolution of Public Education in the US (Washington, DC: The George Washington University Graduate School of Education and Human Development, 2020), https://files.eric.ed.gov/fulltext/ED606970.pdf.

Page 283 3 percent drop in enrollment: Institute of Education Sciences, National Center for Education Statistics, "Nation's Public School Enrollment Dropped 3 Per- cent in 2020–21," news release, June 28, 2021, https://nces.ed.gov/whatsnew/press _releases/06_28_2021.asp.

Page 283 kindergarteners . . . largest declines in enrollment: Thomas Dee, "Public School Enrollment Dropped by 1.2M During the Pandemic," The 74, March 21, 2023, https://www.the74million.org/article/public-school-enrollment-dropped-by-1 -2m-during-the-pandemic/; Daphna Bassok and Anna Shapiro, "Understanding COVID-19-era enrollment drops among early-grade public school students," Brook- ings Institute, February 22, 2021, https://www.brookings.edu/blog/brown-center -chalkboard/2021/02/22/understanding-covid-19-era-enrollment-drops-among -early-grade-public-school-students/.

Page 283 National Association of Independent Schools: National Association of Independent Schools, "About NAIS," accessed January 7, 2024, https://www.nais .org/about/about-nais/.

Page 283 "seeking out schools that are fully in-person": Jessica Dickler, "Families Jump to Private Schools as Coronavirus Drags On," CNBC, November 8, 2020, https://www.cnbc.com/2020/11/08/coronavirus-why-families-are-jumping-to-private -schools.html.

Page 284 half of unenrolled students shifted to homeschool: Gabe Cohen, "No, 2020 Did Not See the Largest Public School Enrollment Decline in US History," Verify (website), August 11, 2021, https://www.verifythis.com/article/news/verify /education-verify/2020-did-not-see-the-largest-public-school-enrollment-decline-in -us-history/536-2b993890-273c-4028-b2b4-1c5745363285.

Page 284 Analysis of 22 jurisdictions for homeschool: Thomas Dee, "Public School Enrollment Dropped by 1.2M During the Pandemic," The 74, March 21, 2023.

Page 284 Urban Institute: Thomas S. Dee, "Where the Kids Went: Nonpublic Schooling and Demographic Change during the Pandemic Exodus from Public Schools," Urban Institute, February 9, 2023, https://www.urban.org/research/publication /where-kids-went-nonpublic-schooling-and-demographic-change-during-pandemic.

Page 285 obligated to attend in person: the teachers who were at great risk, due to age or some other factor, could have been put in charge of teaching the remote students while remaining remote themselves. Furloughs and leaves of absence or early retirements could also have been negotiated. Also remember, per the Swedish study, teachers who worked in person faced no higher risk of infection than average for professionals.

Page 286 Hazard pay: Darsh Singhania, "Hazard Pay Is More Necessary Than Ever for Teachers," The Voice (Irvington High School, Fremont, CA), April 20, 2021, https:// ihsvoice.com/2021/04/20/hazard-pay-is-more-necessary-than-ever/; Ashly McGlone, "Thanks, Incentives, Hazard Pay: More COVID-19 Funds Are Going to School Employees," Voice of San Diego, April 14, 2021, https://voiceofsandiego.org/2021 /04/14/thanks-incentives-hazard-pay-more-covid-19-funds-are-going-to-school -employees/; Laura Gesualdi-Gilmore, "Danger Money: Stimulus Checks for $3K Are Being Given Out to Teachers in Some States as Hazard Pay," Sun (US edition), September 10, 2021, https://www.the-sun.com/news/3638897/stimulus-checks-teachers -3000/.

Michigan: Southfield Public Schools (Southfield, MI), "Teacher and Support Staff COVID-19 Hazard Pay," accessed January 7, 2024, https://www.southfieldk12.org /departments/budget-and-finance/teacher-and-support-staff-covid-19-hazard-pay/; "Teachers Eligible for $500 Hazard Pay for Working During Pandemic," WLNS 6 (Lansing, MI), October 29, 2020, https://www.wlns.com/news/teachers-eligible-for -500-hazard-pay-for-working-during-pandemic/; Teacher COVID-19 Grants and School Support COVID-19 Grants Frequently Asked Questions (FAQs) (Lansing, MI: Michigan Department of Treasury, 2020), https://www.michigan.gov/-/media/Project/Websites /treasury/Uncategorized/2020/2/TSSC19_Grant_Program_FAQs.pdf?rev=2c1e289d

73564c4d87e9ecdea6e7fb72; State of Michigan Office of the Governor, "Executive Order 2020-35: Provision of K–12 Education During the Remainder of the 2019–2020 School Year—Rescinded," April 2, 2020, https://www.michigan.gov/whitmer/news/state-orders-and-directives/2020/04/02/executive-order-2020-35.

Page 286 Joan Tronto: Berenice Fisher and Joan Tronto, "Toward a Feminist Theory of Caring," in, *Circles of Care: Work and Identity in Women's Lives*, ed. Emily K. Abel and Margaret K. Nelson (Albany: SUNY Press, 1990), 35–62; Joan Tronto, interview, Ethics of Care (website), October 16, 2009, https://ethicsofcare.org/joan-tronto/.

Page 287 "Teachers are not babysitters": "Opinion: Teachers Are Not Babysitters and I'm Not Returning Back to School," The Educator's Room, July 27, 2020, https://theeducatorsroom.com/opinion-teachers-are-not-babysitters-and-im-not-returning-back-to-school/; RebelliousByRebel (Rebel Marshall), "Teachers are not babysitters" T-shirt, Etsy.com, listed October 19, 2023, https://www.etsy.com/listing/1416942467/teachers-are-not-babysitters?gpla=1&gao=1&.

Page 287 Zoom in a room in schools around the country: Kyle Stokes, "LAUSD Middle and High School Campuses Are Now Reopening. Here's What To Expect," LAist, April 27, 2021, https://laist.com/news/education/lausd-school-reopening-middle-high-schools-preview-april27.

Spring 2021: Reopen California Schools (@ReopenCASchools), "LAUSD is expanding Zoom-In-A-Room to accommodate teachers with child care issues, even after providing a $500/mo stipend. Some middle and high schoolers won't," Twitter, May 9, 2021, 12:56 pm, https://twitter.com/ReopenCASchools/status/1391436890595753985?s=20.

Page 287 Tronto had been studying: Steven D. Edwards, "Three versions of an ethics of care," *Nursing Philosophy: An International Journal for Healthcare Professionals* 10, no. 4 (2009): 231–40.

CHAPTER 21

Page 290 insinuation that parents who were advocating for schools to open were simply lazy: Andy Slavitt (@ASlavitt), "Some people want their kids back at school to get an education but I think others don't want to be around their kids all day long. They have more passion for the issue," Twitter, July 29, 2020, https://twitter.com/ASlavitt/status/1288622223201370112.

Page 291 "Among parents who have been fighting for open schools all year": Rachel Fremmer: Ginia Bellafante, "Restaurants and Broadway Are Coming Back. What About Our Schools?," *New York Times*, May 7, 2021, https://www.nytimes.com/2021/05/07/nyregion/coronavirus-nyc-public-schools.html.

Page 293 "two case" rule: Alejandra O'Connell-Domenech, "No Update Yet on Changes to 'two Case' Rule for New York City School Closures, Officials Say," AMNY, March 23, 2021, https://www.amny.com/news/no-update-yet-on-changes-to-two-case-rule-for-new-york-city-school-closures-officials/. (New York City dropped the two case rule in early April, 2021.)

Page 296 Governor Newsom dining at an elite restaurant: Jeremy B. White, "Newsom Faces Backlash After Attending French Laundry Dinner Party," *Politico*, November 13, 2020, https://www.politico.com/states/california/story/2020/11/13/newsom-faces -backlash-after-attending-french-laundry-dinner-party-1336419.

DEEP DIVE: HARMS OF SCHOOL CLOSURES

Page 302 Child abuse: This text is drawn from my congressional testimony. See *The Consequences of School Closures: Intended and Unintended: Testimony before the Select Subcommittee on the Coronavirus Pandemic Hearing*, 118th Congress, 1st sess., March 28, 2023 (statement of David Zweig, journalist and author).

Page 302 "Reporting of Child Maltreatment": Eli Rapoport et al., "Reporting of Child Maltreatment During the SARS-CoV-2 Pandemic in New York City from March to May 2020," *Child Abuse & Neglect* 116, Pt 2 (2021): 104719; Katie Kim and Lisa Capitanini, "Doctors Fear Child Abuse Is Underreported During Coronavirus Pandemic," NBC Chicago, May 19, 2020, https://www.nbcchicago.com/news/local /doctors-fear-child-abuse-is-underreported-during-coronavirus-pandemic/2273364/; Richard Winton, "'We Do Not Want Another Gabriel Fernandez': Coronavirus Leads to 'Alarming' Drop in Child Abuse Reports," *Los Angeles Times*, April 21, 2020, https:// www.latimes.com/california/story/2020-04-21/coronavirus-child-abuse-reports -decline; Samantha Schmidt and Hannah Natanson, "With Kids Stuck at Home, ER Doctors See More Severe Cases of Child Abuse," *Washington Post*, April 30, 2020, https://www.washingtonpost.com/education/2020/04/30/child-abuse-reports-coro navirus/; Darren DeRonco: E. Jason Baron et al., "Suffering in Silence: How COVID-19 School Closures Inhibit the Reporting of Child Maltreatment," *Journal of Public Economics* 190 (2020): 104258.

Page 303 school closures and child abuse: Some researchers suggested that the reduction in reports reflected a drop in abuse, that lockdowns prevented abuse through strengthened families. Yet the Wesley Park and Kristen Walsh paper, which compared survey results of self-reported abuse by children during the pandemic with those to a similar survey before the pandemic, shows that self-reported physical abuse doubled: Wesley J. Park and Kristen A. Walsh, "COVID-19 and the Unseen Pandemic of Child Abuse," *BMJ Paediatrics Open* 6, no. 1 (2022): e001553.

Page 303 Individuals with Disabilities Education Act (IDEA): IDEA (Individuals with Disabilities Education Act), "A History of the Individuals with Disabilities Education Act," US Department of Education, last updated November 30, 2023, https://sites.ed .gov/idea/IDEA-History.

Page 304 deaf or hard of hearing: National Institute on Deafness and Other Communication Disorders, "Quick Statistics About Hearing," last updated March 25, 2021, https://www.nidcd.nih.gov/health/statistics/quick-statistics-hearing.

Page 304 These students qualify for an IEP: Nationwide Children's Hospital, "Children with Hearing Loss: Guidelines for Schools," accessed January 7, 2024, https:// www.nationwidechildrens.org/family-resources-education/health-wellness-and -safety-resources/helping-hands/children-with-hearing-loss-guidelines-for-schools.

Page 306 $1,472 a month: Office for Children, Fairfax County, VA, "Supporting Return to School (SRS) Program," https://www.fairfaxcounty.gov/office-for-children/supporting-return-school-program.

Page 306 88 percent of them were not receiving any in-person supports: CommunicationFirst, "National Survey Reveals Students with Communication Disabilities Are Being Denied Safe Access to Education," January 4, 2021, https://communicationfirst.org/national-survey-reveals-students-with-communication-disabilities-are-being-denied-safe-access-to-education/.

Page 306 thousands of cases were filed: ReOpen Class (website), "Frequently Asked Questions," accessed January 7, 2024, https://reopenclass.com/faq/.

Page 306 child suicides in Milwaukee: Amanda Becker, "3 out of 5 teens Who Died by Suicide in Milwaukee County Last Year Cited 'Virtual Learning' as a Stressor," CBS58 (Milwaukee, WI), August 31, 2021, https://www.cbs58.com/news/3-out-of-5-teens-who-died-by-suicide-in-milwaukee-county-last-year-cited-virtual-learning-as-a-stressor.

Page 306 Colorado to Arizona to Washington State: Colorado: Jennifer Brown, "Youth Suicides on the Eastern Plains Spark Political Protest, '7 Is Too Many' Social Media Campaign," *Colorado Sun*, December 17, 2020, https://coloradosun.com/2020/12/17/teen-suicide-on-eastern-plains/. Arizona: Danyelle Khmara, "With Teen Suicide on the Rise, Tucson Educators Struggle to Prioritize Mental Health," *Arizona Daily Star* (Tucson.com), December 27, 2020, https://tucson.com/news/local/with-teen-suicide-on-the-rise-tucson-educators-struggle-to-prioritize-mental-health/article_7db1b000-c0aa-5066-931f-fed3443e0102.html. Washington State: Roman Stubbs, "A Hidden Crisis," *Washington Post*, December 16, 2020, https://www.washingtonpost.com/sports/2020/12/16/teen-athletes-suicide/?arc404=true.

Page 307 not having enough beds for kids with mental health emergencies: Drs. Erin Klein, Hasanga Samaraweera, Michael Bertenthal, Kristie Sparks, and Grace St. Cyr, "Chicago Pediatricians: The Social Isolation of Remote Learning Is Dangerous to Youth," *Sun-Times* (Chicago), January 27, 2021, https://chicago.suntimes.com/2021/1/27/22253057/chicago-pediatricians-remote-learning-social-isolation-suicide-depression-cps-ctu.

Page 307 upward trends in a variety of mental health categories: Frank Edelbut, "Unpacking the effects of Covid," *Journal-Courier* (Jacksonville, IL), February 8, 2023, https://www.myjournalcourier.com/opinion/article/commentary-17762558.php.

Page 307 rates appeared to jump from 2019 to 2021: Centers for Disease Control and Prevention, Division of Adolescent and School Health, National Center for HIV/AIDS, Viral Hepatitis, STD, and TB Prevention, *Youth Risk Behavior Survey: Data Summary and Trends Report, 2011–2021* (Atlanta, GA: Centers for Disease Control and Prevention, 2021), https://www.cdc.gov/healthyyouth/data/yrbs/pdf/YRBS_Data-Summary-Trends_Report2023_508.pdf.

Page 307 In 2020, 581 ten- to fourteen-year-olds year-olds died from suicide; 32 died of COVID: National Institute of Mental Health (website), "Suicide," last updated May 2023, accessed January 7, 2024, https://www.nimh.nih.gov/health/statistics/suicide.

It should be noted that suicides tend to go up when school is in session. So although some kids committed suicide as a result of school closures, in aggregate suicide rates went down. (Needless to say, the solution to some kids tragically committing suicide each year due to the social or academic stresses of school is not to close schools for 50 million children. Conversely, there was no aggregate benefit of closures offsetting the mental health harms they engendered.)

Page 307 eating disorders: Amanda D'Ambrosio, "Eating Disorders: Another Consequence of COVID-19," MedPage Today, March 4, 2021, https://www.medpageto day.com/special-reports/exclusives/91483?vpass=1; Erin Digitale, "Youth at Both Ends of Weight Spectrum Challenged by Global Pandemic," Stanford Medicine News Center, March 17, 2021, https://med.stanford.edu/news/all-news/2021/03/pandemic -worsens-weight-woes-among-young-people.html.

Page 307 body mass index increase: Samantha J. Lange et al., "Longitudinal Trends in Body Mass Index Before and During the COVID-19 Pandemic Among Persons Aged 2–19 Years—United States, 2018–2020," *Morbidity and Mortality Weekly Report* 70, no. 37 (2021): 1278–1283; Susan J. Woolford et al., "Changes in Body Mass Index Among Children and Adolescents During the COVID-19 Pandemic," *JAMA* 326, no. 14 (2021): 1434–1436.

Page 307 CDC published the results of a survey: Jorge V. Verlenden et al., "Association of Children's Mode of School Instruction with Child and Parent Experiences and Well-Being During the COVID-19 Pandemic—COVID Experiences Survey, United States, October 8–November 13, 2020," *Morbidity and Mortality Weekly Report* 70, no. 11 (2021): 369–376.

Page 308 survey of pediatric mental health professionals: The paper was in preparation at time of this writing. The lead author was Peter Duquette at University of North Carolina, co-authors Mary Colvin at Harvard University, Jennifer Reesman at Johns Hopkins University, Tannahill Glenn, a neuropsychologist in private practice, and me.

Page 310 failing grades increased 83 percent: Don Parker, "Students' Failing Grades Increase 83% with Online Learning in Fairfax County Schools," WJLA (Washington, DC), November 24, 2020, https://wjla.com/news/local/fairfax-county-students-failing -grades-online-learningfcps.

Page 311 Vladimir Kogan: Vladimir Kogan and Stéphane Lavertu, "How the COVID-19 Pandemic Affected Student Learning in Ohio: Analysis of Spring 2021 Ohio State Tests," Ohio State University, John Glenn College of Public Affairs 28 (2021): 2021–10, https://glenn.osu.edu/sites/default/files/2021-10/210828_KL_OST_Final_0.pdf.

Page 311 Andrew Ho: Declaration of Andrew Ho, in J Cayla et al. v. State of California et al., August 4, 2023, https://www.documentcloud.org/documents/23923611 -caylaj-andewho-080423

Page 311 Emily Oster: Rebecca Jack, Clare Halloran, James Okun, and Emily Oster, "Pandemic Schooling Mode and Student Test Scores: Evidence from US School Districts," *American Economic Review: Insights* 5, no. 2 (June 2023): 173–190.

Page 312 Harvard University's Center for Education Policy Research: Dan Goldhaber et al., *The Consequences of Remote and Hybrid Instruction During the Pandemic* (Cambridge, MA: Center for Education Policy Research, Harvard University, 2022).

Page 312 Theresa Chapple: Dr. Theresa Chapple (@Theresa_Chapple), "Everyone can think of something bad to say about virtual school. But I asked a group of 10k Black parents what did they like about it. Overwhelmingly, Black parents," Twitter, September 2, 2020, 1:20 p.m., https://twitter.com/Theresa_Chapple/status/1301208 457522151424?s=20.

Page 312 "spared some of the common social pressures": Rory Selinger, "I'm a High School Student. I Don't Want Online Learning to End," Medium, February 22, 2021, https://onezero.medium.com/im-a-high-school-student-i-don-t-want-online-learning -to-end-9a60f6c361ce.

Page 315 staring at a Chromebook was simply not compatible: Monique Hedderson et al., "Trends in Screen Time Use Among Children During the COVID-19 Pandemic, July 2019 Through August 2021," *JAMA Network Open* 6, no. 2 (2023): e2256157.

Page 315 "kids are resilient": Rebecca Mongrain, "9 Crafty, Creative and Educational Things to Do at Home with Kids," Seattle's Child, October 2020, https:// www.seattleschild.com/9-crafty-creative-and-educational-things-to-do-at-home/; Valerie Strauss, "Why Learning Isn't the Most Important Thing Kids Lost During the Pandemic," *Washington Post*, April 23, 2021, https://www.washingtonpost.com /education/2021/04/23/why-learning-isnt-most-important-thing-kids-lost-during -pandemic/. Ron Berger, "Our Kids Are Not Broken," *Atlantic*, March 20, 2021, https:// www.theatlantic.com/ideas/archive/2021/03/how-to-get-our-kids-back-on-track /618269/; Sarah Ferguson, "Getting Students Back to School Safely During the COVID-19 Pandemic," *Forbes*, October 16, 2020, https://www.forbes.com/sites/unice fusa/2020/10/16/getting-students-back-to-school-safely-during-the-covid-19-pandemic /?sh=3eead26b22b9; Holly Burns, "Worried Your Kid Is Falling Behind? You're Not Alone," *New York Times*, July 30, 2020, https://www.nytimes.com/2020/07/30/parenting /online-learning-school-coronavirus.html.

Page 315 Randi Weingarten: "Teachers union president: Kids will be resilient with lost education," Axios, February 21, 2021.

Page 315 Jerome Adams: Jerome Adams (@JeromeAdamsMD), "Question from a recent talk: why is it the young people who lived through the Great Depression (12 years) and WW2 (5+ years) came to be known as our 'greatest generation,'" Twitter, June 20, 2023, 7:36 a.m., https://twitter.com/JeromeAdamsMD/status/16711198074 69551617?s=20.

CHAPTER 22

Page 319 *New York* magazine: David Zweig, "Inside the Schools Open Full Time Right Now," *New York*, October 19, 2020, https://nymag.com/intelligencer/2020/10 /school-openings-covid-19.html. Analysis methodology is explained in a footnote in the article.

Page 321 Emily Oster data on schools: "COVID-19 School Response Dashboard": https://covidschooldashboard.com/

Page 322 "closing schools after widespread influenza-like illness activity did not reduce transmission": Elizabeth S. Russell et al., "Reactive School Closure During Increased Influenza-Like Illness (ILI) Activity in Western Kentucky, 2013: A Field Evaluation of Effect on ILI Incidence and Economic and Social Consequences for Families," *Open Forum Infectious Diseases* 3, no. 3 (Summer 2016).

Page 326 student learning centers: 75,000 students total, 156 schools, over 70% African American: Baltimore City Public Schools, "City Schools at a Glance," accessed January 7, 2024, https://www.baltimorecityschools.org/page/district-overview.

Page 326 1,200 kindergarteners: Erica L. Green, "Plastic Dividers and Masks All Day: What Teaching in a Pandemic Looks Like," *New York Times*, November 28, 2020, https://www.nytimes.com/2020/11/28/us/coronavirus-school-reopening.html. Parents urged to not send kids in: Liz Bowie, "Baltimore Teachers Union says schools aren't safe to send students and teachers back, urges parents to boycott," *Baltimore Sun*, October 15, 2020, www.baltimoresun.com/education/bs-md-teachers-union -city-20201015-hdx3t5n7aveklae6hmtpglimce-story.html. AFT—Maryland (affiliate of the American Federation of Teachers, AFL–CIO): "AFT-Maryland Locals and Other Union Leaders Join for Solidarity Press Conference on Safe School Reopening," press conference news release, November 12, 2020, http://md.aft.org/press/safe -school-reopening-press-conference.

Page 327 "We'd rather have our kids be out of school than dead": Eliza Shapiro, Erica L. Green, and Juliana Kim, "Missing in School Reopening Plans: Black Families' Trust," *New York Times*, February 1, 2021, https://www.nytimes.com/2021/02/01/us /politics/school-reopening-black-families.html.

Page 327 "If you're advocating for opening schools": Derik Chica (@DerikChica), "So if you're advocating for opening schools for the sake of mental health for students, where is your equity lens? Where will you be when students and families," Twitter, January 11, 2022, 5:10 p.m., https://twitter.com/DerikChica/status/1481025827613 691911?s=20.

Page 327 Eleanor Murray tweeted her approval: Ellie Murray (@EpiEllie), "Very excellent thread on schools, covid, and why we should be listening to minority parents & not just rich white influencers," Twitter, April 26, 2022, 8:38 a.m., https://twitter .com/epiellie/status/1518932481386455040?s=10&t=iNLOmqElPvMdFoALTa_ixA; Loretta Torrago (@Loretta_Torrago), "When well-funded schools opened & schools with higher minority shares stayed shut, white influencers decried the inequities. When those schools opened, lagging minority" Twitter, April 25, 2022, 8:32 a.m., https://twitter.com/Loretta_Torrago/status/1518568508744998912.

Page 328 researchers at Michigan State University: Matt Grossmann et al., "All States Close but Red Districts Reopen: The Politics of In-Person Schooling During the COVID-19 Pandemic," *Educational Researcher* 50, no. 9 (2021): 637–648.

Page 328 Michael Hartney and Leslie Finger: Michael Hartney, the political scientist at Boston College, conducted an analysis of a report on the quality of the facilities in California schools cross-referenced with requests by districts to obtain waivers to open. He found that there was no correlation between the quality of school building facilities and its motivation or willingness to open. Moreover, he found that private schools that were most likely to open had the lowest funding. Expensive, elite Manhattan private schools were no more likely to open than other, lower-priced private schools. See Michael Hartney and Leslie Finger: Michael T. Hartney and Leslie K. Finger, "Politics, Markets, and Pandemics: Public Education's Response to COVID-19," *Perspectives on Politics* 20, no. 2 (2022): 457–473.

Page 329 Burbio School Opening Tracker: Burbio, "Burbio's K–12 School Opening Tracker," public dataset accessed January 7, 2024, https://about.burbio.com/school-opening-tracker.

Page 328 Vladimir Kogan, *What's Behind Racial Differences in Attitudes Toward School Reopening (and What to Do About Them)* (Washington, DC: American Enterprise Institute, 2021). It's worth noting that about six months after Kogan's report, he reran his analysis with the latest data. (USC had been continuing its regular surveys after Kogan's report.) This is what's known as an out-of-sample test—if his argument was right, as more schools reopened, we would see public opinion across racial groups converge toward a consensus in favor of in-person learning. That is exactly what he found. "With the additional data, the results were nearly identical," he said, "not only in terms of the direction and signs but also in terms of actual magnitude."

Page 331 Sweden famously never closed: Johan Anderberg, "Sweden Saved Children from Lockdown," UnHerd, Jun3 17, 2022, https://unherd.com/2022/06/sweden-saved-children-from-lockdown/

CHAPTER 23

Page 333 grants awarded by the NIH: Logesvar Balaguru et al., "NIH funding of COVID-19 research in 2020: A Cross-Sectional Study," *BMJ Open* 12, no. 5 (2022): e059041.

Page 335 journal will only publish research that supports current CDC guidelines: Centers for Disease Control and Prevention, *Morbidity and Mortality Weekly Report* (*MMWR*), "Instructions for Authors (Updated June 29, 2023)," https://www.cdc.gov/mmwr/author_guide.html#1.0criteriaforpublication.

Page 336 Widely read feature: Arizona masking study: David Zweig, "The CDC's Flawed Case for Wearing Masks in School," *Atlantic*, December 16, 2021, https://www.theatlantic.com/science/archive/2021/12/mask-guidelines-cdc-walensky/621035/.

Page 337 chief of the Division of Infectious Diseases: cml (@CML915), "New evidence? Must be another Rochelle Walensky who wrote this email to her own mayor saying 3 feet is quite safe back in July. #liar," Twitter, March 19, 2021, 4:52 p.m., https://twitter.com/CML915/status/1373014460261077000?s=20.

Page 337 guidance for summer camps: David Zweig, "Experts: CDC's Summer-Camp Rules Are 'Cruel' and 'Irrational,'" *New York*, Intelligencer (blog), May 4, 2021, https://nymag.com/intelligencer/2021/05/experts-cdcs-summer-camp-rules-are-cruel-irrational.html.

Page 338 two studies, published in the journal *Pediatrics*: David Zweig, "New Research Suggests Number of Kids Hospitalized for COVID Is Overcounted," *New York*, Intelligencer (blog), May 19, 2021, https://nymag.com/intelligencer/2021/05/study-number-of-kids-hospitalized-for-covid-is-overcounted.html. There is utility for health professionals to know how many hospital patients have COVID—for infection control, and epidemiological monitoring—even if the infection is unrelated to the patient's admission. So the numbers are not "wrong" per se. But the way they were presented to the public implied that almost double the number of kids were hospitalized *because* of COVID than was actually the case.

Page 339 *more than 35 percent*: Adi V. Gundlapalli et al., "Death Certificate–Based ICD-10 Diagnosis Codes for COVID-19 Mortality Surveillance—United States, January–December 2020," *Morbidity and Mortality Weekly Report* 70, no. 14 (2021): 523–527.

Page 339 Arizona masking study: David Zweig, "The CDC's Flawed Case for Wearing Masks in School," *Atlantic*, December 16, 2021, https://www.theatlantic.com/science/archive/2021/12/mask-guidelines-cdc-walensky/621035/.

Page 339 Montessori school: David Zweig, "The School That Couldn't Quit COVID," *The Free Press*, April 10, 2023, https://www.thefp.com/p/the-school-that-couldnt-quit-covid.

Page 341 Great Barrington Declaration: I was at the Great Barrington event that spawned the Declaration, and interviewed its three authors. https://gbdeclaration.org/

Page 341 scathing hit pieces: Apoorva Mandavilli and Sheryl Gay Stolberg, "A Viral Theory Cited by Health Officials Draws Fire From Scientists," *New York Times*, October 19, 2020, https://www.nytimes.com/2020/10/19/health/coronavirus-great-barrington.html; Hilary Brueck and Aylin Woodward, "The White House-backed 'Great Barrington Declaration' Calling for Herd Immunity Wouldn't Just Fail—It Could Lead to 640,000 Deaths," *Business Insider*, October 15, 2020, https://www.businessinsider.com/herd-immunity-plan-great-barrington-declaration-wont-work-2020-10; Stephanie M. Lee, "Scientists Are Slamming the Great Barrington Declaration's Call for 'Herd Immunity,'" *BuzzFeed*, October 14, 2020, https://www.buzzfeednews.com/article/stephaniemlee/herd-immunity-great-barrington-backlash-letter; Sonia Sodha, "The Anti-lockdown Scientists' Cause Would Be More Persuasive if It Weren't So Half-Baked," *Guardian*, October 11, 2020, https://www.theguardian.com/commentisfree/2020/oct/11/the-rebel-scientists-cause-would-be-more-persuasive-if-it-werent-so-half-baked; Noah Higgins-Dunn, "Dr. Fauci Says Letting the Coronavirus Spread to Achieve Herd Immunity Is 'Nonsense' and 'Dangerous,'" CNBC, October 15, 2020, https://www.cnbc.com/2020/10/15/dr-fauci-says-letting-the-coronavirus-spread-to-achieve-herd-immunity-is-nonsense-and-dangerous.html; Brian Resnick, "The Great Barrington Declaration Is an Ethical Nightmare," *Vox*, October 16, 2020, https://www.vox.com/science-and-health/21517702/great-barrington-declaration-john-snow-memorandum-explained-herd-immunity; Derrick Z. Jackson, "Herding People to Slaughter: The Dangerous Fringe Theory Behind the Great Barrington Declaration and Push toward Herd Immunity," The Equation (blog of the Union of Concerned

Scientists), October 23, 2020, https://blog.ucsusa.org/derrick-jackson/herding-people
-to-slaughter-the-dangerous-fringe-theory-behind-the-great-barrington-declaration
-and-push-toward-herd-immunity/.

Page 342 "There needs to be a quick and devastating published take down": https://
www.aier.org/wp-content/uploads/2021/12/FirstCollinsEmail.pdf.

Page 342 famous 2006 paper: Thomas V. Inglesby et al., "Disease Mitigation Measures in the Control of Pandemic Influenza," *Biosecurity and Bioterrorism: Biodefense
Strategy, Practice, and Science* 4, no. 4 (2006): 366–375.

Page 342 Susan Sontag: Susan Sontag, *Illness as Metaphor* (New York: Farrar, Straus
and Giroux, 1978).

Page 343 "Sometimes, a scientific consensus is established": Eric Winsberg, "We
Need Scientific Dissidents Now More Than Ever," *The Chronicle of Higher Education*,
August 10, 2023.

CHAPTER 24

Page 346 Duke study: Zimmerman et al., "Incidence and Secondary Transmission
of SARS-CoV-2 Infections in Schools," *Pediatrics*, April 1, 2021. First published
January 8, 2021, https://www.cidrap.umn.edu/covid-19/three-studies-highlight-low
-covid-risk-person-school

Page 346 reason her study got published in *MMWR*: Tracy Høeg (@TracyBethHoeg),
"I was senior author of this WI study & as we said in our paper, because we had no
control group: 'It was not possible to determine the specific roles that mask," Twitter, April 26, 2023, 10:19 pm, https://twitter.com/TracyBethHoeg/status/165141062
2733770752?s=20; Høeg et al., "COVID-19 Cases and Transmission in 17 K–12
Schools—Wood County, Wisconsin, August 31–November 29, 2020," *MMWR*, first
posted January 26, 2021.

Page 347 Norway: Brandal et al., "Minimal Transmission of SARS-CoV-2 from Pae-
diatric COVID-19 Cases in Primary Schools, Norway, August to November 2020,"
Eurosurveillance 26, no. 1 (2021).

Page 347 more than 90 percent: Vladimir Kogan and Vinay Prasad, "New CDC
School Opening Guidelines Fail to 'Follow the Science,'" *Stat*, February 20, 2021,
https://www.statnews.com/2021/02/20/new-cdc-school-opening-guidelines-dont
-follow-the-science/.

Page 349 perfect for a proper study: Branch-Elliman et al., "Effectiveness of 3 Versus
6 ft of Physical Distancing for Controlling Spread of Coronavirus Disease 2019
Among Primary and Secondary Students and Staff: A Retrospective, Statewide Cohort
Study," *Clinical Infectious Diseases* 73, no. 10 (November 2021).

CONCLUSION

Page 353 Cuomo gave an impassioned speech: Office of the Governor of New York
State, "Governor Cuomo Signs the 'New York State on PAUSE' Executive Order," news

release, March 20, 2020, https://www.governor.ny.gov/news/governor-cuomo-signs
-new-york-state-pause-executive-order; https://www.governor.ny.gov/news/video-audio
-photos-rush-transcript-governor-cuomo-signs-new-york-state-pause-executive-order.

Page 353 Florida had a lower excess death rate: The White House, "Excess Mortality
during the Pandemic: The Role of Health Insurance," July 12, 2022, https://www
.whitehouse.gov/cea/written-materials/2022/07/12/excess-mortality-during-the
-pandemic-the-role-of-health-insurance/.

Page 353 Florida's standardized *COVID* death rate: Bollyky et al., "Assessing COVID-
19 Pandemic Policies and Behaviours and Their Economic and Educational Trade-
Offs Across US states from Jan 1, 2020, to July 31, 2022: An Observational Analysis,"
Lancet 401, no. 10385, P1341–1360 (2023).

Page 354 severe cases of appendicitis in kids: David Zweig, "Fear and the Law of
Unintended Consequences," March 11, 2021, https://davidzweig.medium.com/fear
-and-the-law-of-unintended-consequences-21251564b102.

Page 354 "If you're a public health person" Francis Collins: July 10, 2023, YouTube
video, https://www.youtube.com/watch?v=W1eAvh1sWiw.

Page 356 "Not everything that can be counted counts": William Bruce Cameron,
Informal Sociology: A Casual Introduction to Sociological Thinking (New York: Random
House, 1963), 13.

Page 356 Gabriel Radvansky and Jeff Zacks: Gabriel A. Radvansky and Jeffrey M.
Zacks, "Event Boundaries in Memory and Cognition," *Current Opinion in Behavioral
Sciences* 17 (2017): 133–140; Radvansky and Zacks, *Event Cognition* (New York: Oxford
University Press, 2014).

Page 356 Fiona McPherson: Fiona McPherson, "Event Boundaries and Working
Memory Capacity," Mempowered! (website), accessed August 14, 2024, https://www
.mempowered.com/strategies/attention/event-boundaries-and-working-memory
-capacity.

Page 357 "Events require clear demarcations": Christine Rosen, "Technosolution-
ism Isn't the Fix," Hedgehog Review, Fall 2020, https://hedgehogreview.com/issues
/america-on-the-brink/articles/technosolutionism-isnt-the-fix; Institute for Advanced
Studies in Culture, "Christine Rosen" (public profile page), accessed January 3, 2024,
https://iasculture.org/scholars/profiles/christine-rosen.

INDEX